Morgan Greene

Disorders of Motor Speech

This book is printed on recycled paper.

Disorders of Motor Speech

Assessment, Treatment, and Clinical Characterization

edited by

Donald A. Robin, Ph.D.
Department of Speech Pathology and Audiology
National Center for Voice and Speech
University of Iowa
Iowa City, Iowa

Kathryn M. Yorkston, Ph.D.
Department of Rehabilitation Medicine
University of Washington
Seattle, Washington

and

David R. Beukelman, Ph.D.
Department of Special Education and Communication Disorders
University of Nebraska
Lincoln, Nebraska

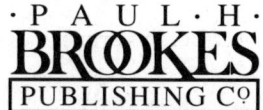

Baltimore • London • Toronto • Sydney

Paul H. Brookes Publishing Co.
Post Office Box 10624
Baltimore, Maryland 21285-0624

Copyright © 1996 by Paul H. Brookes Publishing Co., Inc.
All rights reserved.

Typeset by Brushwood Graphics, Inc., Baltimore, Maryland.
Manufactured in the United States of America by
The Maple Press Company, York, Pennsylvania.

Library of Congress Cataloging-in-Publication Data
Disorders of motor speech : assessment, treatment, and clinical characterization /
   edited by Donald A. Robin, Kathryn M. Yorkston, David R. Beukelman.
       p.   cm.
    Includes bibliographical references and index.
    ISBN 1-55766-223-1
    1. Speech disorders.   I. Yorkston, Kathryn M., 1948–
II. Beukelman, David R., 1943–   III. Title.
RC423.R59   1996   95-24521
616.85'5—dc20   CIP

British Library Cataloguing-in-Publication data are available from the British
Library.

Contents

Contributors ix
Preface xix

SECTION I ISSUES IN MOTOR LEARNING

Chapter 1   New Conceptualizations of Practice:
Common Principles in Three Paradigms
Suggest New Concepts for Training
Richard A. Schmidt and Robert A. Bjork 3

SECTION II PERSPECTIVES ON NORMAL MOTOR SPEECH CONTROL

Chapter 2   Goal-Based Speech Motor Control:
A Theoretical Framework and Some
Preliminary Data
*Joseph S. Perkell, Melanie L. Matthies,
Mario A. Svirsky, and Michael I. Jordan* 27

Chapter 3   Articulated and Inflected Primate Vocalizations:
Developing Animal Models of Speech
Charles H. Brown and Michael P. Cannito 43

SECTION III INTELLIGIBILITY

Chapter 4   Effects of Semantic and Syntactic
Context on Actual and Estimated Sentence
Intelligibility of Dysarthric Speakers
*Carolyn R. Carter, Kathryn M. Yorkston,
Edythe A. Strand, and Vicki L. Hammen* 67

Chapter 5   Top-Down Influences on the Intelligibility
of a Dysarthric Speaker: Addition of
Natural Gestures and Situational Context
Jane Mertz Garcia and Michael P. Cannito 89

Chapter 6   Effects of Insertion of Interword Pauses on
the Intelligibility of Dysarthric Speech
Joanne M. Gutek and Anne Putnam Rochet 105

SECTION IV RELIABILITY AND VALIDITY ISSUES IN ASSESSMENT

Chapter 7 The Multidimensional Nature of Pathologic Vocal Quality
Jody Kreiman, Bruce R. Gerratt, and Gerald S. Berke 123

Chapter 8 Reliability of Auditory–Perceptual Scaling of Dysarthria
Joslin Zeplin and Ray D. Kent 145

Chapter 9 Prosodic Assessment of Dysarthria: Effects of Sampling Task and Issues of Variability
Anja Leuschel and Gerard J. Docherty 155

SECTION V RESPIRATORY INVOLVEMENT IN DYSARTHRIA

Chapter 10 Respiratory Patterning and Variability in Dysarthric Speech
Vicki L. Hammen and Kathryn M. Yorkston 181

Chapter 11 Progression of Respiratory Symptoms in Amyotrophic Lateral Sclerosis: Implications for Speech Function
Kathryn M. Yorkston, Edythe A. Strand, and Robert M. Miller 193

SECTION VI MOTOR SPEECH INVOLVEMENT IN TRAUMATIC BRAIN INJURY

Chapter 12 Differential Patterns of Hyperfunctional Laryngeal Impairment in Dysarthric Speakers Following Severe Closed Head Injury
Deborah G. Theodoros and Bruce E. Murdoch 205

Chapter 13 Laryngeal Airway Resistance Following Traumatic Brain Injury
Monica A. McHenry 229

Chapter 14 Tongue Strength and Endurance: Relation to the Speaking Ability of Children and Adolescents Following Traumatic Brain Injury
Julie A.G. Stierwalt, Donald A. Robin, Nancy Pearl Solomon, Amy L. Weiss, and Jeffrey E. Max 241

SECTION VII PARKINSON'S DISEASE

Chapter 15 Tongue Strength and Endurance in Mild to Moderate Parkinson's Disease
Nancy Pearl Solomon, Daryl M. Lorell, Donald A. Robin, Robert L. Rodnitzky, and Erich S. Luschei 259

Chapter 16 Communication Disability of Parkinson's
Disease: Perceptions of Dysarthric Speakers
and Their Primary Communication Partners
*Kim Antonius, David R. Beukelman, and
Robert Reid*..275

Chapter 17 Maintenance of Speech Changes Following
Group Treatment for Hypokinetic Dysarthria
of Parkinson's Disease
*Marsha D. Sullivan, Patrick J. Brune, and
David R. Beukelman*...............................287

SECTION VIII SPASMODIC DYSPHONIA, INSPIRATORY AIRWAY COMPROMISE, AND APRAXIA OF SPEECH

Chapter 18 Abductor Spasmodic Dysphonia: Acoustic
Influence of Voicing on Connected Speech
*Michael P. Cannito, Laura S. McSwain,
and James P. Dworkin*............................311

Chapter 19 Effects of Inspiratory Airway Impairment
on Continuous Speech
*James A. Till, Mehdi Jafari,
Roger L. Crumley, and Cindy B. Law-Till*.............329

Chapter 20 Phonemic Retrieval in Apraxia of
Speech: Is There More Than One Type
of Impairment?
*Monica Strauss Hough and
Salvatore DeMarco*...............................341

Index...357

Contributors

The Editors

Donald A. Robin, Ph.D., Department of Speech Pathology and Audiology, National Center for Voice and Speech, University of Iowa, Iowa City, IA 52242

Donald A. Robin is Associate Professor of Speech Pathology and Audiology at the University of Iowa and an investigator with the National Center for Voice and Speech. He teaches, conducts research, and treats patients in the area of neurogenic communication disorders. His research interests include disorders of speech motor control, central auditory processing, and language.

Kathryn M. Yorkston, Ph.D., Department of Rehabilitation Medicine, Box 356490, University of Washington, Seattle, WA 98195-6490

Kathryn M. Yorkston is Head of the Division of Speech Pathology and Professor in the Department of Rehabilitation Medicine and Adjunct Professor of Speech and Hearing Sciences at the University of Washington. She is board certified by the Academy of Neurologic Communication Disorders and Sciences. Her publications have focused on clinical research in acquired neurologic communication disorders in adults. She has written and edited texts that include *Clinical Management of Dysarthric Speakers* and *Management of Speech and Swallowing Disorders in Degenerative Disease*.

David R. Beukelman, Ph.D., 202F Barkley Memorial Center, University of Nebraska, Lincoln, Lincoln, NE 68583-0732

David R. Beukelman is Barkley Professor of Communication Disorders and Director of the Barkley Augmentative Communication Center, Department of Special Education and Communication Disorders at the University of Nebraska, Lincoln. He is Director of Research and Education of the Communication Disorders Division of the Meyer Rehabilitation Center, University of Nebraska Medical Center. Dr. Beukelman's primary research and clinical interests have been in the areas of dysarthria and augmentative communication.

The Chapter Authors

Kim Antonius, M.S., SLP, The Hugh MacMillan Rehabilitation Centre, The Augmentative Communication Service, 350 Rumsey Road, Toronto, Ontario M4G 1R8, CANADA

Kim Antonius is a speech-language pathologist working at The Augmentative Communication Service of The Hugh MacMillan Rehabilitation Centre in Toronto, Ontario. Her current research interests include the development of a tool to measure the communication competency of individuals who use augmentative and alternative communication, measurement of intervention outcomes, and the examination of the disability associated with various communication impairments.

Gerald S. Berke, M.D., Division of Head and Neck Surgery, School of Medicine, University of California–Los Angeles, CHS 62-132, Los Angeles, CA 90095-1624

Gerald S. Berke is Professor and Chief in the Division of Head and Neck Surgery at the School of Medicine, University of California–Los Angeles. His research focuses on laryngeal biomechanics and on the acoustics and aerodynamics of normal and disordered phonation.

Robert A. Bjork, Ph.D., Department of Psychology, University of California–Los Angeles, Los Angeles, CA 90095-1563

Robert A. Bjork is Professor of Psychology at the University of California, Los Angeles, and editor of *Psychological Review*. He earlier served as Professor at the University of Michigan and has held visiting appointments at the Rockefeller University, University of California, San Diego, Bell Laboratories, and Dartmouth College. His interests focus on how information is encoded and accessed in human memory and on the implications of that research for training and instruction. He is a recipient of UCLA's Distinguished Teaching Award. His other national responsibilities include editing *Memory & Cognition* (1981–1985) and chairing a National Research Council Committee on Techniques for the Enhancement of Human Performance (1988–1994). He is a fellow of the Society of Experimental Psychologists, the American Psychological Association, and the American Psychological Society.

Charles H. Brown, Ph.D., Department of Psychology, University of South Alabama, Mobile, AL 36688

Charles H. Brown is Professor of Psychology and Adjunct Professor of Speech Pathology and Audiology at the University of South Alabama, where he teaches courses on the psychobiological aspects of sensation, perception, and communication. His current research interests include comparative vocal motor control, comparative perception, and neurolinguistics.

Patrick J. Brune, M.S., Meyer Rehabilitation Institute, Department of Speech-Language Pathology, 600 South 42nd Street, Omaha, NE 68198-5450

Patrick J. Brune is a speech-language pathologist at the Meyer Rehabilitation Institute. His primary research interests are in motor speech disorders and augmentative communication.

Michael P. Cannito, Ph.D., School of Audiology and Speech-Language Pathology, The University of Memphis, 807 Jefferson Avenue, Memphis, TN 38105

Michael P. Cannito is Associate Professor of Speech-Language Pathology at The University of Memphis, where he teaches courses on the neurologic aspects of normal and disordered communication. His current research interests include disorderd speech motor control and neurolinguistics.

Carolyn R. Carter, M.S., St. Joseph Medical Center, Tacoma, WA 98401

Carolyn R. Carter is a speech-language pathologist at St. Joseph Medical Center. She has recently completed a master's degree thesis on the topic of intelligibility of dysarthric speech at the University of Washington, Seattle.

Roger L. Crumley, M.D., University of California, Irvine, 101 The City Drive, South Orange, CA 92668

Roger L. Crumley is Professor and Chairman of the Department of Otolaryngology–Head & Neck Surgery, University of California Irvine College of Medicine. His current clinical work is in laryngology and speech disorders. His research interests focus on the innervation and re-innervation of the larynx. He is known for his work with microsurgical nerve anastomosis in the treatment of laryngeal paralysis.

Salvatore DeMarco, Ph.D., Department of Communication Sciences and Disorders, East Carolina University, Greenville, NC 27858

Salvatore DeMarco is Associate Professor in the Department of Communication Sciences and Disorders at East Carolina University in Greenville, North Carolina. Previous work settings include nonprofit clinics and medical centers. He is former Coordinator of the Scottish Rite Child Language and Dyslexia Clinic. His research interests include word and phonemic retrieval skills in various populations, preschoolers at risk for learning disabilities, and language learning disabilities.

Gerard J. Docherty, Ph.D., Department of Speech, King George VI Building, University of Newcastle, Queen Victoria Road, Newcastle upon Tyne NE1 7RU, UNITED KINGDOM

Gerard J. Docherty is Senior Lecturer in Phonetics in the Department of Speech at the University of Newcastle upon Tyne. He has worked for 10 years on the acoustic analysis of speech. His main research interests lie in the areas of instrumental and experimental phonetics with a particular focus on clinical phonetics and on the nature of the interface between phonetics and phonology.

James P. Dworkin, Ph.D., Department of Otolaryngology–Head and Neck Surgery, Wayne State University, 5E-UHC, Detroit, MI 48201

James P. Dworkin is Professor in the Department of Otolaryngology at Wayne State University in Detroit, Michigan. He also serves as Director of the speech pathology program's Physiology Laboratory. Since completing a postdoctoral fellowship at the Mayo Clinic in 1978, his clinical research has focused on neurogenic communication disorders.

Jane Mertz Garcia, M.S., Department of Speech Pathology and Audiology, University of South Alabama, Mobile, AL 36688

Jane Mertz Garcia is a doctoral candidate in Communication Sciences and Disorders at the University of South Alabama. Her clinical emphasis has focused on acquired neurologic communicative disorders in adults for over 10 years. Her research interests are in the areas of motor speech disorders and neurolinguistics.

Bruce R. Gerratt, Ph.D., Division of Head and Neck Surgery, School of Medicine, University of California–Los Angeles, 31-24 Rehab Center, Los Angeles, CA 90095-1794

Bruce R. Gerratt is Professor in Residence of Head and Neck Surgery at the School of Medicine, University of California–Los Angeles, and Chief of Audiology and Speech Pathology at the UCLA Medical Center. His research interests include the physiology of normal and disordered laryngeal function and the relation of physiology to acoustic and perceptual measures of the sounds produced.

Joanne M. Gutek, M.S., Department of Speech Pathology, St. Paul's Hospital, 1702 20th Street West, Saskatoon, Saskatchewan S7M 079 CANADA

Joanne M. Gutek is a speech-language pathologist at St. Paul's Hospital in Saskatoon, Saskatchewan, where she works with the rehabilitation of head and neck surgery patients as well as with the assessment and treatment of adults with neurogenic communication disorders. Her master's thesis, "Effects of the insertion of interword pauses on the intelligibility of dysarthric speech," was supported by the Province of Alberta Scholarship and was supervised by Dr. Anne Putnam Rochet.

Vicki L. Hammen, Ph.D., Department of Audiology and Speech Sciences, 1252 Heavilon Hall, Purdue University, West Lafayette, IN 47907

Vicki L. Hammen is Assistant Professor of Speech-Language Pathology in the Department of Audiology and Speech Sciences at Purdue University. Her areas of emphasis for research, teaching, and clinical service are motor speech disorders and voice. Dr. Hammen's research interests focus on the relationships between physiologic, acoustic, and perceptual features of both motor speech and voice disorders.

Monica Strauss Hough, Ph.D., Department of Communication Sciences and Disorders, East Carolina University, Greenville, NC 27858

Monica Strauss Hough is Associate Professor in the Department of Communication Sciences and Disorders at East Carolina University. She has been a practicing clinician for over 15 years in various clinical settings specializing in the treatment of patients with neurogenic communication disorders. Her areas of particular interest are semantic categorization and retrieval in brain-damaged populations, apraxia of speech, and contextual influences on aphasia and right hemisphere communication disorders.

Mehdi Jafari, Ph.D., Speech Research Laboratory (126), Department of Veterans Affairs Medical Center, 5901 East Seventh Street, Long Beach, CA 90822

Mehdi Jafari is a research scientist at the Speech Research Laboratory, Department of Veterans Affairs Medical Center in Long Beach/Department of Otolaryngology–Head & Neck Surgery, University of California–Irvine. He has a doctorate in biomedical engineering from University of Texas Southwestern Medical Center at Dallas/University of Texas at Arlington. His background is in electrical and control systems engineering.

Michael I. Jordan, Sc.D., Department of Brain and Cognitive Sciences, Room E10-034D, Massachusetts Institute of Technology, Cambridge, MA 02139

Michael I. Jordan is Associate Professor of Brain and Cognitive Sciences at the Massachusetts Institute of Technology. He is author of numerous publications.

Ray D. Kent, Ph.D., Waisman Center, University of Wisconsin–Madison, 1500 Highland Avenue, Madison, WI 53705-2280

Ray D. Kent is Professor of Communicative Disorders at the University of Wisconsin–Madison. His research on motor speech disorders focuses on impairments of intelligibility and quality, especially in the dysarthrias associated with amyotrophic lateral sclerosis, Parkinson's disease, cerebellar disease, stroke, and cerebral palsy. Other research interests include vocal development in infants, developmental aspects of vocal tract anatomy and motor function, acoustic analyses of speech, and theories of speech production.

Jody Kreiman, Ph.D., Division of Head and Neck Surgery, School of Medicine, University of California–Los Angeles, 31-24 Rehab Center, Los Angeles, CA 90095-1794

Jody Kreiman is Assistant Professor in Residence of Head and Neck Surgery at the School of Medicine, University of California–Los Angeles. Her research focuses on the perception of normal and disordered voice quality and the relationship between perceived quality, acoustics, and laryngeal physiology.

Cindy B. Law-Till, M.A., 3780 Wisteria Street, Seal Beach, CA 90740

Cindy B. Law-Till is a speech-language pathologist with 10 years of experience treating adults with speech and language disorders. She has coauthored articles appearing in the *Journal of Speech and Hearing Disorders*, *Journal of Voice*, and *Archives of Otolaryngology*. She currently is a consultant for medical chart review and specializes in third-party payment issues.

Anja Leuschel, Department of Speech, King George VI Building, University of Newcastle, Queen Victoria Road, Newcastle upon Tyne NE1 7RU, UNITED KINGDOM

Anja Leuschel is a speech-language pathologist whose doctoral work in the Department of Speech at the University of Newcastle upon Tyne has focused on investigating an instrumental acoustic basis for the assessment of prosody in dysarthria.

Daryl M. Lorell, M.S., Department of Speech Pathology and Audiology, University of Iowa, Iowa City, IA 52242-1012

Daryl M. Lorell is currently a speech-language pathologist in Des Moines, Iowa. She assisted with this project while in the doctoral program in the Department of Speech Pathology and Audiology at the University of Iowa. Her primary research interests are the effects of strength and endurance training on dysarthric speech. Previously, Ms. Lorell worked as a speech-language pathologist at the Cleveland Clinic Foundation, Cleveland, Ohio.

Erich S. Luschei, Ph.D., Department of Speech Pathology and Audiology, National Center for Voice and Speech, University of Iowa, Iowa City, IA 52242

Erich S. Luschei is Professor of Speech Pathology and Audiology at the University of Iowa. He is a neurophysiologist who studies the neuromuscular and sensory processes that control the larynx, tongue, and mandible. Dr. Luschei uses experimental approaches in his work, which ranges from the study of tongue strength in normal and disordered speakers to basic neurophysiologic studies of laryngeal control in anesthetized animals.

Melanie L. Matthies, Ph.D., Speech Communication Group, Research Laboratory of Electronics, Room 36-543, Massachusetts Institute of Technology, Cambridge, MA 02139

Melanie L. Matthies is Research Scientist at the Massachusetts Institute of Technology. She is the author of numerous publications.

Jeffrey E. Max, M.B.B.Ch., Department of Psychiatry, University of Iowa, Iowa City, IA 52242

Jeffrey E. Max is Assistant Professor of Psychiatry and Director of the Child and Adolescent Consultation–Liaison Psychiatry Service. He teaches general child and adolescent psychiatry and focuses on pediatric consultation-liaison psychiatry. Research and clinical interests and activities include the neuropsychiatric outcome following child and adolescent brain injury and psychopharmacology of childhood psychiatric disorders.

Monica A. McHenry, Ph.D., Galveston Institute of Human Communication, 1528 Post Office Street, Galveston, TX 77553

Monica A. McHenry is a speech scientist at the Galveston Institute of Human Communication. Dr. McHenry integrates her clinical and research interests through instrumentation-based analysis of speech production. She is particularly interested in the effect of sensory, motor, and psychological variables on intelligibility.

Laura S. McSwain, M.S., Department of Speech Pathology and Audiology, University of South Alabama, Mobile, AL 36688

Laura McSwain is a certified speech-language pathologist. Her clinical interests include adult neurogenic disorders and voice disorders.

Robert M. Miller, Ph.D., Audiology and Speech Pathology (126), VAMC, 1660 South Columbia Way, Seattle, WA 98108

Robert M. Miller is Chief of Audiology and Speech Pathology at the Veterans' Administration Medical Center, Seattle, Washington. He holds the position of Clinical Associate Professor in the departments of Rehabilitation Medicine; Speech and Hearing Sciences; and Otolaryngology, Head and Neck Surgery at the University of Washington, Seattle. Dr. Miller has authored numerous chapters and articles related to swallowing disorders and medical speech pathology.

Bruce E. Murdoch, Ph.D., Department of Speech and Hearing, The University of Queensland, Brisbane, Queensland 4072, AUSTRALIA

Bruce E. Murdoch is Professor and Head of the Department of Speech and Hearing at The University of Queensland and Director of the Motor Speech Research Unit within the Department of Speech and Hearing. His research interests are in the area of acquired neurogenic communication disorders in children and adults with a specific focus on the assessment and treatment of motor speech disorders. He has written and edited texts that include *Acquired Speech and Language Disorders: A Neuroanatomical and Functional Neurological Approach* and *Acquired Neurological Speech-Language Disorders in Childhood*.

Joseph S. Perkell, Ph.D., D.M.D., Speech Communication Group, Research Laboratory of Electronics, Room 36-591, Massachusetts Institute of Technology, Cambridge, MA 02139

Joseph S. Perkell is Senior Research Scientist at the Massachusetts Institute of Technology and Lecturer at the Harvard School of Dental Medicine. He is a Fellow of the Acoustical Society of America and author and volume editor of numerous publications.

Robert Reid, Ph.D., Department of Special Education and Communication Disorders, University of Nebraska, Lincoln, Lincoln, NE 68583

Dr. Reid is Assistant Professor in the Department of Special Education and Communication Disorders at the University of Nebraska, Lincoln. His research interests lie in the areas of attention deficits and cognitive strategy instructions.

Anne Putnam Rochet, Ph.D., Department of Speech Pathology and Audiology, University of Alberta, Edmonton, Alberta, T6G 2E1 CANADA

Anne Putnam Rochet is Professor in the Department of Speech Pathology and Audiology and Associate Dean for Graduate Studies and Research in the Faculty of Rehabilitation Medicine at the University of Alberta, Edmonton. She received postdoctoral training in San Francisco at the Speech Research laboratory of the Veterans Administration Hospital as an NINCDS Postdoctoral Fellow at the University of California. Subsequently, she held an NINCDS Teacher-Investigator Award in the Department of Speech and Hearing Sciences at the University of Arizona, Tucson. At the University of Alberta, Dr. Rochet supervises graduate student research and teaches graduate coursework.

Robert L. Rodnitzky, M.D., Department of Neurology, University of Iowa Hospitals and Clinics, Iowa City, IA 52242

Robert L. Rodnitzky is Professor and Vice Chairman of the Department of Neurology at the University of Iowa College of Medicine and Director of the Movement Disorders Clinic at the University of Iowa Hospitals and Clinics.

Richard A. Schmidt, Ph.D., Department of Psychology, University of California–Los Angeles, Los Angeles, CA 90095-1563

Richard A. Schmidt has held faculty positions at the University of Maryland, the University of Michigan, and the University of Southern California. He is the author of 4 books and 110 articles, has had his work funded by the National Science Foundation and the U.S. Army Research Institutes, and was the founder and editor of the *Journal of Motor Behavior*. He is currently on leave as Professor in the Department of Psychology at UCLA, working as a Principal Scientist in the area of human factors at the consulting firm of Failure Analysis Associates, Inc., in Los Angeles.

Nancy Pearl Solomon, Ph.D., Department of Communication Disorders, University of Minnesota, Minneapolis, MN 55455

Nancy Pearl Solomon is Assistant Professor in the Department of Communication Disorders at the University of Minnesota. She conducted this study at the University of Iowa in her position as Assistant Research Scientist for the National Center for Voice and Speech. Dr. Solomon's research interests relate to the motor control of speech, especially regarding breathing, phonation, and articulation, in normal and neurologically disordered individuals.

Julie A.G. Stierwalt, M.A., Department of Speech Pathology and Audiology, University of Iowa, Department of Neurology, University of Iowa Hospitals and Clinics, Iowa City, IA 52242

Julie Stierwalt shares a joint appointment with the Department of Speech Pathology and Audiology at the University of Iowa and the Department of Neurology at the University of Iowa Hospitals and Clinics in Iowa City, Iowa. She supervises graduate interns and treats patients in the areas of neurogenic communication and swallowing disorders. Her research interests include the exploration of speech, language, and cognition in individuals following neurologic insult/trauma.

Edythe A. Strand, Ph.D., Department of Speech and Hearing Science, Box 354875, University of Washington, Seattle, WA 98195-4875

Edythe A. Strand is Assistant Professor in the Department of Speech and Hearing Science at the University of Washington. Dr. Strand holds a doctoral degree from the University of Wisconsin–Madison. She is board certified by the Academy of Neurologic Communication Disorders and Sciences. Her primary research involves the acoustic and physiologic study of motor speech disorders, with a primary emphasis on the dysarthrias associated with neuromuscular disease.

Marsha D. Sullivan, M.A., Meyer Rehabilitation Institute, Department of Speech-Language Pathology, 600 South 42nd Street, Omaha, NE 68198-5450

Marsha Sullivan is Associate Director of Speech-Language Pathology at Meyer Rehabilitation Institute and an Instructor in Pediatrics at the University of Nebraska Medical Center. Her primary research interests are in motor speech, voice, and head and neck speech disorders.

Mario A. Svirsky, Ph.D., Speech Communication Group, Research Laboratory of Electronics, Room 36-525, Massachusetts Institute of Technology, Cambridge, MA 02139

Mario A. Svirsky is Research Scientist at the Massachusetts Institute of Technology. He received his Ph.D. from Tulane University and is author of numerous publications.

Deborah G. Theodoros, Ph.D., Department of Speech and Hearing, The University of Queensland, Brisbane, Queensland 4072, AUSTRALIA

Deborah G. Theodoros is Lecturer in Speech Pathology in the Department of Speech and Hearing at The University of Queensland. Her research and clinical interests are primarily in the area of the assessment and rehabilitation of motor speech disorders associated with traumatic brain injury, Parkinson's disease, and cerebrovascular accidents.

James A. Till, Ph.D., Speech Research Laboratory (126), Department of Veterans Affairs Medical Center, 5901 East Seventh Street, Long Beach, CA 90822

James A. Till is Director of the Speech Research Laboratory of the Department of Veterans Affairs Medical Center, Long Beach, California. He is Associate Clinical Professor and Director of the Speech and Voice Laboratory, Department of Otolaryngology–Head & Neck Surgery, University of California, Irvine. His current work concentrates on computer-assisted evaluation of disordered speech and analyses of diagnostic profiles.

Amy L. Weiss, Ph.D., Department of Speech Pathology and Audiology, University of Iowa, Iowa City, IA 52242

Amy L. Weiss is Associate Professor of Speech Pathology and Audiology at the University of Iowa. She teaches courses in the areas of language development and disorders as well as clinical intervention in speech-language pathology. She is currently completing a research project focusing on the conversational patterns of school-age children who stutter.

Joslin Zeplin, M.S., Queens Hospital Center, New York Health and Hospitals Corporation, 82-68 164th Street, Jamaica, NY 11432

Joslin Zeplin is a speech-language pathologist at Mount Sinai Services-Queens Hospital Center. Research projects have included work on perceptual scaling of dysarthria and comparison of dementia-related test batteries.

Preface

Disorders of Motor Speech: Assessment, Treatment, and Clinical Characterization is a compilation of articles written for speech-language clinicians, clinical and basic scientists interested in motor speech control and its disorders, and students. The book also has information of interest to related health care professionals who may use it as a resource on motor speech disorders. The book contains peer-reviewed research contributions on a wide range of topics and disorders such as basic motor speech control, assessment and treatment of motor speech disorders, and clinical characterization of specific disorders.

Disorders of Motor Speech is based on selected papers presented at the Conference on Motor Speech held in 1994 at Sedona, Arizona. This conference focuses on two topics: normal motor speech control and motor speech disorders. The majority of the contributions are from the Motor Speech Disorders program. However, for the first time, we have included some selections from the normal motor speech control program and have reprinted a publication that captures some of a presentation on motor learning by Richard A. Schmidt, our featured speaker at the meeting. The meeting was part of a tradition of biennial conferences focusing on motor speech disorders that began in 1982. The intent of the early meetings was to draw together clinicians and researchers with interest in the area of motor speech disorders to discuss their most recent thinking. The first conference, in 1982, was devoted mainly to dysarthria, and the resultant publication, *Clinical Dysarthria* (Berry, 1983), was edited by Bill Berry. Following this initial conference, Dave Beukelman and Kathy Yorkston established an organizational structure that has continued in an informal but careful way. There have been three well-received books of papers from the meeting: *Recent Advances in Clinical Dysarthria* (Yorkston & Beukelman, 1989), *Dysarthria and Apraxia of Speech: Perspectives on Management* (Moore, Yorkston, & Beukelman, 1991), and *Motor Speech Disorders: Advances in Assessment and Treatment* (Till, Yorkston, & Beukelman, 1993).

The present book follows the trend of previous volumes, exploring advances in motor speech disorders from a variety of perspectives. The current volume presents up-to-date information on intelligibility and how intelligibility of individuals with motor speech disorders changes based on contextual and situational variables. The reader will also discover the most recent information on perceptual ratings scales that should assist in the diagnostic and therapeutic process. The ever-evolving interest in quantification of speech and intelligibility is well reflected in the contributions to this book. There is valuable information on respiratory abilities of dysarthric speakers and on the dysarthria of Parkinson's disease and motor speech disorders following traumatic brain injury. Normal motor speech control is covered as well. All of the chapters have potential for affecting clinical practice.

The book is organized into eight sections: Issues in Motor Learning; Perspectives on Normal Motor Speech Control; Intelligibility; Reliability and Validity Issues in Assessment; Respiratory Involvement in Dysarthria; Motor Speech Involvement in Traumatic Brain Injury; Parkinson's Disease; and Spasmodic Dysphonia, Inspiratory Airway Compromise, and Apraxia of Speech. The lead-off chapter by Richard A. Schmidt and Robert A. Bjork on motor learning represents a portion of Schmidt's seminar at the meeting. In this chapter, we learn that factors we commonly think have a positive effect on learning may in fact not facilitate long-term learning of movement patterns. This beginning work is most appropriate for the book, as the issues discussed have immediate relevance to the clinical enterprise and cause us to ask questions about how we treat motor speech disorders.

The second section presents current models of normal speech motor control. Joseph S. Perkell, Melanie L. Matthies, Mario A. Svirsky, and Michael I. Jordan present a theoretical framework for the study of goal-based speech motor control with information on variability and preliminary data on acoustic goals for speech. Charles H. Brown and Michael P. Cannito review primate models of vocalizations and critically review the role of animal models for speech production.

The third section provides important information on intelligibility. Carolyn R. Carter, Kathryn M. Yorkston, Edythe A. Strand, and Vicki L. Hammen report their latest research findings on the effects of semantic and syntactic context on the intelligibility of dysarthric speakers. Following a similar vein, Jane Mertz Garcia and Michael P. Cannito provide a detailed study of "top-down" influences on intelligibility of a dysarthric speaker. They focus on natural gestures and situational context. Joanne M. Gutek and Anne Putnam Rochet discuss the effects of interword pauses on dysarthric speech.

The fourth section comprises new studies on perceptual measures of motor speech disorders and prosody. Jody Kreiman, Bruce R. Gerratt, and Gerald S. Berke present a multidimensional scaling study of abnormal vocal quality that is sure to assist us in further refinements when using perceptual means of rating vocal characteristics. Joslin Zeplin and Ray D. Kent reanalyze the original tapes from the Darley, Aronson, and Brown (1975) studies and provide us with detailed data on the reliability of perceptual rating scales for dysarthria. Anja Leuschel and Gerard J. Docherty focus on the assessment of prosody in dysarthria with specific information on the task used and variability.

The fifth section focuses on respiration and begins with a study by Vicki L. Hammen and Kathryn M. Yorkston that examines respiratory patterns and variability in dysarthric speakers. This is followed by a study by Kathryn M. Yorkston, Edythe A. Strand, and Robert M. Miller that details changes in respiration as a function of disease progression in amyotrophic lateral sclerosis.

The sixth section presents current information on the motor speech disorders found in patients with traumatic brain injury. Deborah G. Theodoros and Bruce E. Murdoch provide information on differential patterns of laryngeal impairment in speakers with traumatic brain injuries. Monica A. McHenry then presents a study of laryngeal resistance in this population with interesting results. Julie A.G. Stierwalt, Donald A. Robin, Nancy Pearl Solomon, Amy L. Weiss, and Jeffrey E. Max end this section with a detailed study of tongue strength and endurance in relation to speech in patients with traumatic brain injury.

The seventh section supplies up-to-date information on the speech disorder of Parkinson's disease. Nancy Pearl Solomon, Daryl M. Lorell, Donald A. Robin, Robert L. Rodnitzky, and Erich S. Luschei provide data showing that tongue strength is reduced in patients with mild Parkinson's disease. Kim Antonius, David R. Beukelman, and Robert Reid provide an important discussion of communication disability in Parkinson's disease focusing on the perceptions of dysarthric speakers and their primary communication partners. Marsha D. Sullivan, Patrick J. Brune, and David R. Beukelman round out this section with a detailed examination of and outcome data on group therapy for Parkinson's disease. They provide important information on maintenance effects of group therapy.

The final section contains information about a variety of different motor speech disorders. Michael P. Cannito, Laura S. McSwain, and James P. Dworkin report detailed data on the acoustic influence of voicing during connected speech in abductor spasmodic dysphonia. James A. Till, Mehdi Jafari, Roger L. Crumley and Cindy B. Law-Till present a carefully controlled study of inspiratory airway impairments on continuous speech. Finally, Monica Strauss Hough and Salvatore DeMarco present an intriguing argument for the presence of multiple types of apraxia of speech.

This book has been made possible through the efforts and immense help of many individuals. Kathryn Yorkston and Christy Ludlow were excellent conference co-chairs and have along with Dave Beukelman been the driving force behind the conference. The individual program committees are to be commended for their work in recruiting excellent presentations and organizing the details of the meeting. The Motor Speech Control committee was chaired by Vince Gracco and consisted of Kevin Munhall and Elaine Stathopoulous. The Motor Speech Disorders program committee was chaired by Don Robin and consisted of Joe Duffy, Carlin Hageman, Vicki Hammen, and Jen Hoit. The local arrangements for the conference were made by Chick LaPointe and Jim Case and their team and were superb. The authors of the volume were professional and met timelines and revised with good cheer, making editing the volume a pleasure. Special thanks are extended to Paul H. Brookes Publishing Co. and a particular thanks to Melissa Behm for all the help in publishing this book and their continued support of the conference. Eileen Finnegan and Erich Luschei of the University of Iowa are acknowledged for their assistance in reviewing some of the submissions. Finally, a thanks goes out to Mary Jo Yotty for her superb logistic and secretarial support at the University of Iowa.

REFERENCES

Berry, W. (1983). *Clinical dysarthria*. Boston: College-Hill Press.
Darley, F., Aronson, A., & Brown, J. (1975). *Motor speech disorders*. Philadelphia: W.B. Saunders.
Moore, C.A., Yorkston, K.M., & Beukelman, D.R. (1991). *Dysarthria and apraxia of speech: Perspectives on management*. Baltimore: Paul H. Brookes Publishing Co.
Till, J.A., Yorkston, K.M., & Beukelman, D.R. (1993). *Motor speech disorders: Advances in assessment and treatment*. Baltimore: Paul H. Brookes Publishing Co.
Yorkston, K., & Beukelman, D. (1989). *Recent advances in clinical dysarthria*. Boston: College-Hill Press.

Disorders of Motor Speech

SECTION I

ISSUES IN MOTOR LEARNING

Chapter 1

New Conceptualizations of Practice
Common Principles in Three Paradigms Suggest New Concepts for Training

Richard A. Schmidt and Robert A. Bjork

> **Editors' Note:** We were fortunate to have Richard A. Schmidt, Ph.D., as an invited speaker at the 1994 Conference on Motor Speech. Dr. Schmidt was invited because of his expertise in motor control and learning. He presented two seminars, one on motor programs and one on issues in motor learning. His discussion on motor learning focused on how the motor system learns and the clinical implications of such information. Dr. Schmidt's presentations were excellent. Moreover, much of what he presented had potential applicability to treatment of motor speech disorders. A particularly intriguing aspect of Dr. Schmidt's presentation on motor learning concerned common misconceptions about how we learn movement skilled routines or actions. Because these ideas have the potential to affect how clinicians approach therapy when treating patients with motor speech disorders, we were anxious to include in this volume some of the ideas presented by Dr. Schmidt at the conference. Dr. Schmidt and his colleague Robert A. Bjork have graciously allowed us to reprint a paper they co-authored on motor learning. The paper contains many of the ideas presented at the conference and should provide food for thought for those of us working in the area of motor speech control and its disorders.

Reprinted with minor revisions from *Psychological Science*, 3(4), 207–217, 1992, by permission of the authors and the American Psychological Society.
This chapter was based in part on a concept paper submitted to the U.S. Army Research Institute (ARI), Basic Research (Schmidt & Bjork, 1989), and was supported in part by Contract No. MDA 903-85-K-0225 from ARI to R.A. Schmidt and D.C. Shapiro.
Thanks to William Estes and Tim Lee for valuable comments on an earlier draft, and to Jack Adams for pointing us to the research on % ORMs.

OVER THE PAST several years, through the normal process of conducting our own individual research programs (in movement learning and human memory, respectively), and as a consequence of listening to and reading reports of each other's work, we have repeatedly encountered research findings that seem to violate some basic assumptions about how to optimize learning in real-world environments. For example, increasing the frequency of information presented to learners about performance errors during practice improves performance during training, yet can degrade performance on a test of long-term retention or transfer. Increasing the amount of task variability required during practice, in contrast, depresses performance during training, yet facilitates performance on later tests of the ability to generalize training to altered conditions. Such findings challenge common views of skill learning. Compared with some baseline training condition, how can a factor that enhances performance in practice interfere with retention or transfer performance? Even more intriguing, how can another factor that degrades performance in practice enhance retention performance?

These findings—and others we discuss below—are obtained from diverse research paradigms that employ several different verbal and motor tasks, and the theoretical motivations guiding those research efforts are often different as well. Taken together, however, these findings suggest that certain conceptualizations about how and when to practice are at best incomplete, and at worst incorrect. These findings also have some theoretical implications with respect to the processes involved in practice, particularly as they relate to the acquisition of real-world skills.

In this chapter, we first describe what we regard as some of the viewpoints, assumptions, and paradigms that, implicitly or explicitly, have provided the foundation for the typical procedures that guide practice and skill acquisition. These views of learning, although flawed in our opinion, have had a strong influence on the design of learning environments in educational, industrial, and military contexts. We then illustrate those flaws with examples from three different research paradigms, and we argue for a set of processes occurring during practice that can, at least in general terms, account for such findings.

SOME COMMON ASSUMPTIONS ABOUT PRACTICE

When researchers conduct studies of practice and learning, they generally ask learners to engage in practice at some task in an *acquisition phase*, and some independent variable is manipulated. The independent variable of interest can be of various types, such as the nature of instructions, the type of feedback, or the scheduling of practice, and the performance on some task is typically charted as a function of practice trials for groups operating with different levels of this variable. The logic of such paradigms, of course, is that those acquisition conditions that speed the rate of improvement, or cause subjects to reach criterion more quickly, or in general result in more effective performance in practice, are expected to be the most effective for learning this particular task. Learning, after all, can be indexed by the improvements in skill across practice; it seems unavoidable, therefore, to conclude that those conditions in acquisition that speed gains in performance have done so because they have enhanced the processes of learning in some way. There are two related problems with this view of the learning process.

**Problem 1: Acquisition Performance
Is an Imperfect Indicator of Learning**

In the recent era of research on the processes of learning, memory, and performance, researchers seem to have lost track of a critical distinction between the momentary strength or accessibility of a response and the underlying habit strength of that response. The major learning theorists of an earlier era recognized decades ago that experimental variables applied during training can have two distinct kinds of effects (see, e.g., Estes, 1955; Guthrie, 1952; Hull, 1943; Skinner, 1938; Tolman, 1932). First, of course, such variables can have the relatively permanent effects that are the usual focus when learning is examined. That is, these variables might speed the development of some relatively permanent capability for responding (the usual definition of learning, and the one we use here), so that a group of subjects with more of this capability will usually perform more effectively during practice than a group with less of this capability. Second, however, there may also be temporary effects of such experimental manipulations—effects that exaggerate or diminish performance differences while the variables are operating, with these performance differences vanishing or being markedly altered as soon as the subjects are allowed to rest, or when the manipulation is removed. Such performance effects can be mediated by a host of factors, such as the elevating effects of motivational instructions or the administration of feedback, as well as the depressing effects of physical (or mental) fatigue and boredom. A given experimental manipulation can have either or both of these learning and performance effects.

This important distinction has been mostly ignored since the late 1950s (see, e.g., Salmoni, Schmidt, & Walter, 1984, in the area of feedback and skill learning), and it is interesting to speculate why that might be the case. In our opinion, the information-processing metaphor, which has dominated much of the modern era of research, has led theorists away from such a distinction. That metaphor, based as it is on the architecture of the typical digital computer, does not readily suggest the kind of dual memory representation implied by, for example, habit strength and reaction potential (Hull, 1943). (For more on these and related arguments, see Bjork, 1989, and Bjork & Bjork, 1992.)

For present purposes, the important point is that only certain kinds of performance changes can qualify for the label *learning effects*. For us to agree that one level of some variable has produced more learning than another, we usually demand that these differences have some permanence across time, or that the differences be able to survive the removal of the manipulation in question. The problem is to discover which of many possible practice variables produce learning effects in the sense just defined—that is, to determine whether a given independent variable has effects that are relatively permanent or are merely transitory.

Testing Posttraining Retention and Transfer The standard approach to this problem is to use various kinds of transfer or retention tests as a means of evaluating the extent to which true learning has taken place. Assume that two groups of subjects practice under different levels of some independent variable during an acquisition phase. For example, they might be learning foreign vocabulary words, with frequency of feedback being manipulated (after every trial vs. after every fifth trial). Differences between groups during the acquisition phase could reflect differences in learning or performance (or both). It is critical, therefore, to add a *retention phase* (sometimes called a *transfer phase*), conducted after an interpolated interval that is long enough to ensure that any temporary effects of the independent variable have been dissipated. If subjects are then tested on the same (or a similar) task again under equated levels of the independent variable (so that differential temporary effects cannot reappear across trials), relative performance differences between the two groups can be viewed with some confidence as reflecting differential learning that occurred during the acquisition phase.

Special Considerations in Real-World Training Measuring the actual level of learning that results from a training regimen of some kind may not seem to be a particularly serious problem for scientists or scientifically trained professionals involved in training, as these issues have been (or should have been) familiar to us for several decades. But the problem is far more serious for the typical person who is actually doing the training in some real-world environment. Here, it is easy to imagine that trainers would make every effort to adjust the training context to maximize the learner's performance in training (measured as either speed of acquisition—that is, the trials or time necessary to reach some specified performance goal—or the level of performance achieved after a fixed amount of training time or trials). Without even giving the matter much thought, trainers might easily assume that maximizing performance during training is their major goal; trainers may themselves even be evaluated in terms of their trainees' performance during training.

Two other considerations exacerbate the problem in real-world environments. First, while instructors have ample opportunity to view their students during practice, they frequently do not have a chance to examine their learners on the transfer or retention tests that are the real goal of training. Such posttraining performance is often delayed or in a different location than the original training. Second, instructors can also be misled by their own trainees: In a study of learning keyboard skills under different practice schedules (Baddeley & Longman, 1978), for example, the schedules that were most preferred by subjects produced the least learning.

Problem 2: Acquisition and Retention Phenomena Are Not Separable

Learning Processes Versus Retention Processes Our basic argument is that the relative amount learned should be measured by performance on retention tests of various kinds, and that performance levels in acquisition are "flawed," or at least ambiguous, with respect to the amount learned. Note that this is quite a different view from that often taken in educational and training environments, where learning and retention are seen as two different phenomena. *Learning* is assumed to refer to that set of processes occurring during the actual practice on the tasks of interest, as assessed by performance measures taken at that time, whereas *retention* is seen to involve the set of processes that occur after practice is completed, during some retention interval, and prior to a retention test. Because learning and retention are thought to be different phenomena, they tend to be studied with separate methods, by different scientists, and even in different laboratories. Rather than viewing learning and posttraining retention as separable phenomena, however, we argue that the effectiveness of learning is revealed by, or measured by, the level of retention shown.

Criteria Against Which Training Should Be Evaluated In most educational, military, and industrial environments, the effectiveness of a training program can be evaluated by several criteria, depending on what we would like our learners to be able to do. Certainly, one of the most important of these is posttraining performance: We want trainees to be able, many months after the training program is completed, to perform well, or at least adequately. This criterion is especially important in times of natural disasters and human-made emergencies, when key people must perform critical functions in situations that reoccur, typically, only after very great delays. A crisis in a nuclear power plant would be a prime example. This criterion is also important in minimizing the time and money spent on retraining or refresher courses.

Another criterion is generalization. Whereas it is important to be able to perform the specific skill acquired in practice some months later in a retention test, it is also important to be able to *generalize* to variations of that skill, perhaps to be performed in contexts different from those experienced in acquisition. For example, the trainee might have to generalize the skill acquired under quiet, controlled conditions in a classroom to a noisy, hot, and cluttered environment in the workplace. The capability to perform in the presence of stress, sleep loss, or fatigue may be critical in some situations, and the need to perform a simultaneous secondary task effectively may be important as well. There may also be a need to have learning generalize to other learning environments, allowing new tasks to be learned more quickly and easily. The acquisition condition that is most effective—given these criteria—is the one leading to the highest performance on a novel version of the task, or on a task performed or practiced under novel conditions. Thus, rather than thinking of learning and generalizability as separate concepts—as is often done—we interpret the capability to generalize as one measure of learning and as a basis for selecting among various training conditions.

It is perhaps not new to suggest that there are several goals of training and instruction, such as long-term retention, generalizability, and resistance to altered contexts. What is new, however, is the notion that the training conditions to achieve these training goals are not necessarily those that maximize performance in the acquisition phase. In fact, as we show next, there can be conditions for which the effectiveness of training—as measured by one or another of these alternative criteria—is best achieved by a condition that produces relatively poor performances during training.

INTRODUCING DIFFICULTIES FOR THE LEARNER CAN ENHANCE TRAINING: THREE ILLUSTRATIONS

In this section, we discuss three broad situations in which, relative to a "standard" practice condition, some condition in acquisition that slows the rate of improvement or decreases performance at the end of practice nonetheless yields enhanced posttraining performance. One of these examples involves variations in the way tasks can be ordered for practice, with the focus on the criterion of producing effective skill retention. A second example involves variations in the nature and scheduling of feedback for learning, again with the emphasis on enhancing a retention criterion. Finally, a third example involves inducing variation among versions of the tasks to be practiced, with the focus on a criterion of generalizability.

Scheduling of Tasks During Practice

Consider the general problem in which several different tasks or items are to be learned in a practice session of a fixed length. How should the practice on these tasks or items be organized to maximize learning and retention?

Experiments with Motor Tasks Many variations in practice scheduling are possible. J.B. Shea and Morgan (1979) contrasted random and blocked schedules of practice, two schedules that differ substantially in terms of what Battig (1966) referred to as "contextual interference." In Shea and Morgan's study, blocked practice involved sequential trials at Task 1, Task 2, and Task 3, with all trials for a given task being completed before moving on to the next. Random practice, in contrast, involved the same number of trials at the three tasks, but the order was randomized so that a given task was never practiced on successive trials. Thus, blocked practice resembles what we usually term *drill*. The tasks required rapid, multiple-component arm movements, with the goal of minimizing response time, and different tasks had different patterns. After practice in an acquisition phase, retention tests were given after 10 minutes and 10 days. These retention tests were given under either random or blocked conditions. The experiment therefore was designed to assess the effect of random versus blocked practice on performance measured under blocked or random conditions.

The results are shown in Figure 1. During the acquisition phase, at the left, there was a clear advantage for the subjects who practiced under the blocked conditions, especially in the initial phases of practice, but continuing until the last acquisition block. Amount of learning, however, as measured by the tests of posttraining retention, tells a different story. Consider first the tests given under the random conditions, shown as the filled and open squares. There was a strong advantage for retention for the subjects who practiced under the random conditions in acquisition. That is, even though the random conditions were less effective during the acquisition phase, they were better than the blocked conditions on the random retention test. These differences are especially impressive given the ecological validity of random tests; that is, most real-world behaviors are not produced in blocked contexts.

An alternative interpretation of the advantage of random practice for random retention conditions is that the practice conditions in the acquisition and test phases were identical for the random subjects, but were different for the blocked subjects. This is, in effect, a kind of "identical elements," specificity-of-learning, or similarity argument. This relatively uninteresting interpretation cannot, however, explain the retention performance observed under the blocked conditions (shown as open and

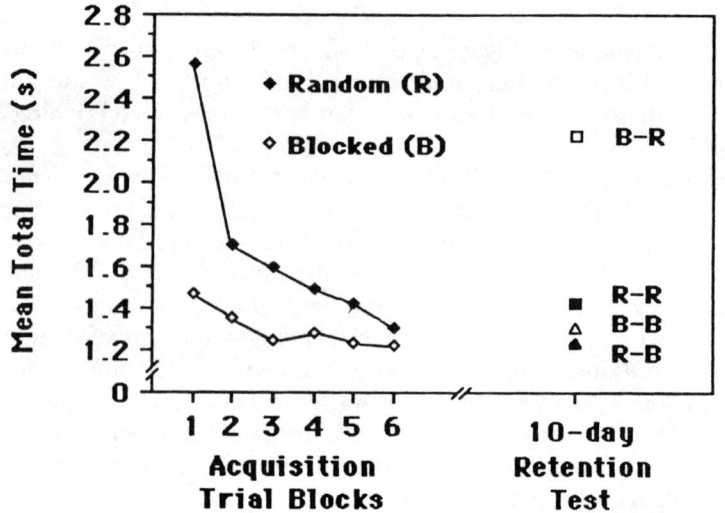

Figure 1. Performance on movement speed tasks under random (R) and blocked (B) conditions in acquisition and, after 10 days, in retention tests under random or blocked conditions. In retention, the first letter indicates the acquisition condition and the second represents the retention condition.

filled triangles). Once again, there was an advantage—although much reduced—for the subjects who practiced under random conditions during acquisition.

Regardless of whether the retention test was itself random or blocked, then, it was always more effective to have practiced under random conditions than under blocked conditions. Remarkably, this was the case even though the random condition was detrimental to performance during acquisition. Relative to blocked practice—a schedule that most people would feel was "natural" or optimal—random practice is, then, a first example of a manipulation that degrades performance in acquisition, yet enhances performance at retention and contributes to the capability to perform in different contexts (see also Wulf & Schmidt, 1988).

Similar effects have been found in several other experiments using real-world skills (serving in badminton, Goode & Magill, 1986; keyboard skills, Baddeley & Longman, 1978), as well as laboratory tasks (Lee, 1988; Lee & Magill, 1983). One exception is that, at minimal levels of practice, blocked practice produces better retention than does random practice, but this effect is reversed with additional levels of practice (C.H. Shea, Kohl, & Indermill, 1990). These phenomena, and various theoretical interpretations thereof, have been reviewed by Magill and Hall (1990).

Experiments with Verbal Tasks The effects of blocked versus random practice in the motor skills literature are analogous to certain verbal-learning phenomena typically studied under the heading of *spacing effects* (Melton, 1967). Here, the general problem is that distinct items presented serially are to be learned, and the question is how the study trials on a given item should be interleaved with the study trials on other items to generate maximal retention. In general, spacing of repetitions yields better long-term retention than does massing of repetitions—often much better. If the final retention interval is short, however, massed repetitions can yield better performance than spaced repetitions. (For examples of such interactions involving intervals ranging from seconds to minutes to days, respectively, see Bahrick, 1979; Glenberg, 1979; Glenberg & Lehmann, 1980; Peterson, Hillner, & Saltzman, 1962.) The interaction of spacing interval and retention interval may again mislead people responsible for training; on the basis of performance during acquisition alone, massed repetitions may appear to be superior to spaced repetitions.

In a variety of real-world situations, the question is not how one should distribute the repetitions of items, but rather how one should distribute one's effort to practice the retrieval of those items. Two experiments (Landauer & Bjork, 1978) examined how such retrieval efforts should be scheduled to optimize long-term retention. In the first experiment, subjects were asked to learn a number of names of hypothetical people. During the study phase, a given name was presented once and then tested three times (by presenting the first name as a cue for the last name or the last name as a cue for the first name). The intervals from the initial presentation of a given name to each successive test of that name were filled with different numbers of intervening presentations and tests of other names. Following the study phase, there was a 30-minute retention interval filled with a distracting activity prior to a final retention test for all the names.

Two aspects of the results of this experiment are of interest. First, as shown in Figure 2, the conditions that yielded optimal performance on the tests during acquisition yielded the poorest long-term retention. In a condition with zero items intervening between successive tests, performance on those tests averaged about 95%, but performance dropped to 33% on the final retention test. Other uniform-spacing conditions, with four or five intervening items between successive tests, yielded poorer performance during acquisition (about 43% correct), but better final retention (41% correct). Second, an expanding sequence of intervals prior to each successive test on a given name during acquisition (0, 3, and 9 intervening items, or 1, 4, and 10 items) appeared to yield optimal retention performance (48% correct).

In the second experiment, subjects were asked to memorize a first and last name corresponding to each of a set of facial photographs. During the acquisition phase, after an initial pairing of a given name and face,

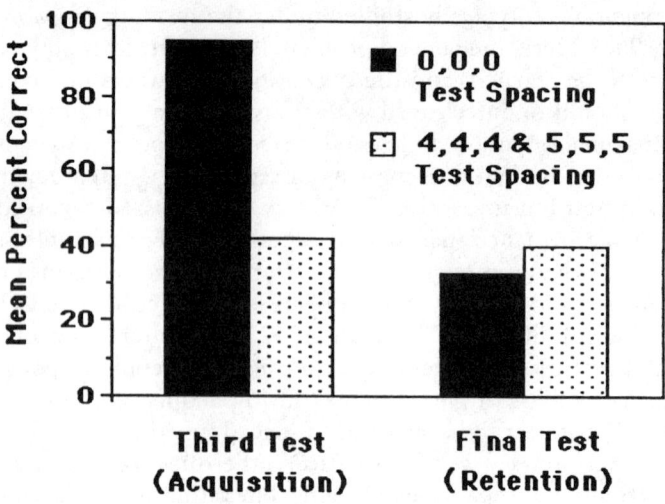

Figure 2. Percentage correct name recall on the third of three tests embedded in a study phase and on a 30-minute delayed retention test, as a function of the spacing of the three study-phase tests.

there were four subsequent tests of that face–name combination, each of which consisted of presenting the face and the first (or second) name as a cue for the missing name. The intervals separating the successive tests of a given name formed an expanding sequence (0, 1, 3, and 8 intervening events) or a uniform sequence with the same average interval length (3, 3, 3, and 3 intervening items), and there was again a test of final retention after a 30-minute delay. On the final test, each face was shown alone, and subjects were asked to recall both the first and last name corresponding to that face.

Once again, an expanding sequence was more effective than a uniform sequence for long-term retention. In fact, for the expanding condition, the retention of a name presented only once (and tested four times) was greater than retention of a name presented—together with a given face—five times (66% vs. 58% correct). This result illustrates the general principle that tests are potent learning events—often more potent than presentations—particularly when the tests are difficult enough to constitute a type of retrieval practice with respect to the criteria retention test. There are analogous results in the motor memory literature. For example, Hagman (1983), using an arm-positioning task, found that four test trials that involved attempting to repeat a once-presented position were more effective for retention than were four presentation trials in which the subject moved to a stop defining the target position.

In terms of the goal of enhancing long-term retention, expanding-interval retrieval practice may well be an important component of an optimal training program. Rea and Modigliani (1985), for example, have gone on to show that expanding retrieval practice is about twice as effective as massed practice in children's memorization of multiplication facts and spelling words. Such effects of expanding-interval retrieval practice in the verbal domain seem quite closely related to another effect we discuss in the next major section—namely, the scheduling of the number of practice trials between presentations of feedback in skill learning.

Common Principles In each of the foregoing paradigms, the condition that produced the best retention performance seemed to have the characteristic that it provided added "difficulty" for the learner during the acquisition phase, reflected in poorer performance at that time. Thus, as we view it, random practice serves to keep the performer from generating a stable "set" for a particular task, and forces the learner to retrieve and organize a different outcome on every trial. Similarly, the spacing of repetitions may prevent superficial massed rehearsal.

These notions suggest that retrieval practice (Bjork, 1975, 1988), in which the learner is actually given practice at the process of retrieving information from memory, may be an important factor in all of these paradigms. Indeed, other information-processing activities that cause forgetting of the to-be-remembered information, and thus require practice at retrieving it again on a subsequent trial, are beneficial for retention (Bjork & Allen, 1970; Cuddy & Jacoby, 1982).

We view retrieval practice as a specific case of transfer-appropriate processing (Morris, Bransford, & Franks, 1977); practice at retrieving in acquisition is appropriate for the need to retrieve during retention or transfer tests. Consistent with this view, there are results in the literature (Allen, Mahler, & Estes, 1969; Hogan & Kintsch, 1971) suggesting that tests as learning events—relative to presentations as learning events—become more effective as 1) the retention interval preceding a criterion test is increased and 2) the criterion test stresses recall rather than recognition.

It is clearly too extreme to argue that every manipulation causing difficulty for the learner during practice will enhance retention performance (see, e.g., J.B. Shea & Upton, 1976, who showed that interpolated processing tasks degrade performance both during practice and on retention tests), but, if the manipulation demands other kinds of information processing—such as retrieval practice—that are also needed for retention performance, then such added difficulty can be expected to enhance retention performance.

Feedback During Skill Acquisition

A second illustration involves the nature and scheduling of feedback presented to learners during an acquisition phase. It has generally been understood that any variation of feedback in practice that makes the information more immediate, more accurate, more frequent, or more useful for modifying behavior will contribute to learning, as measured during the acquisition phase. This view of the relationship of feedback and learning has served as the basis for instructional practice in many settings, as well as for the design of simulators. Recent evidence, however, suggests that this generalization must be qualified.

Experiments with Motor Tasks In one study (Schmidt, Young, Swinnen, & Shapiro, 1989), subjects were asked to learn a relatively complex arm movement in which the subject was to produce two reversals in direction such that the time of the action was as close to a set goal as possible. In one condition, feedback about the movement–time error was given after each trial, a more or less standard schedule typically thought to optimize learning. Feedback was also given in *summary* form (see Lavery, 1962), in which the subject received feedback about each of a set of trials (e.g., five) only after the last trial in the set was completed. This feedback was given in the form of a graph of performance against each of the trials in the set, so that the subject could see the error on each of the previous trials. The summary length—the number of trials summarized on the graph—was either 1 (the every-trial feedback condition mentioned earlier), 5, or 15 trials. After practice under these conditions in an acquisition phase, subjects were given tests of posttraining retention (without any feedback) after 10 minutes and 2 days.

The results of this experiment are shown in Figure 3. In the acquisition phase, subjects in the one-trial summary condition performed more accurately throughout practice than the other groups, with generally larger errors being produced as the summary length increased. It is clear that increased summary length interfered with performance during training, both in slowing the rate of approach to the asymptote and in generating larger errors near the end of practice. However, when performance was evaluated on the delayed retention test, the most effective performance was generated by the 15-trial group, with generally increasing errors as the summary length in the acquisition phase decreased. That is, there was a clear negative relationship between the level of performance in acquisition and the level of performance in retention. These data tend to contradict the long-held view that making feedback more useful is effective for learning, as the 15-trial condition seemed to provide difficulties in relating the feedback received in the graph to the error on the trial to which it referred (see also Schmidt, Lange, & Young, 1990).

Similar effects were obtained when feedback was given in acquisition either on every trial (100% condition) or on only half of the trials (Winstein & Schmidt, 1990; see also Wulf & Schmidt, 1989). In the latter, 50% condition, the feedback was *faded*, such that feedback was given on every

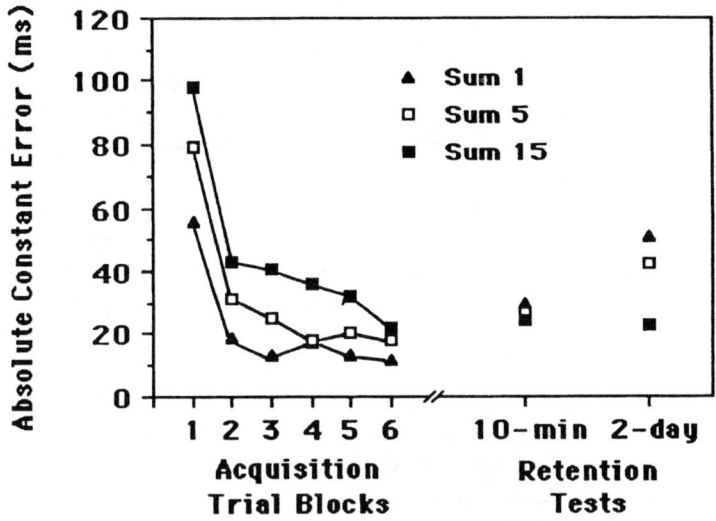

Figure 3. Mean errors in a movement-patterning task for three different summary-feedback lengths in acquisition, and on no-feedback retention tests given after 10 minutes or 2 days.

trial early in practice and gradually withdrawn across practice. Retention performance was measured after 10 minutes and 2 days, either with or without feedback being presented (in separate experiments). In both experiments, the 100% and 50%-faded groups were essentially similar in the acquisition phase, but, on the posttraining retention tests, the 50%-faded group had more effective performance, with the differences becoming larger as the retention interval increased. These data contradict traditional views of feedback operation in that providing half the number of feedback presentations in acquisition produced more effective retention performance. The general finding that expanded spacing of feedback presentations enhanced retention is analogous to the finding (Landauer & Bjork, 1978) that expanded spacing of repetitions was more effective for name learning, suggesting again that some common features underlie these two paradigms.

Experiments with Verbal Tasks During the 1960s, a dozen or so paired-associate experiments were conducted in which the proportion of responses that received feedback was manipulated during the acquisition phase. The percentage of occurrence of response members (% ORM) was defined by the percentage of trials on which the correct response term was shown after the subject had responded to the stimulus term. All of these studies, unfortunately, have characteristics that prevent them from being compared directly with the work just mentioned on motor behavior. For example, practice was always provided until a particular criterion was reached (e.g., 100% correct); because improvement in acquisition was faster with more frequent feedback, this procedure confounded the percentage feedback in acquisition with the amount of practice. Also, delayed retention tests were never given, which is unfortunate in view of the motor findings that the benefits of infrequent feedback seem to increase with longer retention intervals (see, e.g., Figure 3). Even so, several of these studies suggest that reducing the percentage feedback in acquisition—in some cases from 100% to 0%—has negligible effects on performance in immediate retention (Krumboltz & Weisman, 1962; Schultz & Runquist, 1960), suggesting a rough parallel to the work in motor behavior.

Recently, Schooler and Anderson (1990) examined feedback frequency effects in learning the computer language LISP, showing that (relative to frequent feedback) decreasing the number of feedback presentations depressed performance in acquisition but facilitated retention performance. This work suggests that these effects might be generalizable to a variety of cognitive activities as well as to the motor behaviors discussed in the previous section.

Common Principles One interpretation of this work is that frequent feedback during the acquisition phase provides several advantages, one of which is guidance toward the correct behavior. But it also provides some disadvantages (see Schmidt, 1991a). One possibility is that frequent feedback comes to be a part of the task, so that performance is disrupted in retention when the feedback is removed or altered. Also, frequent feedback could block information-processing activities that are important during the acquisition phase for acquiring the capability to produce effective performance at retention. One possibility is that frequent feedback blocks the processing of response-produced (kinesthetic) feedback, leading to less effective error-detection capabilities for use in retention (Schmidt et al., 1989). Another possibility is that frequent feedback makes performance too variable during practice, preventing the learning of a stabilized representation of the kind necessary to sustain performance on a later retention test.

Notice that, except for the particular terminology used, these accounts are very similar to those offered with respect to the spacing paradigms in the previous section. The general point is that certain "difficult" training conditions may foster various kinds of processing activities that are required for effective retention performance.

Induced Variability of Practice

A final example involves the intentional variation, along a single dimension, of the task to be learned in acquisition. In this case, the criterion test performance typically requires performance on some novel variation not experienced in the acquisition session. The question is whether this intentional variation during practice, versus a consistent practice schedule, is effective for transfer to some novel retention test.

Experiments with Motor Tasks Numerous experimenters have dealt with this issue, but Catalano and Kleiner (1984) made the point very well. They used a coincident-timing task in which subjects responded to a simulated moving object by pressing a button when it reached a predefined coincidence point. Subjects received either constant practice at one target speed (either 5, 7, 9, or 11 mph) or variable practice at all four of these speeds for the same number of total trials. Learning was evaluated on a retention test in which novel speeds that lay outside the range of the subjects' previous experiences were presented (1, 3, 13, and 15 mph).

In acquisition, performance in the variable condition was generally less accurate than performance in the constant condition (52 vs. 38 ms absolute error, on average), perhaps reflecting the common view that performing one thing repeatedly is generally more effective than performing four different things. But results for the retention test of generalization to novel speeds, shown in Figure 4, show the variable group was more accurate than the constant group.

Many other experiments in the motor skills literature demonstrate similar findings (see Shapiro & Schmidt, 1982, for a review), with especially strong effects for children. For example, Kerr and Booth (1978) had 8-year-old subjects toss beanbags to targets 2 feet and 4 feet away (variable group) or only to a target 3 feet away (constant group). On a subsequent

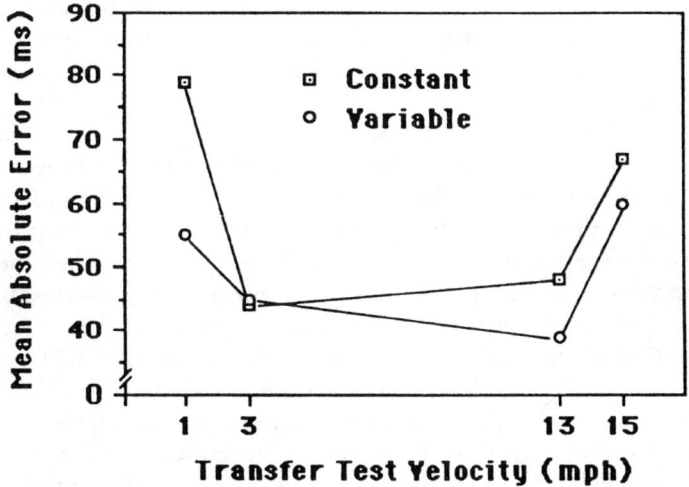

Figure 4. Mean timing error for transfer tests to novel target speeds after variable or constant practice in the acquisition phase.

test using the 3-foot target—the distance practiced by the constant group, but never practiced by the variable group—the variable group performed with greater accuracy than the constant group. This result suggests that learning how to modulate the relationships among the target distances was more important for a test at any one target distance than was specific experience, even at the particular target distance used at testing.

This collection of results about variable practice is usually interpreted in terms of schema theory (Schmidt, 1975; Wulf & Schmidt, 1988). The idea is that practice variability enhances the effectiveness of rules (schemata) that relate the external task requirements to the internal movement commands. But in terms of the arguments raised in the present chapter, these experiments suggest that variable practice alters the practice context to force a change in behavior from trial to trial, encouraging additional information-processing activities about the lawful relationships among the task variants. The result is learning that contributes to performance on the test of retention or generalizability, even though these activities detract from momentary performance during the acquisition phase.

Experiments with Verbal Tasks Several investigations in the concept formation literature provide analogous findings to those seen in the motor literature. For example, Nitsch (1977; see Bransford Franks, Morris, & Stein, 1979) had subjects learn novel concept words (e.g., to "crinch" was to offend someone) by providing several uses of the word that were in either a constant context (all in a restaurant) or a variable context (in numerous settings). Constant contexts were more effective than variable contexts for enabling subjects to identify the concept in the same context as it was presented earlier and were probably more effective in the acquisition phase as well. However, when the subjects were asked to recognize novel examples of the concept, variable practice was more effective than constant practice.

With a different paradigm, Mannes and Kintsch (1987) asked subjects to study a passage of text, preceded by an outline that was in either the same or a different organization as the text materials. The different-organization outline can be thought of as a kind of variable practice and the same-organization outline a form of constant practice. When the subjects were asked to recall the original text materials, the same-organization outline was more effective. But when the subjects were asked to do creative problem-solving tasks that required a deeper understanding of the text materials, the different-organization outline was more effective.

Both of these examples, together with the motor examples discussed above, suggest that, even though constant practice may lead to more effective performance in the acquisition phase, and often more accurate verbatim recall of the materials presented, constant practice produces less effective capabilities to generalize knowledge to novel situations than does variable practice.

CONCLUSIONS

A fundamental concern here has been the characterization of learning, its measurement, and the interpretations that are to be drawn from investigations of acquisition phenomena. Learning is obscured during the acquisition (or practice) phase because relatively permanent effects may be confounded with temporary performance effects that disappear quickly after the practice session is finished, or when the test conditions are changed. We advocate, therefore, the use of various kinds of transfer or retention tests on which (and only on which) the relatively permanent effects of the conditions in acquisition are evaluated. We have provided three experimental variations of practice in which conditions that facilitate performance during the acquisition phase are ineffective for learning as measured on a retention or transfer test. In each of those cases, there appear to be analogous effects across markedly different motor- and verbal-learning paradigms.

We are struck by the common features that underlie these counterintuitive phenomena in such a wide range of skill-learning situations. At the most superficial level, it appears that systematically altering practice so as to encourage additional, or at least different, information-processing activities can degrade performance during practice, but can at the same time have the effect of generating greater performance capabilities in retention or transfer tests. If these processing activities are selected so that they are also needed for success at a test of retention or generalizability, then such conditions will facilitate learning.

What are the processes underlying these empirical effects? We have only begun to ask this question, and answers are necessarily very tentative at present. Many possible information-processing activities have been postulated in the different tasks and paradigms mentioned here, such as the need to retrieve information that has faded from memory in name learning, the need to evaluate one's own response-produced feedback in motor learning, and the need to associate various different facts or actions into a single concept or schema. Other such processes have been suggested as well, and each of these paradigms has an active literature in which these various possibilities are argued and contrasted.

This perspective is distinct from the earlier viewpoints about the specificity of encoding (Tulving & Thomson, 1971) or specificity of abilities (Henry, 1968), in which the overlap of the objective acquisition and test conditions is the critical variable for learning. Whereas this overlap is undeniably of some importance for test performance, there is ample evidence presented here and elsewhere that this is not the only factor, and perhaps is not even the major factor, for test performance: For example, if the test is given under a blocked condition, random practice in acquisition is more effective for this test than is practice with the identical blocked condition (J.B. Shea & Morgan, 1979; see Figure 1 here). Also, even if the test is given under 100% feedback conditions, a 50%-faded condition in acquisition is better at testing than practice under the identical 100% condition (Winstein & Schmidt, 1990, Experiment 3). Finally, when test performance requires a beanbag toss of 3 feet, varied practice at 2- and 4-foot distances is better than practice at the identical 3-foot distance. All of these examples—taken from each of the paradigms mentioned here—tend to violate the specificity view that the simple overlap of conditions between acquisition and test contexts determines test effectiveness.

We prefer to suggest that the more important principle is the overlap of the processes necessary for performance on the test and the processes practiced during acquisition, refined from the ideas of transfer-appropriate processing (Bransford et al., 1979). Note that the overlap of relevant processes does not necessarily mean that there is overlap of the objective conditions of practice, as we have shown here several times already. If certain acquisition conditions force the learner to engage in processes that are also critical for test performance, then those conditions will be judged as effective for learning (because they facilitate test performance), even though they may exhibit different superficial conditions. Also, these conditions that maximize learning may not be very effective for performance during the acquisition phase, as they provide various "difficulties" for the learners. Random practice, reduced feedback, and variable practice all degrade performance during practice relative to more "ideal" conditions in acquisition, yet all can be argued to exercise information-processing activities that are critical for performance at the test. In other words, these conditions can be considered as effective for learning because they prepare the learner for the processing that will be required at testing.

Certainly, then, no single type of extra information-processing activity will be expected to underlie all of the tasks and paradigms discussed here. Even so, these data suggest a new conceptualization, or framework, for learning and training that has broad implications for educational practice (see, e.g., Christina & Bjork, 1991). From a practical perspective, this framework would stress that a trainer's major goal is to focus clearly on the criterion performance, and to understand what kinds of processes are required for its proficiency. Then, practice activities that exercise these particular processes could be designed (see, e.g., Schmidt, 1991b, Chapter 11). The criterial version of many tasks, for example, involves the execution of an essentially novel response that cannot have been practiced previously, such as the solution of a particular mathematical word problem on the job, or the execution of a basketball shot from a location never before experienced. In such cases, practice could be organized in a way to facilitate transfer and generalization, and a form of variable practice would be recommended. Other practice conditions would optimize performance in other contexts, as we have argued here.

REFERENCES

Allen, G.A., Mahler, W.A., & Estes, W.K. (1969). Effects of recall tests on long-term retention of paired associates. *Journal of Verbal Learning and Verbal Behavior, 17*, 573-585.

Baddeley, A.D., & Longman, D.J.A. (1978). The influence of length and frequency of training session on the rate of learning to type. *Ergonomics, 21*, 627-635.

Bahrick, H.P. (1979). Maintenance of knowledge: Questions about memory we forgot to ask. *Journal of Experimental Psychology: General, 108*, 296-308.

Battig, W.F. (1966). Facilitation and interference. In E.A. Bilodeau (Ed.), *Acquisition of skill* (pp. 215-244). New York: Academic Press.

Bjork, R.A. (1975). Retrieval as a memory modifier. In R. Solso (Ed.), *Information processing and cognition: The Loyola Symposium* (pp. 123-144). Hillsdale, NJ: Lawrence Erlbaum Associates.

Bjork, R.A. (1988). Retrieval practice and the maintenance of knowledge. In M.M. Gruneberg, P.E. Morris, & R.N. Sykes (Eds.), *Practical aspects of memory II* (pp. 396-401). London: Wiley.

Bjork, R.A. (1989). Retrieval inhibition as an adaptive mechanism in human memory. In H.L. Roediger & F.I.M. Craik (Eds.), *Varieties of memory and consciousness: Essays in honor of Endel Tulving* (pp. 195-210). Hillsdale, NJ: Lawrence Erlbaum Associates.

Bjork, R.A., & Allen, T.W. (1970). The spacing effect: Consolidation or differential encoding? *Journal of Verbal Learning and Verbal Behavior, 9*, 567-572.

Bjork, R.A., & Bjork, E.L. (1992). A new theory of disuse and an old theory of stimulation fluctuation. In A.F. Healy, S.M. Kosslyn, & R.M. Shiffrin (Eds.), *From learning processes to cognitive processes: Essays in honor of William K. Estes* (Vol. 2, pp. 35-67). Hillsdale, NJ: Lawrence Erlbaum Associates.

Bransford, J.D., Franks, J.J., Morris, C.D., & Stein, B.S. (1979). Some general constraints on learning and memory research. In L.S. Cermack & F.I.M. Craik (Eds.), *Levels of processing in human memory* (pp. 331-354). Hillsdale, NJ: Lawrence Erlbaum Associates.

Catalano, J.F., & Kleiner, B.M. (1984). Distant transfer and practice variability. *Perceptual and Motor Skills, 58*, 851-856.

Christina, R.W., & Bjork, R.A. (1991). Optimizing long-term retention and transfer. In D. Druchman & R.A. Bjork (Eds.), *In the mind's eye: Enhancing human performance* (pp. 23-56). Washington, DC: National Academy Press.

Cuddy, L.J., & Jacoby, L.L. (1982). When forgetting helps memory: Analysis of repetition effects. *Journal of Verbal Learning and Verbal Behavior, 21*, 451-467.

Estes, W.K. (1955) Statistical theory of distributional phenomena in learning. *Psychological Review, 62*, 369-377.

Glenberg, A.M. (1979). Component-levels theory of the effects of spacing of repetitions on recall and recognition. *Memory & Cognition, 7*, 95-112.

Glenberg, A.M., & Lehmann, T.S. (1980). Spacing repetitions over 1 week. *Memory & Cognition, 8*, 528-538.

Goode, S., & Magill, R.A. (1986). The contextual interference effects in learning three badminton serves. *Research Quarterly for Exercise and Sport, 57*, 308-314.

Guthrie, E.R. (1952). *The pscyhology of learning.* New York: Harper & Row.
Hagman, J.D. (1983). Presentation- and test-trial effects on acquisition and retention of distance and location. *Journal of Experimental Psychology: Learning, Memory, and Cognition, 9,* 334–345.
Henry, F.M. (1968). Specificity vs. generality in learning motor skill. In R.C. Brown & G.S. Kenyon (Eds.), *Classical studies on physical activity* (pp. 331–340). Englewood Cliffs, NJ: Prentice Hall. (Original work published 1958.)
Hogan, R.M., & Kintsch, W. (1971). Differential effects of study and test trials of long-term recognition and recall. *Journal of Verbal Learning and Verbal Behavior, 10,* 562–567.
Hull, C.L. (1943). *Principles of behavior.* New York: Appelton-Century-Crofts.
Kerr, R., & Booth, B. (1978). Specific and varied practice of a motor skill. *Perceptual and Motor Skills, 46,* 395–401.
Krumboltz, J.D., & Weisman, R.G. (1962). The effect of intermittent confirmation in programmed instruction. *Journal of Educational Psychology, 53,* 250–253.
Landauer, T.K., & Bjork, R.A. (1978). Optimum rehearsal patterns and name learning. In M.M. Gruneberg, P.E. Morris, & R.N. Sykes (Eds.), *Practical aspects of memory* (pp. 625–632). London: Academic Press.
Lavery, J.J. (1962). Retention of simple motor skills as a function of type of knowledge of results. *Canadian Journal of Psychology, 16,* 300–311.
Lee, T.D. (1988). Transfer-appropriate processing: A framework for conceptualizing practice effects in motor learning. In O.G. Meijer & K. Roth (Eds.), *Complex motor behaviour: 'The' motor-action controversy* (pp. 201–215). Amsterdam: Elsevier Science.
Lee, T.D., & Magill, R.A. (1983). The locus of contextual interference in motor skill acquisition. *Journal of Experimental Psychology: Learning, Memory, and Cognition, 9,* 730–746.
Magill, R.A., & Hall, K.G. (1990). A review of the contextual interference effect in motor skill acquisition. *Human Movement Science, 9,* 241–289.
Mannes, S.M., & Kintsch, W. (1987). Knowledge organization and text organization. *Cognition and Instruction, 4,* 91–115.
Melton, A.W. (1967). Repetition and retrieval from memory. *Science, 158,* 532.
Morris, C.D., Bransford, J.D., & Franks, J.J. (1977). Levels of processing versus transfer appropriate processing. *Journal of Verbal Learning and Verbal Behavior, 16,* 519–533.
Nitsch, K.E. (1977). *Structuring decontextualized forms of knowledge.* Unpublished doctoral dissertation, Vanderbilt University, Nashville.
Peterson, L.R., Hillner, K., & Saltzman, D. (1962). Time between pairings and short-term retention. *Journal of Experimental Psychology, 64,* 550–551.
Rea, C.P., & Modigliani, V. (1985). The effect of expanded versus massed practice on the retention of multiplication facts and spelling lists. *Human Learning, 4,* 11–18.
Salmoni, A.W., Schmidt, R.A., & Walter, C.B. (1984). Knowledge of results and motor learning: A review and critical reappraisal. *Psychological Bulletin, 95,* 355–386.
Schmidt, R.A. (1975). A schema theory of discrete motor skill learning. *Psychological Review, 82,* 225–260.
Schmidt, R.A. (1991a). Frequent augmented feedback can degrade learning: Evidence and interpretations. In G.E. Stelmach & J. Requin (Eds.), *Tutorial in motor neuroscience* (pp. 59–75). Dordrecht, The Netherlands: Kluwer.

Schmidt, R.A. (1991b). *Motor learning and performance: From principles to practice.* Champaign, IL: Human Kinetics.

Schmidt, R.A., & Bjork, R.A. (1989). *New conceptualizations of practice: Common principles in three research paradigms suggest important new concepts for practice.* Concept paper submitted to the U.S. Army Research Institute for the Behavioral and Social Sciences, Alexandria, VA.

Schmidt, R.A., Lange, C.A., & Young, D.E. (1990). Optimizing summary knowledge of results for skill learning. *Human Movement Science, 9,* 325–348.

Schmidt, R.A., Young, D.E., Swinnen, S., & Shapiro, D.C. (1989). Summary knowledge of results for skill acquisition: Support for the guidance hypothesis. *Journal of Experimental Psychology: Learning, Memory, and Cognition, 15,* 352–359.

Schooler, L.J., & Anderson, J.R. (1990). The disruptive potential of immediate feedback. In *Proceedings of the 12th Annual Conference of the Cognitive Science Society* (pp. 702–708). Cambridge, MA: Cognitive Science Society.

Schultz, R.W., & Runquist, W.N. (1960). Learning and retention of paired adjectives as a function of percentage occurrence of response members. *Journal of Experimental Psychology, 59,* 409–413.

Shapiro, D.C., & Schmidt, R.A. (1982). The schema theory: Recent evidence and developmental implications. In J.A.S. Kelso & J.E. Clark (Eds.), *The development of movement control and co-ordination* (pp. 113–150). New York: Wiley & Sons.

Shea, C.H., Kohl, R., & Indermill, C. (1990). Contextual interference: Contributions of practice. *Acta Psychologica, 73,* 145–157.

Shea, J.B., & Morgan, R.L. (1979). Contextual interference effects on the acquisition, retention, and transfer of a motor skill. *Journal of Experimental Psychology: Human Learning and Memory, 5,* 179–187.

Shea, J.B., & Upton, G. (1976). The effects on skill acquisition of an interpolated motor short-term memory task during the KR-delay interval. *Journal of Motor Behavior, 8,* 277–281.

Skinner, B.F. (1938). *The behavior of organisms.* New York: Appleton-Century-Crofts.

Tolman, E.C. (1932). *Purposive behavior of animals and men.* New York: Century.

Tulving, E., & Thomson, D.M. (1971). Retrieval processes in recognition memory: Effects of associative context. *Journal of Experimental Psychology, 87,* 116–124.

Winstein, C.J., & Schmidt, R.A. (1990). Reduced frequency of knowledge of results enhances motor skill learning. *Journal of Experimental Psychology: Learning, Memory, and Cognition, 16,* 677–691.

Wulf, G., & Schmidt, R.A. (1988). Variability in practice: Facilitation in retention and transfer through schema formation or context effects? *Journal of Motor Behavior, 20,* 133–149.

Wulf, G., & Schmidt, R.A. (1989). The learning of generalized motor programs: Reducing the relative frequency of knowledge of results enhances memory. *Journal of Experimental Psychology: Learning, Memory, and Cognition, 15,* 748–757.

SECTION II

PERSPECTIVES ON NORMAL MOTOR SPEECH CONTROL

Chapter 2

Goal-Based Speech Motor Control
A Theoretical Framework and Some Preliminary Data

*Joseph S. Perkell, Melanie L. Matthies,
Mario A. Svirsky, and Michael I. Jordan*

THE PURPOSES OF this chapter are to present a framework for a theory of speech production and to review some preliminary data that can be interpreted to support a key aspect of the framework. The framework is concerned primarily with "segmental" (as opposed to prosodic) aspects of speech production. According to the framework, the input to the speech motor programming system consists of sequences of goals that are defined in terms of acoustic and articulatory parameters. The goals are correlates of distinctive features that specify lexical items. The inclusion of acoustic parameters in goal definitions distinguishes this framework from articulatory phonology (Browman & Goldstein, 1986), in which the basic underlying units are characterized entirely in articulatory terms. The supporting data consist of findings of trading ("motor-equivalent") relations between lip rounding and tongue-body raising that should help to constrain

---

Reprinted from the *Journal of Phonetics*, 23, 23–25, 1995, by permission of the authors and Academic Press Limited.

This chapter contains material that was presented at the Third Seminar on Speech Production: Models and Data, Old Saybrook, Connecticut (May 11–13, 1993) and at the Conference on Motor Speech, Sedona, Arizona (March 24–28, 1994). This work was supported by National Institute on Deafness and Other Communication Disorders Grants No. DC00075 and DC01925.

We are grateful to Harlan Lane and to Robert Rosenthal, Hal Stern, Donald Rubin, and Douwe Yntema of Harvard University for extensive discussions and advice on statistical analyses, and to Ken Stevens, Alice Turk, Anders Lofqvist, and two anonymous reviewers for their helpful comments.

acoustic variation in production of the vowel /u/. Such data are consistent with the idea that the goals for speech motor programming include acoustic parameters; thus they may provide an experimental basis for differentiating between the two theories. (See Diehl & Kluender, 1989, for a discussion of some of the same issues, but dealing mainly with auditory constraints.)

Theories About the Basis of Sound Patterns of Languages

Our ideas for a theoretical framework come from a number of sources, including two theories about the basis of sound patterns of languages and how lexical items are represented. According to one such theory, lexical items are represented phonologically as sequences of discrete segments, which are characterized in terms of primitives called distinctive features (see Chomsky & Halle, 1968; Jakobson, Fant, & Halle, 1963). The features correspond to a universal set of capabilities that people have to produce and perceive sounds with linguistically distinctive properties. They are described as comprising two categories, articulator bound (i.e., executed by particular articulators—"labial" by the lips, "coronal" by the tongue blade) and articulator free ("continuant," "sonorant"—which have robust acoustic correlates and are not tied to the action of any one articulator) (Halle & Stevens, 1990). Contrasts between classes of speech sounds can be characterized in terms of the features and their correlates. One production-related basis for the features is found in quantal, or nonlinear, relations between articulation and properties of the sound output (Stevens, 1989) or between articulatory displacements and parts of the vocal tract area function (Fujimura & Kakita, 1979). This theory has little to say about the conversion of feature-based representations of utterances to articulatory movements. In particular, timing has to be determined largely by some mechanism "extrinsic" to the specification of utterances in terms of primitive elements (see Fowler, 1980).

In another theory, lexical items are represented by primitives that consist of abstract, dynamic gestures, which are defined in terms of the place and degree of vocal tract constrictions—in effect, spatial configurations of the articulators. The dynamic properties of the abstract gestures determine some aspects of articulatory kinematics and timing (Saltzman & Munhall, 1989), although intergestural coordination (relative timing and magnitude of gestures) is specified by a "gestural score" (Browman & Goldstein, 1986).

In principle, the feature theory and the gesture theory each make claims about a universal inventory of primitive units, subsets of which may be employed to characterize sound patterns of individual languages. Another proposal about the basis of sound patterns claims that the values of acoustic parameters characterizing vowel sounds in any language are determined by two principles: sufficient perceptual contrast and minimal articulatory effort (Lindblom, 1983; Lindblom & Engstrand, 1989). The combination of these principles leads to the prediction that vowel sounds occupy contiguous regions in acoustic space. The shapes and distributions of the regions depend on the number of vowels in the particular language (see also Boë, Schwartz, & Vallée, 1994). This idea, along with the quantal theory, is based on interactions among production, acoustics, and perception, whereas the gesture theory is based primarily in articulation.

Such theories seem to capture important organizational principles of sound patterns; however, none comes near to accounting for their diversity across languages. Observations of sound patterns across many languages reveal enormous variety and richness (see Henton, Ladefoged, & Maddieson, 1992; Ladefoged & Maddieson, 1990), some of which may not be accounted for by quantal, dynamic, or distributional principles. In general, sound systems of languages provide for linguistic contrast with acoustic cues; however, they do so while also incorporating presumably less quantifiable influences, such as factors that influence regional dialects (see Labov, 1986). Since the sound patterns of languages are influenced by a compromise among several organizing principles (Boë et al., 1994), some more difficult to quantify than others, it is not surprising that sound patterns vary and that it is difficult to find robust experimental support for any single principle to the exclusion of others.

Variability in "Listener-Oriented," Reduced Speech
When utterances are produced as sequences of sounds, the sounds are modified by coarticulation. In addition, speakers usually adjust the clarity of utterances, depending on the speaking situation (see Charles-Luce, 1995; Moon & Lindblom, 1994). Less clear utterances are said to be "reduced" (see Kohler, 1991): Some feature-specified acoustic cues are modified or obscured. Utterances can be reduced, because listeners are able to understand them without having access to a lot of detailed acoustic information. Listeners use their knowledge of the world, of syntax, and of the lexicon to fill in missing information in a form of "top-down processing." Thus, the level of clarity (measurable as intelligibility) that a speaker uses in any given situation is "listener oriented" (see Eefting, 1991; Lindblom, 1990). The speaker adjusts clarity according to an ongoing assessment of the listener's ability to understand what is being said. With reduction, some sound segments are dropped and others are changed so that articulatory movements are less complicated or extreme. As a result, the speaker transmits the message more efficiently—in a shorter time with less effort.

Depending on factors such as the amount of noise in the environment, the listener's familiarity with the language, speaker, and subject matter, and whether or not the listener can see the speaker's face, there is a considerable amount of variation in expression of the values of some of the parameters that define sound categories (feature correlates). In extreme cases of reduction, the boundaries of some articulatory and acoustic regions may be crossed or modified. (Perceptual judgments of within-category differences in prototypicality of speech sounds [see Volaitis & Miller, 1992] indicate that the regions may have internal structure, with centers that represent the highest degree of prototypicality and boundaries that are not sharp.) Consequently, the expression of acoustic parameters responsible for sound contrasts is not invariant; articulatory movements are programmed to constrain acoustic variation within situation-specific, perceptually acceptable limits, which may be rather broad. For a given speech sound or utterance, a wide range of acoustic signals may result in a correct percept, due to a combination of linguistically governed sound categorization (by virtue of a compromise among quantal, distributional, and other principles) and top-down predictive processing by the listener.

Goal-Based Speech Motor Control

According to our theoretical framework, lexical items consist of sequences of segments, which are characterized by combinations of contrast-defining features. The features specify how the articulators are to be moved or positioned and/or what acoustic properties are to be achieved by these movements. For some types of segments, such as vowels, features such as [high], [low], and [back] are described primarily in terms of acoustic goals, with the articulators being adjusted to achieve these goals (see Johnson, Ladefoged, & Lindau, 1993). For consonants, some of the features, such as the specification of which articulator is forming the consonantal constriction, are described primarily in articulatory terms. There are, of course, patterns of acoustic properties that signal to the listener what features are being implemented. These acoustic properties may depend on other features that are involved in producing the segment. The generation of a segment usually requires the coordination of movements of several articulators. In the case of a consonant, the segmental (feature) description specifies the major articulator (such as the lips, tongue blade, or tongue body—and its positioning) that forms a constriction in the vocal tract and creates an acoustic discontinuity that serves as a landmark. Other features specify the action of secondary articulators (such as the glottis and velum). The movements of the secondary articulators must be coordinated with the timing of the primary articulation that is generating a landmark so that evidence for the various features is present in the acoustic signal in the vicinity of the landmark (see Stevens, Manuel, Shattuck-Hufnagel, & Liu, 1992).

When feature-specified representations of utterances are converted to sound, the ultimate goals of the articulatory movements are acoustic patterns that will allow the listener to understand what is said. However, for the speaker's production mechanism, the goals may be specified in terms of more than one type of parameter, and they may vary in kind from one sound segment to the next. As noted above, the goals are defined as regions in acoustic and articulatory space by quantal, dynamic, and distributional principles. In the simple vowel-consonant-vowel (VCV) utterance /uku/, the acoustic goal for the /u/ may be a region in formant frequency space; its articulatory goal may be "encoded neurophysiologically in terms of significant area–function information, specifically by information related to cavity configuration at points of maximum constriction" (Gay, Lindblom, & Lubker, 1981, p. 802). For the consonant /k/, two supraglottal articulatory goals may be to have the tongue body produce a complete closure with adequate force in the velopalatal region and to have sufficiently tense vocal tract walls so that the intraoral air pressure built up during the stop will be sufficient to produce a noise burst at the moment of release; one of its acoustic goals is a silent interval.

When an utterance is planned with a certain prosodic specification and degree of clarity, some feature-specified goals may be obscured or modified, affecting the sizes and locations of their regions in articulatory and acoustic space. (If the sequence /uku/ were embedded in a word, the target region of formant values for /u/ might be expanded toward those of a more neutral vowel; the required force of contact for the /k/ might be less.) Based on the resulting modified goal sequence, temporal occurrences of acoustic landmarks and the relative timing of articulatory movements around the landmarks are programmed by a mechanism that uses an internal model of relations between commands to the articulators, their movements, and the acoustic consequences of those movements (Jordan, 1992; Nooteboom, 1970). The internal model is acquired and maintained with the use of auditory and somatosensory feedback (Jordan & Rumelhart, 1992; see also Laboissière, Schwartz, & Bailly, 1991), but, once speech has been learned, auditory feedback is not used in the on-line, moment-to-moment control of articulatory movements (see Lindblom, Lubker, & Gay, 1979). Somatosensory feedback probably is used on line, moment to moment, but at lower levels in a hierarchically organized system of speech motor control (see Gracco, 1987; Gracco & Abbs, 1988; Perkell, 1980).

One important purpose of this hierarchical organization is to reduce the number of degrees of freedom that have to be controlled by higher levels (see Abbs, Gracco, & Cole, 1984; Johnson et al., 1993): It is necessary to control multiple muscles for each articulatory movement, multiple articulators for each vocal tract constriction, and multiple constrictions for some acoustic transfer functions. The articulatory trajectories that result from this control obey a smoothness constraint (Jordan, 1992), which represents an interaction between the serial (discrete) nature of the task on the one hand, and a combination of dynamic response properties of the articulators and an effort-minimizing motor control strategy on the other (see Nelson, 1983).

EXPERIMENTAL SUPPORT FOR ACOUSTIC GOALS IN SPEECH MOTOR PROGRAMMING

In the remainder of this chapter, we review some relevant preliminary evidence for the existence of an acoustic goal for the vowel /u/, in the form of findings of "motor equivalence" at the level of the transformation between the vocal tract area function and the acoustic transfer function. The term *motor equivalence* refers to the observation that the same goal is reached in more than one way (see Hughes & Abbs, 1976). Theoretically, this may occur at more than one level in a control hierarchy. In multiple repetitions, there can be complementary (covarying or trading) contributions of two or more muscles to the same articulatory movement; two or more movements (e.g., of the two lips, or tongue and mandible) to the same constriction; and, in some cases, two different constrictions (e.g., formed with the tongue and with the lips) to the same acoustic transfer function. (For illustrations of the first two types of trading relations, see Abbs et al. [1984] and Abbs & Gracco [1984].) Some research on motor equivalence has been criticized because of insufficiently strong evidence at the muscle-to-movement level and interdependence of correlated parameters at the movement-to-constriction level (see Folkins & Brown, 1987; Sussman, 1980). However, the weakness of evidence at the muscle-to-movement level may be due to the difficulty of sampling adequately all of the muscle activity that contributes to any given movement, and motor equivalence has been shown between articulator displacements by techniques that do not rely on correlations of interdependent parameters (see Maeda, 1991).

Findings of trading relations in muscle-to-movement and movement-to-constriction transformations would be compatible with articulatory phonology and its associated task-dynamic model (Saltzman & Munhall, 1989), as well as with the framework we have outlined above. However, since our framework includes goals that have acoustic components and articulatory phonology and the task-dynamic model do not, a finding of motor equivalence in the transformation between the vocal tract area function and its acoustic transfer function should favor the theory that includes acoustic goals. Theoretically, such trading relations should be possible and testable for sounds such as /u/, /r/, and /ʃ/, whose acoustic transfer functions are determined by two relatively independent degrees of freedom of the area function—constrictions formed by the tongue and by the lips.

Preliminary Findings of Articulatory-to-Acoustic Motor Equivalence

The double-headed arrows in Figure 1 illustrate the motor equivalence hypothesis for production of the vowel /u/ in American English. The /u/ is produced by constricting the area function in the velopalatal region with tongue-body raising, and constricting the area function in the labial region with lip rounding. Because of the many-to-one mapping between vocal tract area functions and the acoustic transfer function (see Atal, Chang, Mathews, & Tukey, 1978), a similar transfer function can be produced with a bit more tongue raising and a bit less lip rounding, and vice versa. So, for example, if some source of variation were to cause the tongue body to be too low, an acceptable /u/ could be produced with increased lip rounding. Such a strategy could be used to help constrain acoustic variability, in effect, to keep the sound output within the appropriate acoustic–phonetic region.

To test the hypothesis, we have made articulatory and acoustic measurements for multiple repetitions of the vowel /u/ by six male speakers of American English. The vowel was embedded in various environments using a carrier phrase, such as "Ma *who* hid it." Movements were transduced with an electromagnetic midsagittal articulometer (EMMA) system (Perkell et al., 1992). As illustrated by the filled circles in Figure 1, we tracked the movements of points on the tongue body (TB), upper and

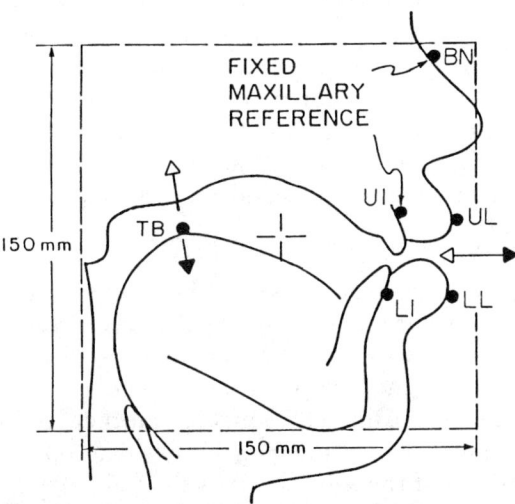

Figure 1. A midsagittal outline of the vocal tract, with filled circles showing the approximate locations of the transducers on the vermillion border of the upper lip (UL) and the lower lip (LL), the gingival papilla between the two lower central incisors (LI), the tongue-body dorsum (TB), the bridge of the nose (BN), and the upper incisors (UI). The double-headed arrows illustrate a trading relation between tongue-body raising and lip rounding.

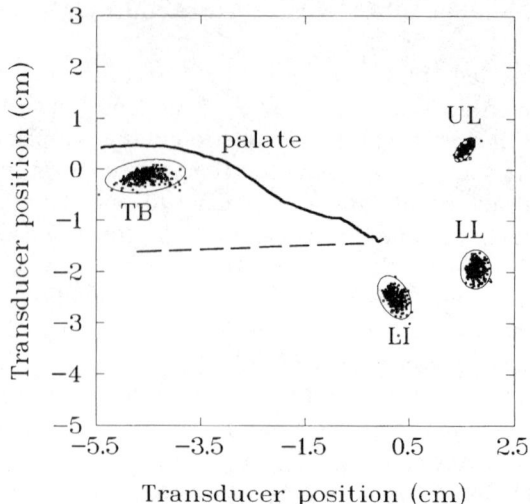

Figure 2. Midsagittal-plane distributions of transducer locations for the vowel /u/ from Subject 2 of Perkell et al. (1993) for the tongue body (TB), lower incisors (LI), lower lips (LL), and upper lips (UL), along with an outline of the hard palate. The dashed line indicates the orientation of the occlusal plane. Ninety-nine percent confidence interval ellipses are drawn around the distribution for each transducer. Anterior is to the right; distances are given in centimeters.

lower lips (UL, LL), and mandible (LI) in a maxilla-based coordinate system. Figure 2 shows scatter plots of the mid-vowel locations of transducers on the tongue body, upper lip, lower lip, and lower incisor for multiple repetitions of /u/ by one of the subjects. Anterior is to the right. The dashed line indicates the orientation of the occlusal plane. Experimental details and results from Subjects 1–4 are presented in Perkell, Matthies, Svirsky, and Jordan (1993); for the current chapter, we are reviewing the results from the first four subjects and are including new results from two more subjects.

To use EMMA data to test the hypothesis, it was necessary to know how the ranges of coordinates observed in Figure 2 translated into vocal tract cross-sectional areas and how those areas might affect the vowel acoustics. Findings of an articulatory trading relation would provide more convincing support of the hypothesis if the ranges of the articulatory variables produced approximately equal magnitudes of change in the acoustics, as opposed to producing highly disproportionate acoustic changes. For three of the subjects (Perkell et al., 1993), we used dental casts of their palates and ranges of EMMA measures of tongue height, along with video recordings of their lips, to derive approximate ranges of cross-sectional areas in the velopalatal and labial regions. The ranges of labial and velopalatal areas were then used in manipulating an articulatory synthesizer to determine their influence on the vowel acoustics. The observed velopalatal and labial area ranges in all three subjects produced approximately equal effects on F_2, so the EMMA data could be used to test the hypothesis. It is important to note that we cannot demonstrate that acoustic variation was reduced when the subjects used a motor equivalence strategy; however, the modeling showed that, with the same ranges of articulatory variation and no trading relation, the amount of acoustic variation was substantially greater.

We have looked for trading relations between measures of tongue-body raising and lip rounding, expressed in the form of negative correlations for multiple repetitions. Across the six subjects, upper lip protrusion has been the component of lip rounding with the largest variance, so we have concentrated on the relation between tongue-body raising and upper-lip protrusion. These two parameters are mechanically independent of one another, and thus they represent two independently controllable degrees of freedom of the vocal tract area function.

We have found statistically significant negative correlations of these two parameters in full data sets from three speakers and in a phonetically defined subset of data from one more, making a total of four out of the six. Table 1 summarizes these correlation results, with significant r values ($p \leq$ .05) shown in boldface. The columns labeled "r", "p," and "n" under "All data" give correlation results from the entire data set from each of the subjects. The next two columns give the standard deviations of tongue-body raising (tbr) and upper-lip protrusion (ulp) in millimeters. The right part of Table 1 shows the correlation results of the subset consisting of stressed /u/ followed by /ɪ/, the phonetic context common to the largest number of the subjects' data sets. Three of the subjects, 2, 3, and 4, show significant negative correlations, and one, Subject 6, shows a significant positive correlation. In the subset, Subject 1 also shows a significant negative correlation. The asterisks indicate that such utterances were not included in the corpora for Subjects 3 and 4. Thus, the results for Subjects 2, 3, and 4 sup-

Table 1. Correlations between tongue-body raising and upper-lip protrusion

Subject	All data[a]					Stressed /u/ followed by /ɪ/		
	r	p	n	SD tbr (mm)	SD ulp (mm)	r	p	n
1	.054	.311	354	1.1	0.5	−.251	.033	72
2	−.262	.002	137	1.1	0.7	−.405	.029	29
3	−.361	.000	290	1.3	1.0	*	*	*
4	−.382	.046	96	0.9	0.7	*	*	*
5	−.046	.391	344	1.1	1.6	−.046	.391	344
6	.349	.000	148	0.6	1.3	.349	.000	148

Adapted in part from Perkell et al. (1993).
[a]SD tbr, standard deviation, tongue-body raising; SD ulp, standard deviation, upper-lip protrusion.
*Utterance not included in corpora for this subject.

port the motor equivalence hypothesis and those from Subject 1 are at least partly consistent with it.

Factors Underlying Findings of Articulatory-to-Acoustic Motor Equivalence

In this section, we address several issues that are raised by the results: 1) why the negative correlations for Subject 1 may be found only in a subset of his data, 2) why there are differences among subjects, 3) whether the results could be an artifact of the selection of times for articulatory data extraction, and 4) why the observed correlations are not stronger.

Findings in Subsets of the Data In Table 1, Subject 1 shows a negative correlation only in the subset stressed /u/ followed by /ɪ/. (The corpora for Subjects 1 and 2 also included subsets containing unstressed /u/ and /u/ followed by /æ/.) The value of F_2 was higher for /u/ followed by /ɪ/ than for /u/ followed by /æ/, so we reasoned that the tokens of stressed /u/ followed by /ɪ/ may have been in danger of sounding insufficiently like the intended sound, by virtue of being near the edge of the vowel's acoustic–phonetic region. A variation-constraining motor equivalence strategy might be most evident when it is really needed, among tokens that occur near the acoustic–phonetic boundary.

To investigate this idea, Perkell et al. (1993) examined correlations for subsets of the data corresponding to different F_2 ranges. For two of the four subjects in Perkell et al.'s (1993) study, there was a tendency for more significant negative correlations to occur at higher F_2 ranges, that is, near the boundary for an acceptable value of F_2 for /u/ where the vowel is least prototypical.

Given such results, we considered the possibility that calculating correlations for subsets of the data would test the hypothesis that, as the /u/ became less prototypical, more motor equivalence might be evident. We were aware of the argument that creating variation-reducing subsets of data could produce a bias toward negative correlations in the subsets (see Folkins & Brown, 1987; Sussman, 1980). However, we assumed that, if subset formation was in the acoustic domain, correlations of articulatory data would be readily interpretable (Perkell et al., 1993), especially since we had observed informally that the range of articulatory data in acoustically defined subsets was not diminished. Subsequent careful examination of the analysis methods and results has convinced us that this assumption was not easily testable and unlikely to be met. The acoustic variables must be a function of the articulatory variables (although the relations are weak due to undersampling of the area function by EMMA data); therefore, the correlations between the articulatory variables are likely to be affected by creating subsets, even according to the acoustic variables. We conclude that it is inappropriate to use acoustically defined subsets in correlations of articulatory data to test the idea that motor equivalence comes into play more near acoustic–phonetic boundaries. Another approach to this idea that we are pursuing is to run additional experiments in which manipulations of phonetic context provide a priori bases for examining subsets that differ in prototypicality.

Differences Among Subjects In one way or another, Subjects 1, 5, and 6 are different from Subjects 2, 3, and 4, who had significant negative correlations in their entire data sets. Table 1 shows that Subject 6 has a positive correlation between tongue-body raising and upper-lip protrusion, indicating that, instead of exhibiting a trading relation, these two parameters acted in a positively coordinated way to produce the vowel /u/. Subject 1 has a negative correlation in the subset but not in the entire data set, and Subject 5 does not have a significant correlation.

Figure 3 shows shapes of the hard palates of the six subjects, obtained from coronal sections of dental casts just behind the second molars. Among the subjects, Subject 6 had the smallest standard deviation of tongue height variation (Table 1) in combination with one of the flattest palates (in the region close to the highest point of the palatal arch). His relatively flat palate means that small vertical tongue movements would produce relatively large percentage changes in the cross-sectional area of the narrow velopalatal constriction and in the resulting acoustics. Although this factor does not explain his positive correlation, it may have something to do with his having developed a different strategy for producing /u/, which includes considerable constraint of tongue height variation. In spite of the fact that Subject 1 also has a flat palate, he used an amount

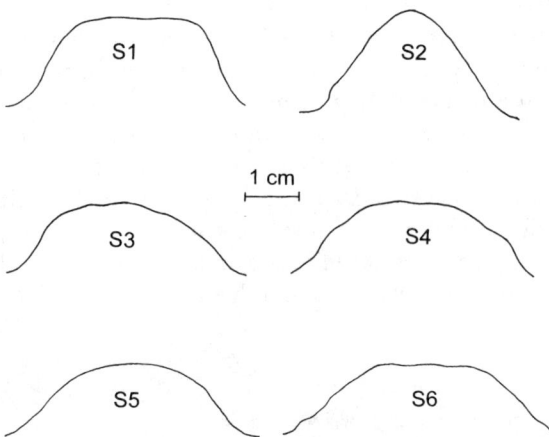

Figure 3. Shapes of the hard palates of the six subjects, obtained from coronal sections of dental casts just behind the second molars.

of tongue height variation that was similar to that of the other subjects (except 6). However, Perkell et al. (1993) observed that Subject 1 was using tongue-body raising in combination with lip rounding to produce a significant articulatory difference between stressed and unstressed tokens. This stress-related strategy may have overridden the possibility of finding motor equivalence in his full data set. We have been unable to identify any such factor for Subject 5 that might account for his lack of a significant negative correlation (although we note that Subject 5, like Subject 6, used a wider range of upper-lip protrusion as compared to tongue-body raising; see Table 1).[1] Thus, attention to physical characteristics and production strategies of individual subjects may help us to understand some, but not all, of the differences among the subjects.

Effect of Times of Articulatory Data Extraction In looking for alternative explanations for the negative correlations, we considered the possibility that they may have arisen from movement asynchrony in combination with our choice of times of data extraction (averaged over the middle third of the vowel), as opposed to actual covariation of articulatory targets (defined as minimum-velocity movement end points). To investigate this possibility, we have compared correlations of data for tongue-body raising and upper-lip protrusion based on extraction of articulatory data at the beginning of the /u/, at the times of the respective velocity minima for the upper-lip protrusion and tongue-body raising gestures, at the time of the tongue-body velocity minimum, and averaged over the middle third of the vowel. All of these results were remarkably similar, indicating that the trajectories are synchronous enough so that the findings are not due to the choice of time points for data extraction.

Strength of the Correlations When considering the relatively low r values of the negative correlations in these studies, the experimental results need to be viewed with respect to the limitations of EMMA data and the wide range of variability in normal speech. Correlation strengths might be increased somewhat with more accurate estimates of vocal tract cross-sectional areas. However, high correlations are not to be expected in any case, mainly because there is usually not a strong requirement to constrain acoustic variability in an absolute sense. Furthermore, if the hypothesized motor equivalence strategy is being used, it is very likely to be only one of a number of factors that are influencing the observed data.

---

[1] An additional, more recent experiment on Subject 5 used utterances containing /u/, /ʃ/, and /r/, with differences in prototypicality induced by phonetic context and speaking condition. Evidence of motor equivalence was found for all three sounds, almost exclusively among less prototypical subsets (Perkell, Matthies, & Svirsky, 1994).

CONCLUSIONS

The theoretical framework we have outlined will need a lot of refinement and testing before it has reached the degree of development that has been achieved by articulatory phonology and the task-dynamic model, which themselves still do not cover some very important aspects of speech production. As alluded to above, it is highly unlikely that there can be a straightforward, unequivocal test of any aspect of a simple theory about speech, which we know is very complicated. So, although these initial motor equivalence findings provide tentative support for the idea that speech motor programming includes acoustic goals, we remain very cautious about this interpretation. A great deal of additional work is needed, and, even then, there may be room for alternative explanations.

REFERENCES

Abbs, J.H., & Gracco, V.L. (1984). Control of complex motor gestures: Orofacial muscle responses to load perturbations of lip during speech. *Journal of Neurophysiology, 51*, 705–723.

Abbs, J.H., Gracco, V.L., & Cole, K.J. (1984). Control of multimovement coordination: Sensorimotor mechanisms in speech motor programming. *Journal of Motor Behavior, 16*, 195–232.

Atal, B.S., Chang, J.J., Mathews, M.V., & Tukey, J.W. (1978). Inversion of articulatory-to-acoustic transformation in the vocal tract by a computer-sorting technique. *Journal of the Acoustical Society of America, 63*, 1535–1555.

Boë, L.-J., Schwartz, J.-L., & Vallée, N. (1994). The production of vowel systems: Perceptual contrast and stability. In E. Keller (Ed.), *Fundamentals of speech synthesis and speech recognition* (pp. 185–213). New York: John Wiley & Sons.

Browman, C.P., & Goldstein, L. (1986). Towards an articulatory phonology. *Phonology Yearbook, 3*, 219–252.

Charles-Luce, J. (1995). Cognitive factors involved in incomplete neutralization. Manuscript submitted for publication.

Chomsky, N., & Halle, M. (1968). *The sound pattern of English*. New York: Harper & Row.

Diehl, R.L., & Kluender, K.R. (1989). On the objects of speech perception. *Ecological Psychology, 1*, 121–144.

Eefting, W. (1991). The effect of "information value" and "accentuation" on the duration of Dutch words, syllables and segments. *Journal of the Acoustical Society of America, 89*, 412–424.

Folkins, J.W., & Brown, C.K. (1987). Upper lip, lower lip and jaw interactions during speech: Comments on evidence from repetition-to-repetition variability. *Journal of the Acoustical Society of America, 82*, 1919–1924.

Fowler, C.A. (1980). Coarticulation and theories of extrinsic timing control. *Journal of Phonetics, 8*, 113–133.

Fujimura, O., & Kakita, X. (1979). Remarks on quantitative description of the lingual articulation. In B. Lindblom & S. Öhman (Eds.), *Frontiers of speech communication research* (pp. 17–24). London: Academic Press.

Gay, T., Lindblom, B., & Lubker, J. (1981). Production of bite-block vowels: Acoustic equivalence by selective compensation. *Journal of the Acoustical Society of America, 69*, 802–810.

Gracco, V.L. (1987). Multilevel control model for speech motor activity. In H.F.M. Peters & W. Hulsijn (Eds.), *Speech motor dynamics in stuttering* (pp. 57–76). New York: Springer-Verlag.

Gracco, V.L., & Abbs, J.S. (1988). Sensorimotor characteristics of speech motor sequences. *Experimental Brain Research, 72*, 1–13.

Halle, M., & Stevens, K.N. (1990). Knowledge of language and the sounds of speech. In J. Sundberg, L. Nord, & R. Carlson (Eds.), *Music, language, speech and brain* (pp. 1–19). Basingstoke, Hampshire, England: MacMillan Press.

Henton, C., Ladefoged, P., & Maddieson, I. (1992). Stops in the world's languages. *Phonetica, 49*, 65–101.

Hughes, O.M., & Abbs, J.H. (1976). Labial-mandibular coordination in the production of speech: Implications for the operation of motor equivalence. *Phonetica, 33*, 199–221.

Jakobson, R., Fant, G., & Halle, M. (1963). *Preliminaries to speech analysis.* Cambridge, MA: M.I.T. Press.

Johnson, K., Ladefoged, P., & Lindau, M. (1993). Individual differences in vowel production. *Journal of the Acoustical Society of America, 94*, 701–714.

Jordan, M.I. (1992). Constrained supervised learning. *Journal of Mathematical Psychology, 36*, 396–425.

Jordan, M.I., & Rumelhart, D.E. (1992). Forward models: Supervised learning with a distal teacher. *Cognitive Science, 16*, 307–354.

Kohler, K.J. (1991). Cognitive-auditory constraints on articulatory reduction. In *PERILUS XIV* (pp. 11–15). Stockholm: University of Stockholm, Institute of Linguistics.

Laboissière, R., Schwartz, J.-L., & Bailly, G. (1991). Modeling the speaker-listener interaction in a quantitative model for speech motor control: a framework and some preliminary results. In *PERILUS XIV* (pp. 57–62). Stockholm: University of Stockholm, Institute of Linguistics.

Labov, W. (1986). Sources of inherent variation in the speech process. In J.S. Perkell & D.H. Klatt (Eds.), *Invariance and variability in speech processes* (pp. 402–422). Hillsdale, NJ: Lawrence Erlbaum Associates.

Ladefoged, P., & Maddieson, I. (1990). Vowels of the world's languages. *Journal of Phonetics, 18*, 93–122.

Lindblom, B. (1983). Economy of speech gestures. In P. MacNeilage (Ed.), *The production of speech* (pp. 217–245). New York: Springer-Verlag.

Lindblom, B. (1990). Explaining phonetic variation: A sketch of the H and H theory. In W.J. Hardcastle & A. Marchal (Eds.), *Speech production and speech modeling* (pp. 403–440). Dordrecht: Kluwer.

Lindblom, B., & Engstrand, O. (1989). In what sense is speech quantal? *Journal of Phonetics, 17*, 107–121.

Lindblom, B., Lubker, J., & Gay, T. (1979). Formant frequencies of some fixed-mandible vowels and a model of speech motor programming by predictive simulation. *Journal of Phonetics, 7*, 147–161.

Maeda, S. (1991). On articulatory and acoustic variabilities. *Journal of Phonetics, 19*, 321–331.

Moon, S.-J., & Lindblom, B. (1994). Interaction between duration, context, and speaking style in the reduction of stressed vowels. *Journal of the Acoustical Society of America, 96*, 40–55.

Nelson, W.L. (1983). Physical principles for economies of skilled movement. *Biological Cybernetics, 46*, 135–147.

Nooteboom, S.G. (1970). *The target theory of speech production* (Progress Rep. No. 5, pp. 51–53). Eindhoven, The Netherlands: Institute for Perception Research.

Perkell, J.S. (1980). Phonetic features and the physiology of speech production. In B. Butterworth (Ed.), *Language production* (pp. 337–372). London: Academic Press.

Perkell, J., Cohen, M., Svirsky, M., Matthies, M., Garabieta, I., & Jackson, M. (1992). Electromagnetic midsagittal articulometer (EMMA) systems for transducing speech articulatory movements. *Journal of the Acoustical Society of America, 92*, 3078–3096.

Perkell, J., Matthies, M.L., & Svirsky, M.A. (1994). Articulatory evidence for acoustic goals for consonants [abstract]. *Journal of the Acoustical Society of America, 96*, 3326.

Perkell, J.S., Matthies, M.L., Svirsky, M.A., & Jordan, M.I. (1993). Trading relations between tongue-body raising and lip rounding in production of the vowel /u/: A pilot motor equivalence study. *Journal of the Acoustical Society of America, 93*, 2948–2961.

Saltzman, E.L., & Munhall, K.G. (1989). A dynamical approach to gestural patterning in speech production. *Ecological Psychology, 1*, 333–382.

Stevens, K.N. (1989). On the quantal nature of speech. *Journal of Phonetics, 17*, 3–45.

Stevens, K.N., Manuel, S.Y., Shattuck-Hufnagel, S., & Liu, S. (1992). Implementation of a model for lexical access based on features. In *ICSLP 92 Proceedings: 1992 International Conference on Spoken Language Processing* (pp. 499–502). Edmonton, Alberta, Canada: University of Alberta.

Sussman, H.M. (1980). Methodological problems in evaluating lip/jaw reciprocity as an index of motor equivalence. *Journal of Speech and Hearing Research, 23*, 699–704.

Volaitis, L.E., & Miller, J.L. (1992). Phonetic prototypes: Influence of place of articulation and speaking rate on the internal structure of voicing categories. *Journal of the Acoustical Society of America, 92*, 723–735.

Chapter 3

Articulated and Inflected Primate Vocalizations
Developing Animal Models of Speech

Charles H. Brown and Michael P. Cannito

ADVANCEMENTS IN NEUROIMAGING and neuroscience techniques have heightened the possibility of identifying the neural mechanisms that underlie normal and disordered speech production (Barlow, 1992). Although cerebral blood flow and metabolism studies (Gilman & Kluin, 1992; Ryding, Bradvik, & Ingvar, 1987) and electrophysiologic stimulation and recording studies of neurons in the human central nervous system (McClean, Dostrovsky, Lee, & Tasker, 1990; Penfield & Roberts, 1959) will continue to contribute to our understanding of the neural control of the vocal tract, the scope of these studies is necessarily constrained by considerations relevant to patient management and by the possibility of death or permanent injury resulting from experimental invasive procedures. Hence, advancements in the understanding of many aspects of neural vocal control will depend to a great extent on the integration of our understanding of the pathophysiology of human speech disorders on the one hand and animal studies of vocal behavior and the neural physiology of vocal performance on the other. Kolb and Wishaw (1990) have suggested that animal models in neuropsychology enhance the understanding of human brain–behavior relationships in three important ways: first, through "understanding of basic mechanisms of brain functions"; second, by producing "models of human neurologic disor-

---

This work was supported in part by National Institutes of Health Grant No. R01 DC00164.

ders"; and, third, by providing "description of phylogenetic development of the brain" (p. 102). Furthermore, Sussman (1989) argued that "similarities in both brain structure and function across species with common stimulus processing requirements motivate the use of findings from neuroethological studies to inspire by analogy realistic models of human neural processing systems" (p. 631). One impediment to the development of sophisticated integrative studies is the absence of recognized animal models with productive and receptive capacities comparable to those underlying speech communication.

Major advancements in the elucidation of upper extremity motor control were achieved through the coupling of sophisticated animal behavior studies and neurobiologic techniques, including single-unit recording, dye injection, selective lesions, pharmacologic manipulations, and histochemical techniques (Evarts, 1980; Kots, 1977). In effect, contemporary neurobiology and behavioral psychology could also elucidate the neural regulation of voice and articulation if even a partial or rudimentary model of speech production analogues existed in animals. Indeed, significant work on the mesencephalic vocalization system has already been accomplished (Jurgens & Ploog, 1970, 1988; Jurgens & Pratt, 1979a, 1979b; Kirzinger & Jurgens, 1982; Larson, 1985; Larson & Kistler, 1986; Larson, Ortega, & DeRosier, 1988; Magoun, Atlas, Ingersoll, & Ranson, 1937). Arguments against the relevance of this "primitive" vocalization pathway for an understanding of speech have been predicated on the view that there was no cortical mechanism for animal social vocalizations comparable to Broca's area and that no animal (including nonhuman primates) produces any vocal output resembling speech (Whitaker, 1976). More recently, however, evidence of cortical mechanisms for call perception and production have begun to emerge (Glass & Wollberg, 1979; Heffner & Heffner, 1984; Jurgens, 1983; Kirzinger & Jurgens, 1982; Muller-Preuss, Newman, & Jurgens, 1980). Moreover, some evidence of rudimentary vocal tract source–filter interaction reminiscent of human speech has begun to emerge for some classes of monkey utterances (Brown & Cannito, in press; Hauser, 1992). Thus, Barlow (1992) suggested that "animal vocalization studies need continued support to firmly establish the neural substrate for propositional and nonpropositional vocal/verbal behavior," and that such efforts strive to include acoustic and perceptual measures of "call quality or 'intelligibility'" (p. 351).

In spite of these advancements, the limited development of animal models may in part continue to stem from the belief that only humans are endowed with the capacity for speech. Speaking presumably requires sophisticated computational systems dedicated to regulating the timing, sequencing, and force of contraction of the motor systems underlying respiration and oral–laryngeal behaviors, and to the subsequent analysis (and potential reconstruction of the sequence of motor events that gave rise to the utterance) by the recipient. This discontinuous view of human and nonhuman communicative capacities has potentially inhibited the search for (and recognition of) useful animal models of communicative processes. Although the full development of vocal communication may be absent in all animals except humans, at some point during the course of human phylogeny speech may have emerged from primate vocal behavior. Given the possibility that speech and primate vocal behavior may share common underlying motor and neural mechanisms, it may be practical to examine two questions: What are the desirable characteristics of an animal model for speech, and, secondarily, to what extent are any of these characteristics met by available animal models?

It is probable that the neural substrate underlying oral–laryngeal behavior is phylogenetically conservative and quite similar across mammals. For example, recent studies have shown that the neurotransmitter norepinephrine regulates the activity of tongue motoneurons in the hypoglossal nucleus (nXII) of probably all mammals (Aldes et al., 1988), and studies of the innervation of the rat tongue are likely relevant for understanding tongue reflexes in monkeys, humans, and other mammals as well. Thus, the findings of primate studies, in conjunction with those from the dog (Alipour, Titze, & Durham, 1987), cat (Buchwald et al., 1988), and rat (Kehoe, 1988) preparations, would likely interrelate with one another and be significant for understanding speech motor control. Nevertheless, species that exhibit motor patterns most similar to human phonation and articulation would most directly model speech, and consequently it is particularly appropriate to examine the status of research in primate communication. The goals of this chapter are to describe the requisite characteristics of an animal model for speech production, to survey some of the recent observations of primate vocal behavior pertinent to model development, and to identify some important directions for future research.

CANDIDATE CHARACTERISTICS OF AN ANIMAL MODEL OF SPEECH

The characteristics of an animal model for speech are enumerated below. To our knowledge, no catalog of the desirable characteristics for such a model has been previously advanced, and the following list is surely not exhaustive. For example, neuroanatomic and phylogenetic characteristics have been intentionally excluded from consideration. Nevertheless, this catalog provides a starting point for evaluating the potential efficacy of animal models.

Criteria of Structural Diversification of Vocalizations and Indices of a Communicative Intent

1. The model would exhibit a rich repertoire of structurally diversified vocalizations.
2. The emission of some vocalizations would be nonvegetative, and the amplitude of the sound would be altered to compensate for changes in the transmission distance to "intended recipients" or for changes in the background noise level.
3. Different vocalizations would be given in response to different social situations.
4. Different vocalizations would "evoke" different classes of behaviors in recipients for some categories of utterances.

Criteria of Repertoire Acquisition, Selection, and "Distinguishability"

5. Some characteristics of the vocal repertoire would be species specific.
6. The physical structure of some sounds would conform to a species-specific acoustic standard and be distinguishable from the similar sounds of competing species.
7. The model would exhibit vocal learning in which both the physical form and the usage of the vocalization would be socially transmitted.

Criteria of Phonation and Articulation

8. The acoustic nucleus of some vocalizations would be produced by voicing.
9. The model would exhibit stability of phonatory control of air flow for a "sufficient" time interval.
10. Voiced sounds would be produced with different vocal tract configurations.
11. Acoustic variations within and between some vocalizations would be produced by changes in articulation.
12. Acoustic variations within and between some vocalizations would be produced by changes in the fundamental frequency (F_0).
13. The model would produce stoppage of air flow at one or more places of articulation.
14. The model would produce frication (air turbulence) by constricting the airway at one or more places of articulation.
15. The model would produce both air flow stopping and frication at the same place of articulation.

16. The model would produce sounds differing in voice onset time (VOT) and voicing duration following release of aperiodic noise.

**Criteria of Perceptual and Behavioral
Validation of Putative Vocal Contrasts and
Vocal Feature Production and Detection**

17. Some patterns of change in articulation, F_0, frication, stops, or VOT (criteria 8–16 above) would be perceptually very salient to conspecific recipients.
18. The model would permit listeners to be trained to provide a score of the intelligibility of normal and abnormal utterances. This may be derived from measures of detection, discrimination, and classification.
19. The model would behave as if vocalizations were designed to conform to an acoustic target, and some experimentally induced (or accidentally produced) deviations in vocal tract length or shape would be compensated by corresponding changes in production.

**Criteria of "Propositional"
Vocal Behavior and Syntax**

20. The model would produce vocalizations in which the *communicative intent* parallels that of "propositional" and "nonpropositional" speech.
21. The model would exhibit rule-governed sequential constraints (syntax) for vocal sequences, and variations in vocal sequences would be perceptually very salient to recipients and influence their reaction to the sequence.

This catalog provides an ambitious list of desirable characteristics for a biologic model of speech communication. The elements on this list underscore the fact that communication is a *behavioral* phenomenon. Animal behavioral research over the past two decades has begun to address questions pertinent to the development of biologic models of speech communication.

PRIMATE COMMUNICATIVE BEHAVIOR

Structural Diversification of
Vocalizations and Indices of Communicative Intent

Criteria 1–4 are necessary to establish the fact that a candidate model species has the capability of varying the structure of its acoustic output and that some classes of acoustic activity exhibit at least rudimentary properties of communicative signals. Both Old World and New World primates produce a broad variety of structurally elaborate and variant vocalizations (Todt, Goedeking, & Symmes, 1988). Thus, Criterion 1 is easily satisfied by a variety of primate species. Although humans are readily able to distinguish vegetative sounds from speech, or discern when sneezes, coughs, or burps may be volitionally issued as a signal, this facility is not objectively extended across species boundaries. Hence, researchers have sought indirect but objective indices of a putative communicative role for various gestures. Vegetative sounds would presumably show no audience effect and would show no consistent variation in form linked to changes in the external environment. Structural changes in the calls of pygmy marmosets (*Cebuella pygmaea*) have been linked to changes in the spacing between interactants, and it is thought that changes in call morphology act to compensate for changes in transmission distance (Snowdon & Hodun, 1981). Furthermore, compensatory changes in the vocal amplitude of pigtailed monkey (*Macaca nemestrina*) coo calls have been found for changes in the ambient noise level (Sinnott, Stebbins, & Moody, 1975). Criterion 2 is exhibited by both Old World and New World monkeys.

Many studies (Gautier & Gautier, 1977; Gouzoules & Gouzoules, 1989; Gouzoules, Gouzoules, & Marler, 1984; Green, 1975; Hauser, 1992; Rowell & Hinde, 1962; Snowdon & Hodun, 1981) have shown that structurally distinguishable vocalizations are given in response to different social situations (Criterion 3) and that these variations may evoke different responses in recipients (Criterion 4). One of the best known examples of this phenomenon is the observation that vervet monkeys (*Cercopithecus aethiops*) produce three different alarm calls on sighting an eagle, leopard, or snake and that these calls evoke different evasive reactions appropriate to each class of predator (Seyfarth, Cheney, & Marler, 1980). The recipients of eagle alarm calls seek the cover provided by a thorny bush or tree, leopard alarm calls stimulate terrestrial recipients to run toward and climb a tree, and snake alarm calls elicit visual searching for the position of the snake. The correct usage of these calls is not innate; rather, it is dependent on some type of social learning process. For example, infant vervet monkeys may initially emit eagle alarm calls on sighting nonpredatory as well as predatory birds (Seyfarth & Cheney, 1986). Gradually, infant monkeys learn to restrict the emission of alarm calls to "appropriate" stimuli, and the reactions of adults to episodes of correct and incorrect alarm call usage are thought to reinforce the development of reliable, selective, socially appropriate usage of these calls (Cheney & Seyfarth, 1990). As is the case for speech, not all vocalizations produce an immediate visible response, and only utterances associated with immediate danger should be expected to produce this pattern of results. Both Old and New World species exhibit these characteristics.

Repertoire Acquisition, Selection, and Distinguishability

Criteria 5–7 are focused on repertoire acquisition issues concerned with how organisms may learn to selectively "attend" to acoustic patterns that are relevant to their own communication system and accordingly ignore potentially similar, yet biologically irrelevant, noises. The questions of species identification (Criterion 5) and signal distinguishability (Criterion 6) are most pressing for organisms living in sympatry with other similar species or that are undergoing the development of new species. That is, whereas humans do not live in ranges overlapping with those of other competing species of hominids, other primates do, and some groups of primates, such as the guenon monkeys, appear to be in various stages of the process of the emergence of new species (Lernould, 1988). In contrast, the question of vocal learning (Criterion 7) is most pressing for species like humans that exhibit the phenomenon of dialects. In all cases, it is unknown how the brain preferentially produces (or selectively attends to) certain combinations of acoustic patterns but not others. Evidence for species identification by voice is provided by field studies showing a vigorous response to playbacks of conspecific calls but not to control broadcasts (Waser, 1975; Whitehead, 1987). However, unlike much of the comparable work with frogs and birds, investigations with primates have tended to restrict the repertoire of control or comparison broadcasts relevant to the question of species identification. Thus, the acoustic features giving rise to species recognition are poorly known for most primates, and it would be desirable for future studies to address this question.

Perhaps the most striking case of the distinguishability of acoustically similar calls is provided by guenon monkeys. Sykes' monkeys (*Cercopithecus albogularis*) and their allies produce chirps as a general alarm call following a sudden movement in the forest or an unexpected noise. These chirps are so similar in form to the chirps of unalarmed sympatric birds that human listeners readily confuse the two. Sykes' monkeys, however, perceive their own alarm calls and those of sympatric guenons as being very similar to one another but quite distinctive from bird chirps (Brown, Sinnott, & Kressley, 1994).

Many of the best examples of vocal learning in primates involve Old World monkeys. Vervet monkeys have been shown to exhibit social learning in the usage of alarm calls, but not in the physical morphology of the call (Cheney & Seyfarth, 1990). In this case, infants, for example, will emit eagle alarm calls in response to sightings of nonpredatory birds as well as eagles and will over time come to restrict the emission of these calls to "appropriate" stimuli. In comparison, the physical morphology of rhesus monkey (*Macaca mulatta*) coo calls has been attributed to vocal learning

(Hauser, 1992). Hence, Old World monkeys may provide appropriate models for Criteria 5–7.

Phonation and Articulation

Because impediments to speech intelligibility are of such fundamental concern, Criteria 8–16 are of particular relevance for the development of animal models. Studies of the acoustics of primate habitats have shown that long-duration calls tend to be susceptible to higher rates of distortion induced by the acoustics of the local habitat than are shorter duration calls (Brown, 1994a; Brown & Gomez, 1992; Brown & Waser, 1988). Hence, it may not be surprising that many primate utterances are short (100–300 ms, about the length of a syllable) and will consequently exhibit correspondingly brief intervals of phonation. Primates, however, have the capacity for sustained phonation (Criterion 9). Sykes' monkey trills, for example, frequently exhibit over 1,000 glottal cycles per call, and differences in the duration of phonation between calls are likely the result of selection for gestures with specific cardinal features rather than any inherent limitation in the capacity to regulate phonation for prolonged intervals.

Although many studies have directly or indirectly implicated voicing as the acoustic source of different utterances (Criterion 8), no investigation has rigorously shown that nonhuman primates alter the vocal tract shape to achieve specific distinguishable vowel-like configurations (Criterion 10). As shown in Figure 1, however, the first formant frequency (F_1) of grey-cheeked mangabey (*Cercocebus albigena*) grunts changes as a function of the degree of lowering of the mandible. In the second grunt, F_1 is raised about 300 Hz relative to that in the first grunt. Future work should examine if grunts cluster into particular formant frequency patterns suggestive of specific vocal tract shapes. This is an area where intensive research is merited because it is important to explore the neural organization that specifies particular vocal tract configurations. Methodologically, however, this is a very challenging area requiring the development of analytical tools and algorithms designed to accommodate the length and shape of the monkey's vocal tract, high rates of phonation, the possibility of diplophonic or polyphonic sources, the potential significance of accessory air sacs, and so forth. Although it is unknown if primates alter the shape of the airway to achieve specific vowel-like configurations, there is good evidence that acoustic variations are produced by changes in articulation (Criterion 11) as well as by variations in F_0 (Criterion 12).

Figure 2 shows an acoustic sound spectrogram (Panel A) of a Sykes' monkey squeal displayed in register with a spectrogram of the Lx wave recorded directly from the monkey's larynx (Panel B). Spectral sections of the acoustic and Lx spectrograms are shown at three corresponding points in the vocalization (Panels D and E). The results show that changes in the

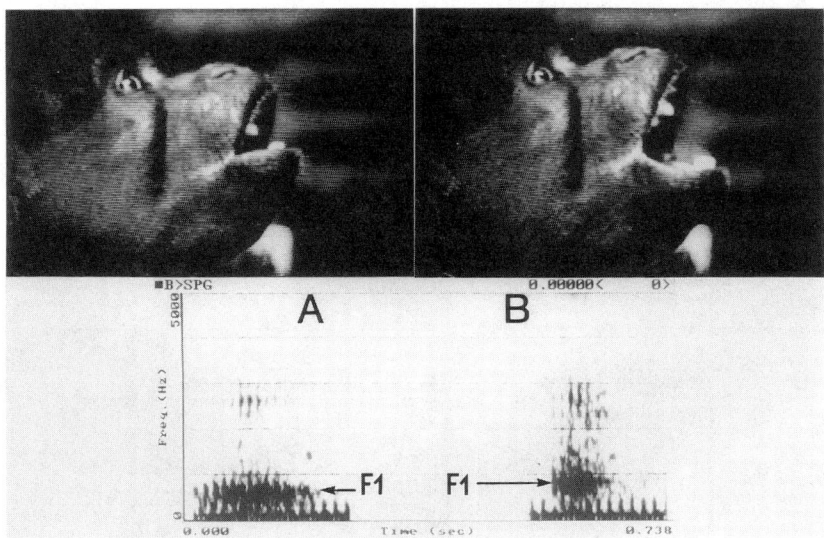

Figure 1. Two grunts given in close succession by a grey-cheeked mangabey. The frequency of the first formant (F_1) is denoted by the arrows in the spectrograms. In the second grunt, the mandible is lowered and F_1 increases in frequency. F_0 is about 100 Hz for both grunts. The filter bandwidth of the spectrogram was 293 Hz.

acoustic signal are not associated with changes in the fundamental frequency, and hence are due to articulation (Class I calls). These calls contrast with utterances in which the pattern of acoustic variation within and between calls is due to changes in the F_0 contour (Class II calls).

Figure 3 shows acoustic (Panel A) and Lx (Panel B) spectrograms of a Class II squeal, and slices of the spectrograms (Panels D and E) are displayed at three points in time. The results show that the fundamental frequency always matches the frequency of the lowest band in the acoustic sound spectrogram, and frequency variations in the audio signal are due to changes in F_0. The monkey is in effect "singing" without changing the shape of its vocal tract.

This contrast between Class I and Class II calls is summarized in Figure 4, which displays the relationship between F_0 and the frequency of the lowest band in the sound spectrogram. In Class I and Class II calls, the frequency of the lowest band in the spectrogram is believed to closely approximate the lowest resonance, or first formant, of the vocal tract (Brown & Cannito, in press). In Class I calls, less than 14% of the variance in the acoustic signal, as indexed by the frequency of the lowest band in the spectrogram, is associated with F_0, whereas, in Class II calls, 99% of the variance in the frequency modulation of the acoustic waveform is associated with changes in F_0. The characteristics of these calls show that monkeys

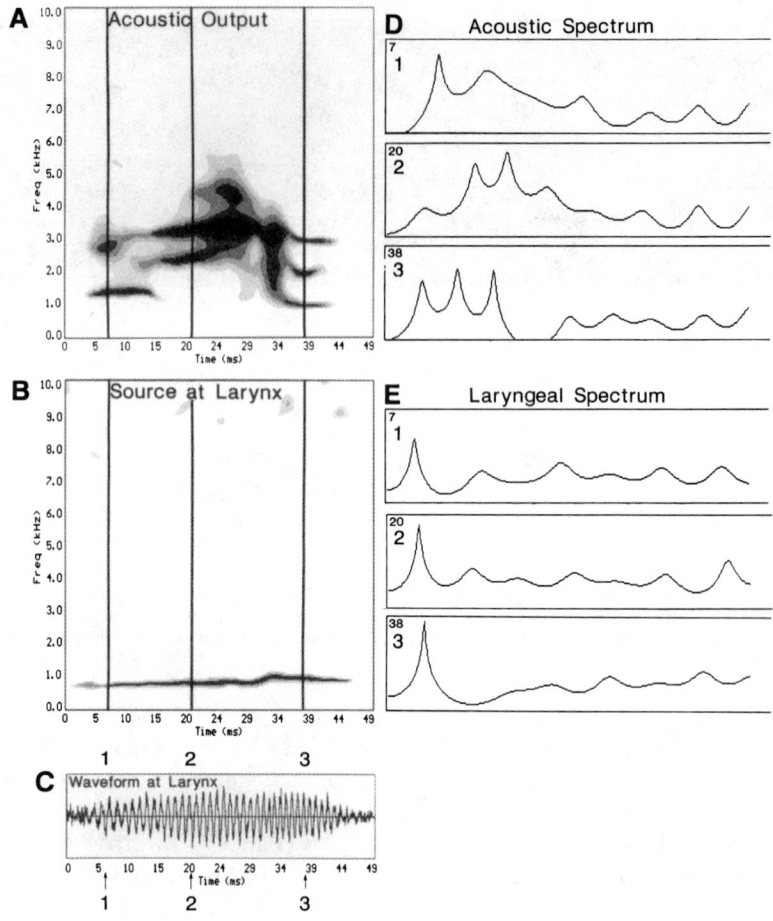

Figure 2. A representative Class I Sykes' monkey vocalization. Sound spectrograms are shown of the acoustic signal (Panel A) and the Lx signal recorded from the larynx (Panel B) in juxtaposition with the Lx waveform (Panel C). The spectrum of the vocal output is shown in Panel D at times 1, 2, and 3, and the corresponding spectrum of the Lx signal is shown in Panel E. The filter bandwidth of the spectrogram was 39 Hz. (Adapted from Brown & Cannito, in press.)

possess the computational hardware to both regulate F_0 in a manner resembling intonation or inflection and produce acoustically significant changes in the shape of the airway (articulation). Although acoustic studies show that vocalizations vary according to these principles, perceptual studies are needed to distinguish those sources or modes of variation that are insignificant from those that are perceptually very salient. Presumably the central nervous system would be designed to finely control perceptually salient variation and to less precisely regulate perceptually irrelevant or less salient vocal parameters.

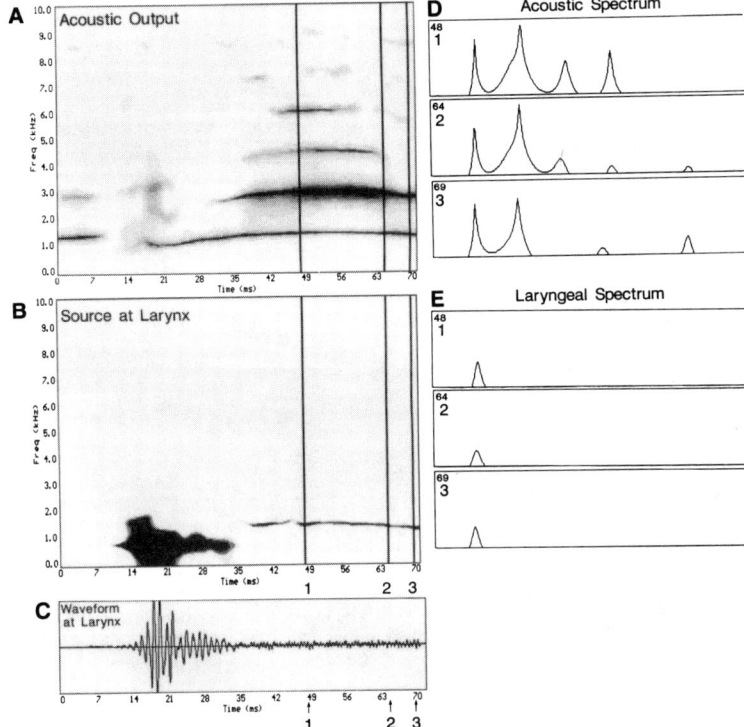

Figure 3. A representative Class II Sykes' monkey vocalization. The panels correspond with those in Figure 1. Note the reduced amplitude of the Lx wave from 35 to 70 ms, implicating changes in the aspect of the vocal folds and a corresponding reduction of the vocal fold contact area during phonation. The vocalization was preceded by an environmental noise visible in the first 7 ms of Panel A. (Adapted from Brown & Cannito, in press.)

Old World monkeys may be trained to serve as subjects in perceptual experiments (Criterion 17). Multidimensional scaling procedures have been used to characterize the relative similarity or dissimilarity of different classes of vocalizations (Brown, Kressley, & Sinnott, 1994). Accordingly, calls that are very distinguishable would occupy a large spatial map, whereas perceptually very similar calls would occupy a very small space. Figure 5 shows perceptual pyramids (tetrahedrons) derived by multidimensional scaling of four exemplars each of Class I and Class II squeals. Tetrahedrons for two additional classes of calls are also shown for comparison. The results show that monkey listeners find both Class I and Class II acoustic variation to be very salient. Human listeners, in contrast, find only Class II variation salient. Relative to human listeners, monkeys are 44 times more sensitive to variations resulting from articulation (Class I calls). This observation suggests that the neural regulation of articulation,

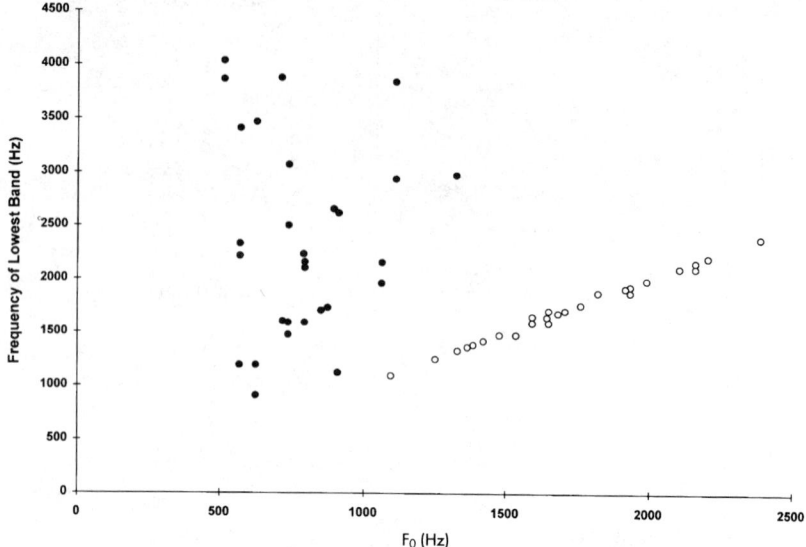

Figure 4. The relationship between F_0 and the lowest frequency band in the sound spectrogram for Class I (solid circles) and Class II (open circles) monkey calls. The lowest frequency band in the spectrogram excites the first formant, but it may not fall at the peak resonance of the formant. (Adapted from Brown & Cannito, in press.)

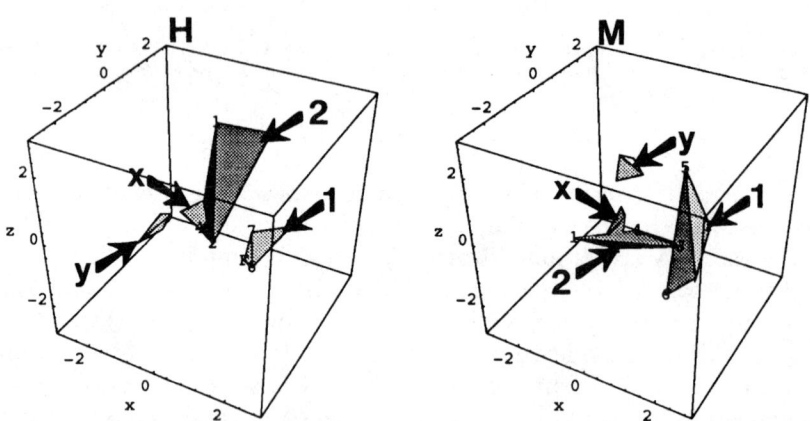

Figure 5. Three-dimensional perceptual maps of vocalizations derived by multidimensional scaling. The four vertices of each tetrahedron correspond to the perceptual location of each of the four test exemplars of a category of sounds. The tetrahedrons corresponding to Class I and II vocalizations (labeled 1 and 2, respectively) are shown with respect to two additional comparison categories (labeled x and y). Four monkey (M) and three human (H) subjects were tested. (Adapted from Brown, Kressley, & Sinnott, 1995.)

as well as F_0 contour, is probably very well developed in primates. In addition, it indicates that judgments by humans of the important dimensions of primate vocalizations may not capture significant parameters that are salient to conspecific listeners. This finding underscores the need for complementary perceptual studies in both conspecific and heterospecific listeners.

Figure 6 shows sound spectrograms of two kinds of chirps occasionally produced by grey-cheeked mangabeys. The chirp in Call A is produced somewhat like a T stop consonant. The tongue is positioned behind the alveolar ridge to occlude the airway, and the tongue and mandible are lowered to release the stop. In Call B, the tongue is elevated near the alveolar ridge, but it does not occlude the airway. The stop in Call B is produced either laryngeally or pharyngeally. Perceptual studies are required to determine if these two chirps are perceived as members of different classes or if they serve as two alternative mechanisms to achieve the same objective. It is possible that monkeys produce both laryngeal and pharyngeal stops. To date, no studies that have explored this possibility. Hence, additional research should focus on the mechanisms of stop production in primates (Criterion 13).

Constrictions of the airway producing turbulence are also very notable features of monkey vocalizations. Figure 7 shows four different Class III squeals that exhibit patterns of abrupt alterations between vocalic (elements produced with an unobstructed airway) and fricativelike (produced

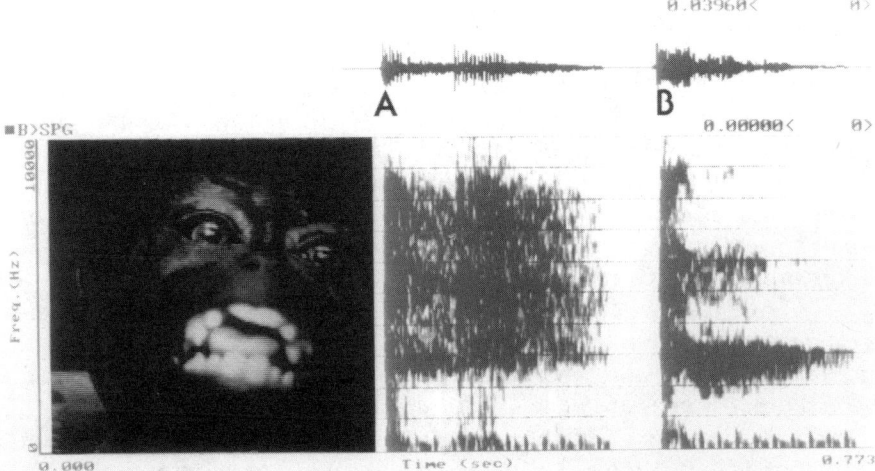

Figure 6. Two chirps with an alveolar place of articulation. Grey-cheeked mangabeys elevate their tongue to produce stopping at the alveolar ridge (Call A) or to constrict the airway, producing frication at the same place of articulation at call onset (Call B). The filter bandwidth of the spectrogram was 293 Hz.

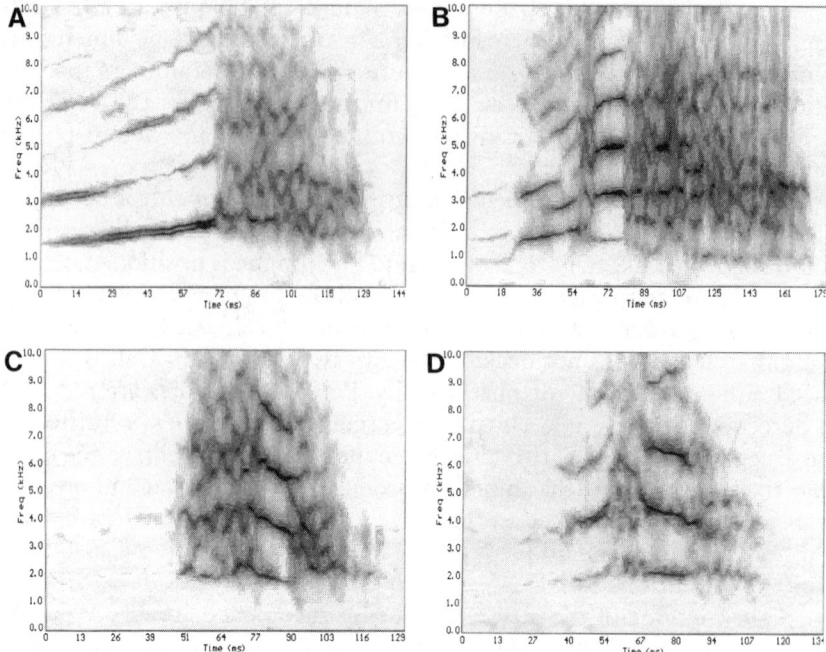

Figure 7. Sound spectrograms for four representative Class III Sykes' monkey calls. Note that the transition between the vocalic and fricative (broadband width) components is usually abrupt, and the fricative component may be positioned in the terminal segment (Panels A and B), initial segment (Panel C), or middle segment (Panel D) of the call. The filter bandwidth of the spectrogram was 39 Hz. (Adapted from Brown & Cannito, in press.)

with a partially obstructed airway) turbulent components. Future research should address whether different places of articulation are employed in the production of fricativelike gestures (Criterion 14). Although the number of places of articulation for fricativelike gestures is unknown, it appears likely that monkeys can finely control airway constriction at one or more places of articulation to produce calls that are distinguished by stopping or frication (Criterion 15).

Figure 8 shows chirps produced by Sykes' monkeys that are acoustically distinguishable by their onset times. Chirp A has an abrupt onset, characteristic of a stop, whereas chirp B has a more gradual fricative onset. Perceptual studies are necessary to determine if this level of variation serves as a distinctive feature or is treated as communicatively insignificant variation within a single class of gestures. If variations in onset time prove to be perceptually salient, field studies should be conducted to explore when different chirp tokens are emitted in natural vocal exchanges.

Figure 9 shows two exemplars of the acoustic and Lx waveforms of Sykes' monkey screams that differ in VOT and the duration of voicing.

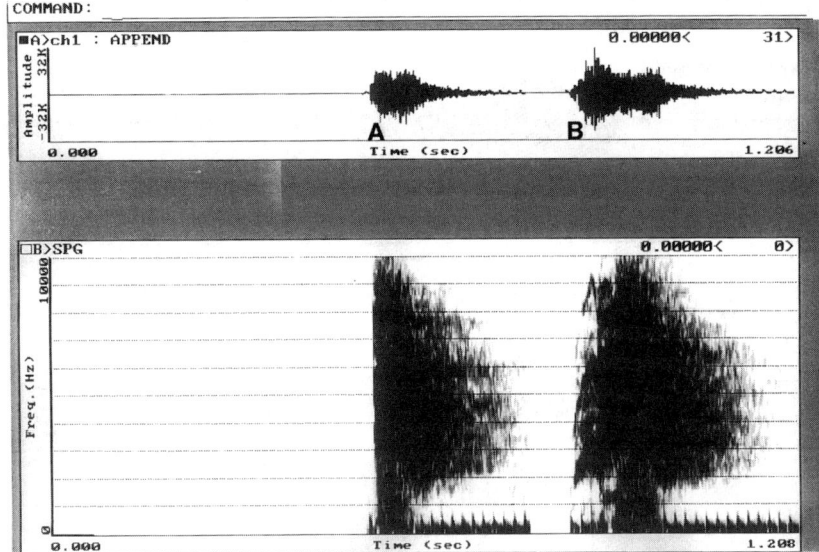

Figure 8. Two Sykes' monkey chirps. Most chirps have an abrupt onset, indicative of a stop (Call A), but some chirps have a more gradual onset (Call B). Unlike the chirps of grey-cheeked mangabeys (Figure 6), the place of articulation for Sykes' monkey chirps is the pharynx or larynx.

This observation raises the possibility that differences in voicing may serve as a distinctive feature in some primate gestures, just as it does in speech (Criterion 16). Future studies should examine patterns of variation in voicing in the production of different calls to determine if VOT or voicing duration tends to cluster into different classes. Furthermore, complementary perceptual studies are necessary to determine if observed variations in voicing are perceptually salient and potentially serve as a distinctive feature.

Perceptual and Behavioral Validation of Putative Vocal Contrasts and Vocal Feature Production and Detection

Advancements in understanding the "vocabulary" of primate vocal repertoires are dependent on interlinked studies of sound production on the one hand and the perception of these sounds on the other (Criteria 17 and 18). Fortunately, methods are now well developed to objectively assess the discrimination and categorization of conspecific and comparison species' vocalizations (Brown et al., 1995; Sinnott, 1995).

Because humans have some ability to produce intelligible speech through compensatory adjustments when the normal mode of production is changed by partial paralysis of the oral musculature, or by the application of bite blocks and other dental appliances, it would be useful if animal models would show some capacity for compensation (Criterion 19).

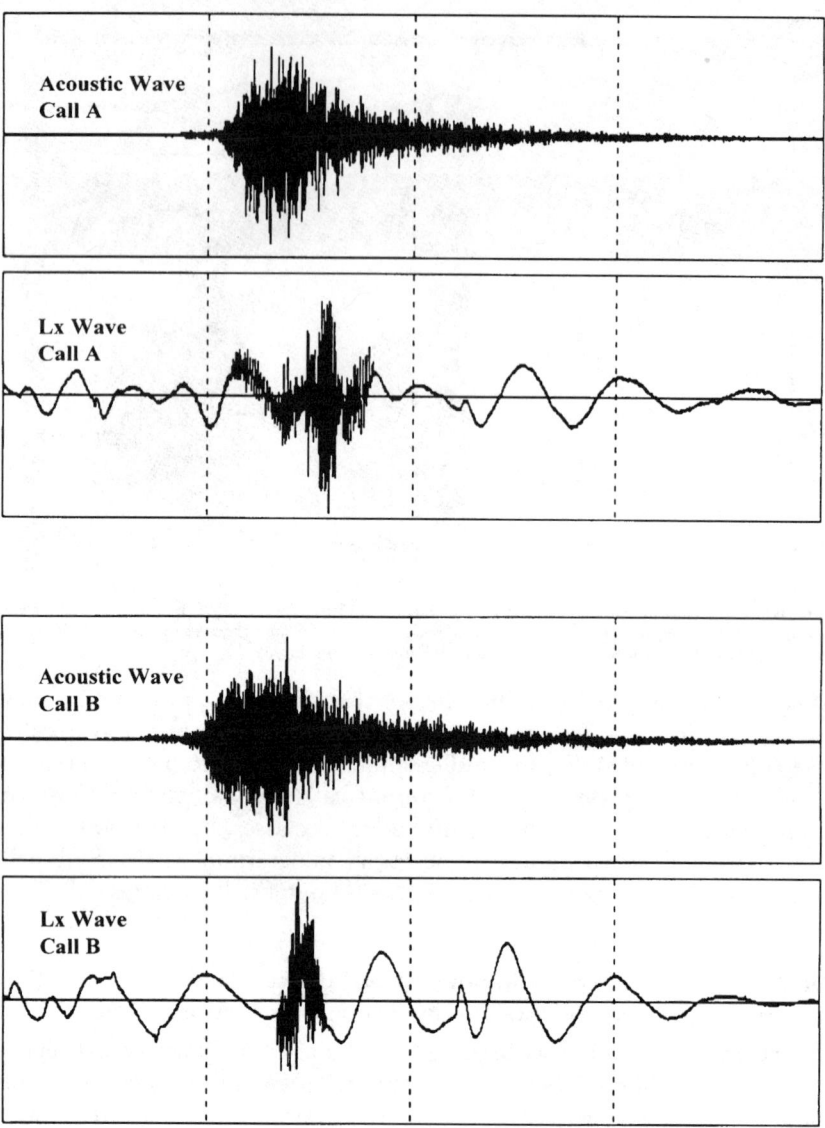

Figure 9. Sykes' monkey screams potentially distinguishable by voicing. In both Call A and Call B, the Lx wave shows a high-amplitude 20-Hz tremor both preceding and following call emission. During intervals between calling bouts, the tremor is not present in the Lx wave. Voicing is denoted by the high-frequency wave superimposed on the low-frequency tremor. In Call A, the voice onset time (VOT) was 11 ms; in Call B, the VOT was 50 ms. In Call B, voicing terminated prior to call termination. The duration of each waveform file was 450 ms.

Hauser and his associates have begun to address this question. Following temporary paralysis of the lips produced by xylocaine injections, rhesus monkeys exhibited acoustic changes in coo vocalizations associated with a reduced vocal tract length caused by an inability to round the lips (Hauser & Schon Ybarra, 1994). Monkeys apparently were unable to overcome the effect of lip paralysis to produce normal calls. However, because xylocaine paralysis only lasts for about 30 minutes, the time course of the study may have been insufficient for monkeys to develop compensatory strategies. In this respect, Hauser and his colleagues have proposed that the possibility of compensation in monkeys could also be explored over a longer time course by using bite blocks, and this idea merits investigation (Hauser & Fitch, in press).

Propositional Vocal Behavior and Syntax

The neural control for propositional and nonpropositional vocal behavior is apparently disassociated in humans. Strokes and other cerebrovascular accidents that may virtually abolish the capacity of the victim to initiate propositional speech will frequently permit subjects to retain the capacity to curse and produce other nonpropositional gestures. Because our understanding of the "speech" of other primates is so limited, it is difficult to distinguish between propositional and nonpropositional vocal behavior in primates other than humans. Are alarm calls propositional gestures or "curses" evoked by a life-threatening situation? The development of innovative new metrics for evaluating the potential for specific information content in vocal and gestural exchanges is necessary for researchers to pursue these difficult questions (Criterion 20).

Human syntax for the ordering of sequences of vocal gestures is important at the phonemic level to produce the correct word and at the morphemic level to produce the correct sentence. As is the case for Criterion 20, our understanding of a possible syntax for primate vocal exchanges is very primitive (Criterion 21). Nevertheless, some gains have been made. Hauser and Fowler (1992) have argued that rhesus monkeys, like humans, use declination in F_0 as a cue to signal when to "take turns" in the alternation of vocal bouts. Furthermore, several studies have shown that sequences of vocal emissions tend to follow a particular order (Cleveland & Snowdon, 1982; Robinson, 1984) and that playbacks of calls in which the natural sequence has been experimentally altered to produce an abnormal "syntax" evoke a heightened number of "disturbance behaviors" in conspecific listeners (Robinson, 1979). These results suggest that it is at least possible that the ordering of these vocal events is meaningful (i.e., segmentally contrastive). Figure 10 shows an example of such a sequence emitted by a Sykes' monkey. Resolution of this issue requires further empirical research, and, for our understanding of the syntax of primate calls

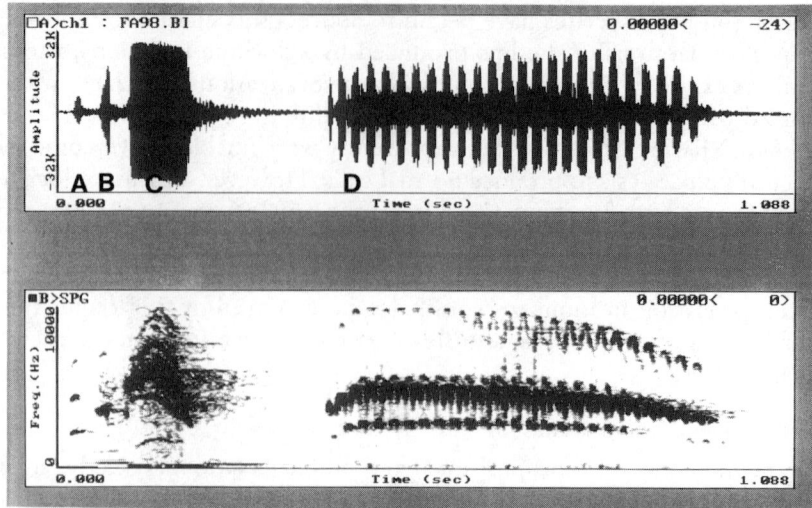

Figure 10. A Sykes' monkey vocal sequence emitted in a single breath. Three acoustically different squeals (A, B, and C) precede a trill (D). The filter bandwidth of the spectrogram was 293 Hz.

to be advanced very far, the question of the propositional employment of these signals needs continued investigation.

CONCLUSIONS

At our present stage of knowledge, animal models (and especially primate models) may have significant potential for contributing to our understanding of normal and disordered regulation of phonation and articulation. This is an area in which a more detailed understanding of the neural regulation of voice, frication, and articulation may assist the development of new therapeutic strategies. For example, stuttering and spasmodic dysphonia are just two of the disorders that are poorly understood at a neurobiologic level and that have been further elucidated by reference to animal models (Cannito, 1991; Rosenfield, 1984). The continued development of animal models may contribute to improvements in treatment strategies for these and other disorders. Multidisciplinary anatomic, physiologic, and behavioral studies hold the greatest promise for advancing our understanding of the mechanics and neural mechanisms giving rise to intelligible speech, and their development merits continued encouragement. Although speech, in its complete form, may occur only in humans, further development of animal models of speech in a variety of species is likely to pay rich dividends in understanding the neurobiologic organization and expression of this most precious of human capacities.

REFERENCES

Aldes, L.D., Chronister, R.B., Shelton, C., Haycock, J.W., Marco, L.A., & Wong, D.L. (1988). Catecholamine innervation of the rat hypoglossal nucleus. *Brain Research Bulletin, 21*, 305–312.
Alipour, F., Titze, I., & Durham, P. (1987). Twitch response in the canine vocalis muscle. *Journal of Speech and Hearing Research, 30*, 290–294.
Barlow, S.M. (1992). Prospects for neurophysiological approaches to the study of speech intelligibility. In R.D. Kent (Ed.), *Intelligibility in speech disorders: Theory, measurement and management*. Philadelphia: John Benjamin Publishing Co.
Brown, C.H. (1994). Ecological constraints for the evolution of primate vocalizations. In J.J. Roeder, B. Thierry, J.R. Anderson, & N. Herrenschmidt (Eds.), *Current primatology, Volume II: Social development, learning, and behavior* (pp. 227–232). Strasbourg: Université Louis Pasteur.
Brown, C.H., & Cannito, M.P. (in press). Modes of vocal variation in Sykes' monkey (*Cercopithecus albogularis*) squeals. *Journal of Comparative Psychology, 109*(4).
Brown, C.H., & Gomez, R. (1992). Functional design features in primate vocal signals: The acoustic habitat and sound distortion. In T. Nishida, W.C. McGrew, P. Marler, M. Pickford, & F.M.B. de Waal (Eds.), *Topics in primatology, Vol. One: Human origins* (pp. 177–198). Tokyo: University of Tokyo Press.
Brown, C.H., Kressley, R.A., & Sinnott, J.M. (1995). *The perception of articulated, inflected and poly-phonic modes of vocal variation in Sykes' monkey* (Cercopithecus albogularis) *utterances*. Manuscript submitted for publication.
Brown, C.H., Sinnott, J.M., & Kressley, R.A. (1994). The perception of chirps by Sykes' monkeys (*Cercopithecus albogularis*) and humans. *Journal of Comparative Psychology, 108*, 243–251.
Brown, C.H., & Waser, P.M. (1988). Environmental influences on the structure of primate vocalizations. In D. Todt, P. Goedeking, & D. Symmes (Eds.), *Primate vocal communication* (pp. 51–66). Berlin: Springer-Verlag.
Buchwald, J.S., Shipley, C., Altafullah, I., Hinman, C., Harrison, J., & Dickerson, L. (1988). The feline isolation call. In J.D. Newman (Ed.), *The physiological control of mammalian vocalization* (pp. 119–135). New York: Plenum Press.
Cannito, M.P. (1991). Neurobiological interpretations of spasmodic dysphonia. In D. Vogel & M.P. Cannito (Eds.), *Treating disordered speech motor control for clinicians by clinicians* (pp. 275–317). Austin, TX: PRO-ED.
Cheney, D.L., & Seyfarth, R.M. (1990). *How monkeys see the world*. Chicago: Chicago University Press.
Cleveland, J., & Snowdon, C.T. (1982). The complex vocal repertoire of the adult cotton-top tamarin (*Saguinus oedipus oedipus*). *Zeitschrift fur Tierpsychologie, 58*, 231–270.
Evarts, E.V. (1980). Brain mechanisms in voluntary movement. In D. McFadden (Ed.), *Neural mechanisms in behavior: A Texas symposium* (pp. 223–259). New York: Springer-Verlag.
Gautier, J-P., & Gautier, A. (1977). Communication in Old World monkeys. In T.E. Sebeok (Ed.), *How animals communicate* (pp. 890–964). Bloomington: Indiana University Press.
Gilman, S., & Kluin, K.J. (1992). Speech disorders in cerebellar degeneration studies with positron emission tomography. In A. Blitzer, M.F. Brin, C.T. Sasaki, S. Fahn, & K.S. Harris (Eds.), *Neurologic disorders of the larynx* (pp. 279–285). New York: Theime Medical Publishers.

Glass, I., & Wollberg, Z. (1979). Lability in the response of cells in the auditory cortex of squirrel monkeys to species specific vocalizations. *Experimental Brain Research*, *34*, 489–498.

Gouzoules, H., & Gouzoules, S. (1989). Design features and developmental modification of pig-tailed macaque, *Macaca nemestrina*, agonistic screams. *Animal Behaviour*, *37*, 383–401.

Gouzoules, S., Gouzoules, H., & Marler, P. (1984). Rhesus monkey (*Macaca mulatta*) screams: Representational signalling in the recruitment of agonistic aid. *Animal Behaviour*, *32*, 182–193.

Green, S. (1975). Variation in vocal pattern with social situation in the Japanese monkey (*Macaca fuscata*): A field study. In L.A. Rosenblum (Ed.), *Primate behavior, Vol. 4: Developments in field and laboratory research* (pp. 1–102). New York: Academic Press.

Hauser, M.D. (1992). Articulatory and social factors influence the acoustic structure of rhesus monkey vocalizations: A learned mode of production? *Journal of the Acoustical Society of America*, *91*, 2175–2179.

Hauser, M.D., & Fitch, W.T. (in press). Vocal production in nonhuman primates: Structure and function. *American Journal of Primatology*.

Hauser, M.D., & Fowler, C.A. (1992). Fundamental frequency declination is not unique to human speech: Evidence from nonhuman primates. *Journal of the Acoustical Society of America*, *91*, 363–369.

Hauser, M.D., & Schon Ybarra, M. (1994). The role of lip configuration in monkey vocalizations: Experiments using xylocaine as a nerve block. *Brain and Language*, *46*, 232–244.

Heffner, H.E., & Heffner, R.S. (1984). Temporal lobe lesions and perception of species-specific vocalizations by macaques. *Science*, *226*, 75–76.

Jurgens, U. (1983). Afferant fibers to the cingular vocalization region in the squirrel monkey. *Experimental Neurology*, *80*, 395–409.

Jurgens, U., & Ploog, D. (1970). Cerebral representation of vocalization in the squirrel monkey. *Experimental Brain Research*, *10*, 532–554.

Jurgens, U., & Ploog, D. (1988). On the motor coordination of monkey calls. In J.D. Newman (Ed.), *The physiological control of mammalian vocalization* (pp. 7–19). New York: Plenum Press.

Jurgens, U., & Pratt, R. (1979a). The cingular vocalization pathway in the squirrel monkey. *Experimental Brain Research*, *34*, 499–510.

Jurgens, U., & Pratt, R. (1979b). Role of periaqueductal grey in vocal expression of emotion. *Brain Research*, *167*, 367–378.

Kehoe, P. (1988). Ontogeny of adrenergic and opioid effects on separation vocalizations in rats. In J.D. Newman (Ed.), *The physiological control of mammalian vocalization* (pp. 301–320). New York: Plenum Press.

Kirzinger, A., & Jurgens, U. (1982). Cortical lesion effect and vocalization in the squirrel monkey. *Brain Research*, *233*, 299–315.

Kolb, B., & Wishaw, I.Q. (1990). *Fundamentals of human neuropsychology*. New York: W.H. Freeman & Co.

Kots, Y.M. (1977). *The organization of voluntary movement: Neurophysiological mechanisms* (E.V. Evarts, Trans.). New York: Plenum Press.

Larson, C.R. (1985). The midbrain periaqueductal gray: A brainstem structure involved in vocalization. *Journal of Speech and Hearing Research*, *28*, 241–249.

Larson, C.R., & Kistler, M.K. (1986). The relationship of periaqueductal gray neurons to vocalization and laryngeal EMG in the behaving monkey. *Experimental Brain Research*, *63*, 596–606.

Larson, C.R., Ortega, J.D., & DeRosier, E.A. (1988). Studies on the relation of the midbrain periaqueductal gray, the larynx and vocalization in awake monkeys. In

J.D. Newman (Ed.), *The physiological control of mammalian vocalization* (pp. 43–65). New York: Plenum Press.

Lernould, J.-M. (1988). Classification and geographical distribution of guenons: A review. In A. Gautier-Hion, F. Bourliere, J.-P. Gautier, & J. Kingdon (Eds.), *A primate radiation: Evolutionary biology of the African guenons* (pp. 54–78). Cambridge, England: Cambridge University Press.

Magoun, H.W., Atlas, D., Ingersoll, E.H., & Ranson, S.W. (1937). Associated facial, vocal and respiratory components of emotional expression: An experimental study. *Journal of Neurology and Psychopathology, 17*, 241–255.

McClean, M., Dostrovsky, J.O., Lee, L., & Tasker, R.R. (1990). Somatosensory neurons in human thalamus respond to speech-induced orofacial movements. *Brain Research, 513*, 343–347.

Muller-Preuss, P., Newman, J.D., & Jurgens, U. (1980). Anatomical and physiological evidence for a relationship between the 'cingular' vocalization area and the auditory cortex in the squirrel monkey. *Brain Research, 202*, 307–315.

Penfield, W., & Roberts, L. (1959). *Speech and brain mechanisms*. Princeton, NJ: Princeton University Press.

Robinson, J.G. (1979). An analysis of the organization of vocal communication in the titi monkey (*Callicebus moloch*). *Zeitschrift fur Tierpsychologie, 49*, 381–405.

Robinson, J.G. (1984). Syntactic structures in the vocalizations of wedge-capped capuchin monkeys (*Cebus olivaces*). *Behaviour, 90*, 46–79.

Rosenfield, D.B. (1984). Stuttering. *CRC Critical Reviews in Clinical Neurobiology, 1*, 117–139.

Rowell, T.E., & Hinde, R.A. (1962). Vocal communication by the rhesus monkey (*Macaca mulatta*). *Symposium of the Zoological Society of London, 138*, 279–294.

Ryding, E., Bradvik, B., & Ingvar, D.H. (1987). Changes of regional bloodflow measured simultaneously in the right and left hemisphere during automated speech and humming. *Brain, 110*, 1345–1358.

Seyfarth, R.M., & Cheney, D.L. (1986). Vocal development in vervet monkeys. *Animal Behaviour, 34*, 1640–1658.

Seyfarth, R.M., Cheney, D.L., & Marler, P. (1980). Monkey responses to three different alarm calls: Evidence for predator classification and semantic communication. *Science, 210*, 801–803.

Sinnott, J.M. (1995). Methods to assess the processing of speech sounds by animals. In R. Dooling, R. Fay, G. Glump, & W.C. Stebbins (Eds.), *Methods in comparative psychoacoustics* (pp. 281–292). Zurich: Birkhauser.

Sinnott, J.M., Stebbins, W.C., & Moody, D.B. (1975). Regulation of voice amplitude by the monkey. *Journal of the Acoustical Society of America, 58*, 412–414.

Snowdon, C.T., & Hodun, A. (1981). Acoustic adaptations in pygmy marmoset contact calls: Location cues vary with distance between conspecifics. *Behavioral Ecology and Sociobiology, 9*, 295–300.

Sussman, H.M. (1989). Neural coding of relational invariance in speech: Human language analogs to the barn owl. *Psychological Review, 96*, 631–642.

Todt, D., Goedeking, P., & Symmes, D. (1988). *Primate vocal communication*. Berlin: Springer-Verlag.

Waser, P.M. (1975). Experimental playbacks show vocal mediation of intergroup avoidance in a forest monkey. *Nature, 255*, 56–58.

Whitaker, H.A. (1976). Neurobiology of language. In E.C. Carterette & M.P. Friedman (Eds.), *Handbook of perception, Vol. VII: Language and speech*. (pp. 121–144). New York: Academic Press.

Whitehead, J.M. (1987). Vocally mediated reciprocity between neighboring groups of mantled howling monkeys, *Aloutta palliata palliata*. *Animal Behaviour, 35*, 1615–1627.

SECTION III

INTELLIGIBILITY

Chapter 4

Effects of Semantic and Syntactic Context on Actual and Estimated Sentence Intelligibility of Dysarthric Speakers

Carolyn R. Carter, Kathryn M. Yorkston, Edythe A. Strand, and Vicki L. Hammen

THE DYSARTHRIAS ARE a group of chronic motor speech disorders characterized by disturbed muscle control resulting from damage to the central or peripheral nervous systems or to the speech musculature. Paralysis, weakness, abnormal tone, or incoordination may lead to impaired function of the speech musculature and may affect the parameters of direction, range, force, endurance, timing, and regulation of movements in the muscles responsible for respiration, phonation, articulation, resonance, or prosody. One potential disability brought about by these impairments is reduced intelligibility of the dysarthric speaker.

Intervention with dysarthric speakers may help them to improve their motoric capacity for intelligible speech. Yet because of the nature of the neurophysiologic disorders causing dysarthria, significant improvements in motor capability are often not realistic treatment goals for some speakers. An alternative strategy for enhancing communication effectiveness is to compensate for the unintelligible speech by directing intervention efforts toward other variables in the communication environment. There are many possible compensatory strategies that could be proposed. This study focused on one: Perhaps the intelligibility of a dysarthric speaker could be improved by intervening with the listeners to enhance their abilities to understand distorted speech and thus to compensate for the speech signal distortion of the speaker.

The degree to which such a compensation is successful may depend on the skills, attributes, and information available to both the speakers and listeners. One type of information is prior knowledge of the context of the utterance, which might provide a frame of reference from which listeners can interpret the speech signal. Three context conditions were explored in this study: no context, semantic context, and syntactic context.

Context is the knowledge shared by communication partners about the time, place, topic, purpose, or any other feature of an utterance or the setting in which the utterance occurs. The context may include but is not confined to information contained in the speech signal. Context may take many forms, including semantic, syntactic, suprasegmental, and pragmatic. This concept of total context includes the sum of all conditions surrounding a communication event (Miller & Selfridge, 1950). The purpose of this study was to partition this total context into its components and to investigate two specific types of context: semantic and syntactic.

Semantic context is closely related to the concept of total context in that it incorporates information from the speech signal and the environment to provide cues about the intended meaning of an utterance or the intent of a speaker. The traditional form of semantic context is a cue word or phrase that conveys information about the meaning of a stimulus item (Dongilli, 1994; Dowden, 1992; Hammen, Yorkston, & Dowden, 1991; Kalikow, Stevens, & Elliot, 1977; Pierce and Beekman, 1985; Waller and Darley, 1978; Zwitserlood, 1989). In general, semantic context has been demonstrated to have a significant effect in increasing the single-word intelligibility of dysarthric speakers for words presented in isolation (Dongilli, 1994; Dowden, 1992; Hammen et al., 1991). Semantic context has also been demonstrated to increase the intelligibility of target words presented at the end of a sentence, although the effects of context in this condition were not as large as they were on isolated words (Dongilli, 1994). In all studies, there have been interactions between the effects of context and dysarthria severity. Hammen et al. (1991) found that the greatest improvement in intelligibility from the effects of context was demonstrated by severely dysarthric speakers, followed by moderately and then profoundly dysarthric speakers. Dongilli (1994) also concluded that the greatest effects were seen in moderately and severely dysarthric speakers. Semantic context was not as beneficial for profoundly dysarthric speakers. In all studies, there appeared to be a point of impaired intelligibility below which speech was so profoundly distorted that intelligibility could not be improved with contextual support.

The definition of syntactic context is less clear than that of semantic context. For this study, syntactic context was defined as knowledge of the grammatical structure of a sentence that rendered components of the utterance predictable to listeners based on their knowledge of the rule-governed construct of the language. In this study, grammatical structure included functor words, such as articles and conjunctions, as well as identification of the location and number of content or meaning words within the sentence. Syntactic context specified the number of words, the placement or boundaries of words, and the role of each word as either a content or grammatical functor word. However, syntactic context did not yield any semantic information about the meaning or intent of the utterance.

Researchers have applied different interpretations of syntactic context in their investigations. For example, the effects of syntactic context have been studied by testing the intelligibility of grammatical versus agrammatical strings of words (Ellis & Fucci, 1991; Goodman, McClelland, & Gibbs, 1981; Miller & Isard, 1963). In general, the grammatical word strings were understood with greater accuracy and speed than the agrammatical strings under a variety of testing conditions. Another technique for examining the effects of syntactic context has been to compare the intelligibility of key words in isolation versus when embedded in sentences (Dongilli, 1994; Kalikow et al., 1977; McAllister, 1988; Miller, Heise, & Lichten, 1951; O'Neill, 1957; Sitler, Schiavetti, & Metz, 1983). These researchers found that key words were more intelligible in the sentence context than in isolation. Again, intelligibility was improved only for those speakers who were already somewhat intelligible even without context. Speakers who had a baseline intelligibility of less than 30% did not benefit from added contextual support when words were presented in sentences compared to presentation in isolation (Sitler et al., 1983).

Studies such as those described above have often been interpreted as investigating syntactic context. However, they have actually tested the influences of both semantic and syntactic context combined. Placing a target word in a complete sentence does provide syntactic context by supplying grammatical structure. However, a well-formed sentence also provides semantic context because other content words in the sentence identify the meaning or intent of the sentence with which a stimulus word must agree. A meaningful grammatical sentence must also be semantically appropriate, and vice versa. A sentence cannot be considered well formed unless both semantic and syntactic elements are correct (Goodman et al., 1981). Therefore, semantic and syntactic contexts are very difficult to separate. The interaction between these elements has not been sufficiently controlled in previous studies using grammatical versus agrammatical stimuli and isolated words versus sentence stimuli to provide definite conclusions as to the role of purely syntactic context on intelligibility.

Recognizing this interdependence of semantic and syntactic context, many researchers have returned to the more general concept of overall verbal context that incorporates semantic and syntactic context as well as any other linguistic information about an utterance. Studies show that this overall context improves intelligibility of target words (Duffy & Giolas, 1974; Miller et al., 1951; Zwitserlood, 1989).

In summary, there is consensus that overall verbal context can significantly improve the intelligibility of target words in a variety of test conditions. When global verbal context is partitioned into semantic and syntactic context, each type of context appears to improve intelligibility. There is general agreement among researchers as to the definition of semantic context and its significant effects on the intelligibility of single words. Although there are statements in the literature suggesting that syntactic context also enhances intelligibility, these findings should be considered with caution because of the various interpretations of syntactic context in the literature as well as the difficulties in isolating syntactic context from semantic context to study each separately.

In addition to the different interpretations of what constitutes semantic and syntactic context, there are also various theories as to the mechanisms by which context affects intelligibility. Context may restrict the field of plausible responses to those options that would be semantically or syntactically appropriate in relation to the stimuli (Miller & Isard, 1963; Miller et al., 1951; Pierce & Beekman, 1985; Yorkston & Beukelman, 1978, 1980). Thus, context renders the target items more predictable (Duffy & Giolas, 1974). Another theory is that context increases the redundancy of information available to listeners (Waller & Darley, 1978) and therefore decreases the need for listeners to rely solely on the acoustic signal for information (Kalikow et al., 1977; Miller et al., 1951). These two processes of increasing the predictability of stimuli and decreasing the need to rely on the acoustic signal are most likely complementary in that they both contribute to the integrative process during which contextual cues are combined with acoustic input and memory to assist in comprehension. Zwitserlood (1989) supported this integrative hypothesis by suggesting that context does not influence a listener's preparatory set or initial lexical access, but instead promoted recognition of words and integration of ideas at a higher level of linguistic representation. A final theoretical mechanism specific to syntactic context is the identification of the boundaries of linguistically meaningful units in the speech signal, such as word or phrase boundaries. Demarcation of these boundaries might help listeners identify the correct units for linguistic processing.

Although context appears to have significant effects on the intelligibility of dysarthric speakers, it may also affect other factors, such as the confidence that listeners have in their ability to understand that speech. Listeners must often rely on their own intuitions and interpretations to replace information missing from the distorted speech signal. Listeners who are overconfident may attend more to their own interpretations than to the information that is available from the speaker or context. Thus, they may not use repair strategies and seek the input they need from the speaker or the environment to be sure their interpretations match the intent of the speaker. In contrast, underconfident listeners may place too great a burden on the speaker by not being assertive enough in supplying their own interpolations to compensate for information the speaker cannot provide. The confidence of listeners may be affected by many variables, such as the overall quality of the stimuli (Nelson, Gerler, & Narens, 1992), experience with the speaker or task, feedback (Dowden, 1992), support received from context and other resources, and the listeners' own attitudes.

On various memory and comprehension tasks, research has shown that subjects tend to overestimate their performance, thus demonstrating overconfidence (Glenberg, Wilkenson, & Epstein, 1992; Koriat, Lichtenstein, & Fischhoff, 1992). Koriat et al. (1992) suggested that such overestimation may stem from the tendency for subjects to rely on their own biases or interpretations instead of attending to concrete evidence in the stimuli. For example, listeners who hear the beginning of a sentence incorrectly may interpret the remainder of the sentence so that it is syntactically and semantically appropriate in relation to their initial perceptions instead of attending to the actual speech signal to determine what is truly being said.

Few studies have examined listener confidence in speech comprehension tasks. Barefoot, Bochner, Johnson, and vom Eigen (1993) found that listeners were able to provide valid judgments of the degree to which they had understood hearing-impaired speakers. Dowden (1992) suggested that listeners were fairly accurate in evaluating the correctness of their responses on word transcription tasks for dysarthric speakers because listeners reported higher confidence on items that they transcribed correctly than on items transcribed incorrectly. Subjects in the Dowden (1992) study were also more confident on the stimulus words presented with semantic context than on words without context.

The goal of this study was to contribute to the body of knowledge about dysarthria by exploring the effects of semantic and syntactic context on the sentence intelligibility of dysarthric speakers and on the confidence and perceptions of the listeners who interact with them. Another purpose of the study was to provide recommendations for improving intervention with dysarthric speakers and their communication partners by highlighting strategies that boost intelligibility even when the speech signal itself cannot be improved. To achieve these goals, the following questions were defined and explored:

- What are the effects of semantic and syntactic context on the intelligibility of sentences produced by dysarthric speakers? How do these effects vary as a function of dysarthria severity?
- What are the effects of semantic and syntactic context on the abilities of listeners to evaluate how well they understand dysarthric speakers? How do these effects vary as a function of dysarthria severity?

Previous studies of the effects of context on the intelligibility of dysarthric speakers have focused on the transcription of single words in a variety of conditions. No study has examined the effects of context on the sentence as a whole. This study extended the investigation of the role of context in the intelligibility of dysarthric speakers to sentence stimuli, thus providing a more realistic measure of functional communication than the single-word stimuli. Previous researchers have purported to study the effects of syntactic context on the intelligibility of dysarthric speakers. However, as discussed earlier, these efforts have not succeeded in isolating syntactic from semantic context in a manner that would allow a comparison of the two. This experiment introduced a new method of defining syntactic context in an attempt to separate it from semantic context and to thus allow a comparison of the two types of context and their individual influences on the intelligibility of dysarthric speakers.

Previous studies also have suggested that listeners are fairly accurate in evaluating the success with which they understand dysarthric speakers (Dowden, 1992) and hearing-impaired speakers (Barefoot et al., 1993). However, a collection of studies outside of the field of communication disorders explored subject confidence on various memory and comprehension tasks and revealed consistent overconfidence in subjects (Glenberg et al., 1992; Koriat et al., 1992). Additional studies are needed to objectively compare listeners' actual performance with their interpretations of their performance when attempting to comprehend dysarthric speakers. This study explored that comparison in an attempt to contribute to the body of knowledge about dysarthria by addressing variables that influence communication with dysarthric speakers but that traditionally have not been included in other studies of intelligibility.

METHODOLOGY

Speakers

Recorded samples from six dysarthric speakers were used in this study. The recordings of all six speakers were available from previous research conducted at the University of Washington Medical Center. These six samples were chosen according to their baseline sentence intelligibility as determined by prior studies. The goal for sample selection was to create two distinct groups, one to represent moderate dysarthria and the other to represent severe dysarthria. Speakers 1–3 were included in the moderate group, with intelligibility scores ranging from approximately 70%–83%. The severe group consisted of Speakers 4–6, whose intelligibility scores ranged from 35% to 39%. Table 1 presents the demographic information for each speaker.

The purpose of forming two distinct groups of speakers was to determine if the effects of context on intelligibility varied depending on the severity of dysarthria. Although the entire range of dysarthria severity that occurs in the general population was not represented in the study, the speakers were selected to represent the two extremes of a range of intelligibility in which context is expected to have the most impact. Speakers with greater than 90% intelligibility were not selected because, although their speech may sound unnatural or distorted, intelligibility is still almost complete. There is little or no additional information that context could provide. Research has shown that context also has very little effect below 30% intelligibility (Sitler et al., 1983), so samples with scores below this level were not chosen.

Sentence Stimuli

The stimulus materials were randomly generated samples of the Computerized Assessment of Intelligibility of Dysarthric Speakers (CAIDS) (Yorkston, Beukelman, & Traynor, 1984). Each speaker's sample consisted of 11 sentences containing a total of 110 words. Sentences ranged in length from 5 to 15 words, with one sentence of each length per sample. Each speaker produced different sentences. However, all samples were equated in length, the frequency of word occurrence in the language, and the variety of semantic and syntactic forms represented. Therefore, although each sample was unique in its content, all samples were equivalent in construct to allow comparison of results across speakers. The sentences had been recorded on reel-to-reel tapes in a quiet clinical environment.

Table 1. Speaker characteristics

	Age (gender)	Etiology	Dysarthria type	Sentence intelligibility (%)
Moderate group				
S1	32 (F)	Cerebrovascular accident	Ataxic/flaccid	81.2
S2	56 (M)	Parkinsonism	Hypokinetic	82.3
S3	71 (M)	Parkinsonism	Hypokinetic	70.6
Severe group				
S4	45 (M)	Traumatic brain injury	Ataxic	34.5
S5	73 (F)	Parkinsonism	Hypokinetic	37.9
S6	39 (M)	Tumor	Ataxic	38.7

Context Generation

Semantic Context The semantic context was developed by two independent sets of judges, including the examiner (the first author) and staff in the Division of Speech Pathology, Department of Rehabilitation Medicine at the University of Washington Medical Center. Two sets of judges were used to ensure that unusual or idiosyncratic semantic context would be eliminated through multiple reviews. Judges in the first set ($N=3$) were asked to independently read each of the stimulus sentences and to write down four words that each represented the meaning or semantic context of the sentence. The judges received no instructions about how to select context other than to avoid words actually contained in the sentences. Judges in the second set ($N=5$), none of whom had participated in the first set, were then presented with the proposals for semantic context that had been generated by the first set of judges. Proposals were listed in random order with duplicates omitted. Judges in the second set were asked to independently read each sentence and the proposed contexts and then to select and rank their top three choices for the word that best represented the meaning of the sentence. That item that received the most first-place rankings was selected as the semantic context for that sentence. The following is an example of semantic context for one sentence:

- *Stimulus sentence:* The police said the collision was not my fault.
- *Semantic context:* ACCIDENT

The semantic context was printed on response forms to be read by listeners while they transcribed the sentences.

Syntactic Context Syntactic context was defined as those components of a sentence that provided the grammatical structure of the sentence without revealing any semantic content. Thus, the syntactic context consisted of the grammatical or functor words and the identification of their positions in a sentence relative to the content words. Functor words (conjunctions, prepositions, articles, pronouns) were determined according to a list compiled by Yorkston, Dowden, Honsinger, Marriner, and Smith (1988).

The syntactic context was printed on listener response forms. For each sentence, the form presented the sentence structure such that the functor words were provided and blank lines were drawn to indicate missing content words in the appropriate places in each sentence. The blank lines were all of uniform length, so they did not yield any clues as to the length of the missing word. The following is an example of syntactic context using the same sentence that was presented above with semantic context:

Syntactic context: The _____ _____ the _____ was not my _____.
Stimulus sentence: The police said the collision was not my fault.

Listening Tasks

Listeners Thirty-six listeners participated in the study. This number allowed for the presentation of all possible combinations of speakers ($N=6$), intelligibility levels ($N=2$), and context conditions ($N=3$). Testing all possible permutations reduced the threat of any potential effects of presentation order or context–speaker combination from influencing the results.

All listeners included in the study met the following criteria: 1) adults in the age range of 18–40 years, 2) high school or general equivalency diploma graduates, and 3) native speakers of American English. Listeners were excluded from the study if they presented with any of these five variables: 1) a history of hearing loss, 2) a history of language disorders, 3) a history of extensive experience interacting with dysarthric speakers, 4) a history of experience with the CAIDS stimuli, or 5) a history of formal study in the academic disciplines of speech and hearing sciences or linguistics beyond the introductory level. Listeners were paid for their participation. Table 2 provides a description of the listener population in this study.

Listener Orientation and Training The entire procedure was completed in a single 2-hour session for each listener. The listener was seated at a table in a quiet clinic room where he or she transcribed the speech samples. The samples were played on a TEAC A-2340SX reel-to-reel tape player, and the listener wore headphones adjusted to a comfortable loudness level. Breaks were provided during the sessions to prevent fatigue.

Listeners were provided with written instructions and verbal clarification regarding the transcription task. Listeners were instructed to write down as much of the sentences as they could understand. Guessing on the transcriptions was allowed, although listeners were instructed to guess only on the basis of what they thought they heard. All sentences were presented twice to ensure uniform exposure to the stimuli for all listeners. No time restrictions were imposed on the listeners, and they were allotted as much time as they needed to transcribe sentences.

The experimental session began with a training exercise to familiarize the listener with dysarthric speech and the CAIDS procedure. The training protocol was similar to that published in the CAIDS manual (Yorkston et al., 1984). The training speech sample was identical in construct but different in content than the experimental samples. The training speech sample was from the CAIDS training tape and was not from a speaker from one of the six experimental samples. The listener was presented with

Table 2. Listener characteristics

	Number	Percentage
Age (years)		
18–25	24	67
26–30	3	8
31–35	4	11
36–40	5	14
Gender		
Male	17	47
Female	19	53
Occupation		
Student	27	75
Secretary	3	8
Other	6	17
Education		
Some college	20	56
Bachelor's degree	7	19
Master's degree	9	25
Foreign language experience (years)		
0–5	29	81
6–10	5	14
11–20	2	6

each sentence twice, after which he or she transcribed the sentence using English orthography. After completion of the entire sample, the listener's transcription score was calculated according to the CAIDS procedure. If the listener's practice score was within a predetermined range of intelligibility recommended in the CAIDS manual (Yorkston et al., 1984), the listener was considered to be reliable and to have successfully completed the training. Only one candidate was dismissed from the study and replaced by another listener as a result of unsatisfactory performance on the training task. Listeners were shown the results of their training sample, but not the results of the experimental tasks that followed.

Experimental Procedure The experimental tasks were similar to the training task except for the presentation of the different context conditions. Each listener transcribed all six speech samples. Each sample was presented to each listener only once. Each listener transcribed one moderately dysarthric speech sample and one severely dysarthric speech sample in each of the three context conditions (none, semantic, syntactic). The order of presentation of samples and the assignment of speech samples to the context conditions were counterbalanced across all 36 listeners so that all possible combinations of speaker–context–order were tested. Each listener was randomly assigned to one such combination.

In the no-context condition, the instructions and procedures were identical to those of the training task. In the semantic-context condition, the listeners were presented with the appropriate response forms as described above. They were instructed to read the semantic context and to use it to help them understand the sentences. For the syntactic context condition, the listeners were provided with the appropriate response forms as described above. They were instructed that portions of each sentence had been provided for them on the forms and that their task was to fill in the missing words as designated by the blank lines.

Listeners were also asked to evaluate the accuracy of their transcriptions. Immediately following each sentence in all three context conditions, listeners were told to write down the number of words in that sentence that they believed they had transcribed correctly. Listeners were instructed to include in their evaluations only those words that they felt confident were correct and not those words that were guesses.

Analysis of Data

All response forms were scored by the examiner according to the CAIDS protocol (Yorkston et al., 1984). In the no-context and semantic-context conditions, the percentage of the total number of words transcribed correctly in the sentences was calculated. In the syntactic-context condition, the percentage of the total number of content words transcribed correctly was calculated because listeners had the opportunity to transcribe content words only.

The listeners' estimates were scored by adding the number of words each listener estimated to be correct for that sample and determining the percentage that estimate represented of the total number of words that could have been transcribed for that sample. A two-factor repeated-measures analysis of variance (ANOVA) was applied for data analysis.

Reliability

The reliability of the examiner in scoring the transcriptions and the estimates was assessed when the examiner repeated the scoring procedure with 17% of the response forms approximately 2 months following the original data analysis. Pearson product correlations ranged from 0.999 to 1.000 and indicated highly reliable scoring.

RESULTS

Question 1: Speaker Intelligibility

Figure 1 illustrates speaker intelligibility as a function of the three context conditions for both the moderate and severe groups of speakers. The

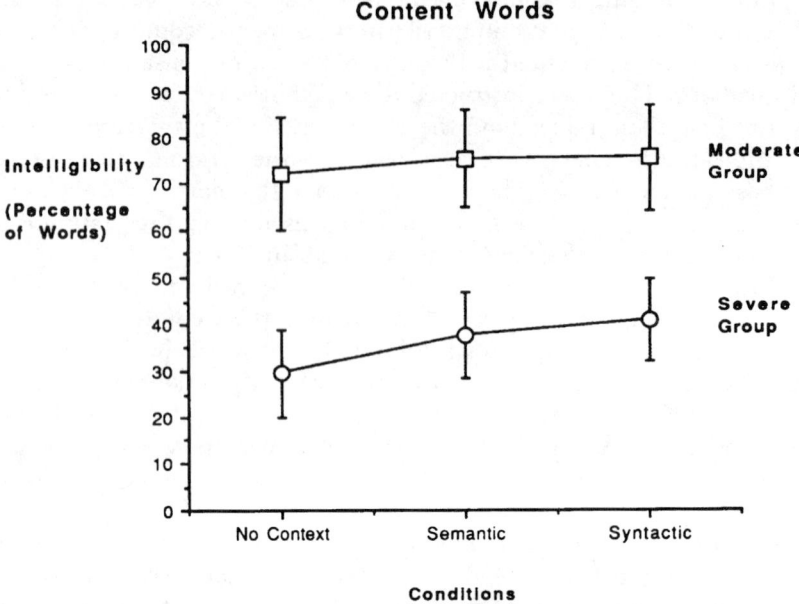

Figure 1. Intelligibility scores, with standard deviations, for moderately and severely dysarthric speakers as a function of context.

mean percentages for the moderate group were: no context, 72.2% (standard deviation [SD] = 12.1%); semantic context, 75.3% (SD = 10.7%); and syntactic context, 75.5% (SD = 11.2%). The mean percentages for the severely dysarthric group of speakers were: no context, 29.4% (SD = 9.5%); semantic context, 37.7% (SD = 9.2%); and syntactic context, 40.8% (SD = 8.9%).

The results of a two-factor repeated-measures ANOVA indicated that the moderate and severe groups were significantly different from each other ($p < .001$). The context conditions produced a significant effect ($p < .001$), and post hoc analysis using Tukey's Honestly Significant Difference (HSD) test was conducted to identify the significant pairwise comparisons. This post hoc analysis revealed no significant difference among the three context conditions for the moderate group of speakers. However, for the severely dysarthric speakers, Tukey's HSD analysis indicated a significant difference between the no-context and semantic-context scores ($p = .003$) and between the no-context and syntactic-context scores ($p < .001$). The difference between semantic and syntactic context scores was not significant in the severe group. There was no significant interaction between context and dysarthria severity.

Question 2: Listener Evaluation Ability

Figure 2 presents a comparison of the estimated versus actual transcription scores as a function of the three context conditions for both the moderate and severe groups of speakers. The listeners' evaluations, expressed as the mean percentages of words estimated to be correct for the moderate group, were: no context, 82.3% ($SD = 9.4\%$); semantic context, 84.9% ($SD = 8.4\%$); and syntactic context, 80.5% ($SD = 9.5\%$). The listeners' evaluations in terms of the mean percentages of words estimated to be correct for the severe group were: no context, 46.6% ($SD = 14.6\%$); semantic context, 55.0% ($SD = 11.5\%$); and syntactic context, 48.5% ($SD = 9.8\%$).

A two-factor repeated-measures ANOVA with post hoc testing revealed no significant difference between the transcription scores and the listener evaluations in the no-context condition for the moderate group of speakers. However, all other comparisons were significant. Listener evaluations were significantly higher than the actual transcription scores for semantic context ($p = .026$) and syntactic context ($p = .048$) in the moderate group. Listener evaluations were significantly higher than the actual transcription scores in all three context conditions for the severely dysarthric speakers: no context ($p = .002$), semantic context ($p < .001$), and syntactic context ($p = .001$).

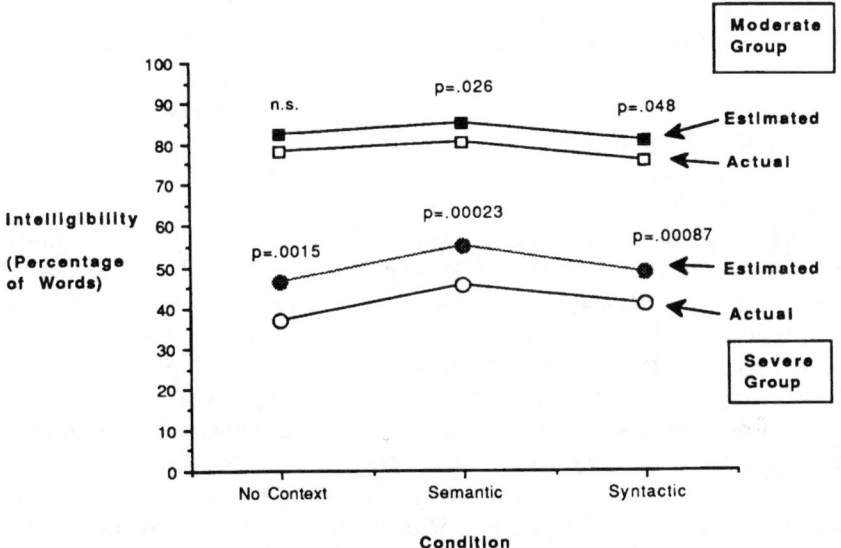

Figure 2. A comparison of actual and estimated intelligibility scores for both moderately and severely dysarthric speakers as a function of context.

DISCUSSION

Speaker Intelligibility

Results of this study indicated that the effects of semantic and syntactic context on sentence intelligibility vary depending on the severity of dysarthria. Neither semantic nor syntactic context affects the intelligibility of moderately dysarthric speakers, but both forms of context significantly improve the intelligibility of severely dysarthric speakers. There was no significant difference between semantic and syntactic context for either group of speakers.

For the moderate group, the results revealed no significant difference in the intelligibility scores between the no-context and semantic-context conditions. Thus, semantic context does not improve the intelligibility of moderately dysarthric speakers on sentence stimuli. This conclusion does not concur with related discussions in the literature. Hammen et al. (1991), Dowden (1992), and Dongilli (1994) all found that the intelligibility of moderately dysarthric speakers on single-word stimuli improved in the presence of semantic context. There are three possible reasons for these different conclusions.

The first possible reason why the results from this study differ from prior related research is that perhaps the investigators did not define and implement semantic context in the same way. This explanation is not satisfactory for two reasons. First, although the procedures for creating the context varied slightly for each researcher, the semantic context appears to be very similar in nature among the three prior studies and the present investigation. Second, if the semantic context in the current study truly was less effective, it probably would not have caused the significant effects evident in the severe group, as discussed below.

The second explanation for the rejected hypothesis is possible disparity between single-word transcription and sentence transcription, and what this might reveal about the effects of semantic context on functional connected speech. Dongilli (1994) suggested that the difference between words and sentences should be considered. In his study, the effects of semantic context on intelligibility were greater for isolated words than for target words presented in sentences. Transcription of single words is a more controlled environment for semantic context because the context can define specific semantic categories that clearly constrain the choice of potential words. For example, the context "days of the week" clearly restricts the target word to one of seven choices. However, there are no restricted inventories of sentences from which a listener can select a response to fit semantic context. Language is flexible in that there are a seemingly infinite number of word sequences that can be combined in a sentence to convey even one meaning. Semantic context may cue the listener as to the general meaning of a sentence. Yet even with highly specific context, the choice and sequence of specific words cannot be controlled completely. Therefore, the ability to generate vast numbers of sentences prevents context from having a powerful influence over the intelligibility of sentences compared to words, which truly can be categorized into limited inventories with more clearly defined contextual boundaries.

Another theory relating to the difference between word and sentence transcription tasks is that the sentences inherently convey context through the other words in them. The extra-context cue may not provide additional useful information beyond that already present in the sentence. With word transcriptions there is no internal context, and all contextual information must come from the provided cue.

As with the first rationale, this explanation contributes to our understanding but is inadequate to account for the findings of this study. If semantic context was truly not effective in improving the intelligibility of sentences produced by dysarthric speakers, there would not have been a significant increase in intelligibility in the severe speakers in this study.

This leads to the third and most plausible explanation for the results of this study. Although the possible contributions of the theories above are recognized, it appears that the severity of dysarthria must play a key role in determining how context affects intelligibility. There appears to be a general consensus that, within the range of moderate to severe dysarthria, context exerts a more powerful influence as the speech becomes less intelligible. However, slight variations in the interpretation of the range of moderate to severe dysarthria may lead to different conclusions. Among the four studies in comparison here, there were slight variations in the classification of baseline intelligibilities that were considered moderately severe. The speakers used in the current study were skewed more toward the higher end of the range of intelligibilities accepted as moderate dysarthria. This skew may have been created by the scoring format used to determine baseline intelligibility, because research has shown that sentence transcription scores tend to be higher than word transcription scores (Yorkston et al., 1984). However, if the speakers in this study truly did have a higher baseline intelligibility than those in previous studies, this disparity may account for the different conclusions regarding moderate dysarthria reached by various investigators. If the listeners were able to understand 70%–83% of the sentence material at baseline, they were probably already gleaning the main semantic information from the stimuli on their own without the aid of external context.

For the severe group, semantic context significantly improved the sentence intelligibility scores. This finding is consistent with the conclusions of related studies in the literature. Apparently, when dysarthria is severe, listeners have difficulty interpreting the topic of the sentence based on information in the speech signal itself. Semantic context provides additional information about the meaning of the sentence that listeners then use to better understand the speaker.

The mechanism by which semantic context improves intelligibility has been discussed in the literature and addressed above. Previous researchers (Miller et al., 1951; Miller & Isard, 1963; Pierce & Beekman, 1985; Yorkston & Beukelman, 1978, 1980) have suggested that semantic context affects intelligibility by limiting the inventory of plausible responses from which a listener can choose. Semantic context cannot limit the number of possible sentences because of the enormous number of word combinations that can form a sentence related to a particular topic. However, this study shows that semantic context must at least orient the listener toward the topic of a sentence such that the listener can recognize words or phrases that have a higher probability of occurring in the sentence as a result of their semantic association with the context. Semantic context may increase the probability of correctly identifying the content words in sentences, thus creating a significant change in intelligibility for severely impaired speakers.

For the moderate group, no significant difference in the intelligibility scores was found between the no-context and syntactic-context conditions. The conclusion is that syntactic context does not affect the sentence intelligibility of moderately severe dysarthric speakers. Several of the possible reasons for this outcome are similar to those presented for semantic context. For example, perhaps the manner in which syntactic context was defined and utilized was not effective. This study introduced a new method for presenting syntactic context, and it is possible that syntactic context, defined as it was for this study, does not affect the intelligibility of dysarthric speakers. Yet this statement would not account for the results discussed below for the severely dysarthric speakers, whose intelligibility was improved by syntactic context. Once again, this points to the conclusion that it is the baseline intelligibility of the speakers that is the key factor in determining the influence of syntactic as well as semantic context in intelligibility. Apparently, the speakers in the moderate group were already intelligible enough that the listeners were able to understand the syntactic structure of the sentence without the support provided by the context.

For the severely dysarthric speakers, syntactic context significantly improved sentence intelligibility scores. The finding that syntactic context is just as effective as semantic context in improving intelligibility of severely dysarthric speakers is critical because it brings to attention an important variable for research and clinical intervention.

The mechanism by which syntactic context improves intelligibility is not clear from this study. However, hypotheses that warrant further research can be proposed. One suggestion is that, as with semantic context, syntactic context increases the probability of correct transcription by limiting the words that are likely to occur in the sentence. For example, if the syntactic context provides an article such as "the," a portion of the sentence that follows must include a noun phrase. In this case the syntactic context primes the listener to be alert for a noun to occur—if not as the next word, at least in the near vicinity following any modifiers.

Syntactic context may also improve intelligibility by helping listeners to define the boundaries between words and phrases. Knowledge of these boundaries allows the listener to segment a string of distorted speech into linguistically appropriate units from which meaning can be extracted. Normal speakers place pauses between words, phrases, and sentences to help listeners organize the linguistic information in the signal. If these pauses are not easily discernible in the distortion of dysarthric speech, syntactic context may compensate by clearly marking the grammatical segments of sentences and thus helping the listener to interpret the meaningful linguistic units.

A final plausible mechanism is that of varying degrees of grammatical predictability imposed by syntactic context. This theory emerged from the observation that there were several sentences that received consistently high transcription scores across all listeners. The reliability and accuracy of the transcription of these sentences were remarkable when compared to the average scores and variability in the samples as a whole. The hypothesis was formed that some sentences might be understood better because of the quality of information in the syntactic context. Sentences that were reliably more intelligible might contain greater grammatical predictability in the syntactic context as compared to sentences that were less predictable.

To investigate this question, the data from the no-context condition were analyzed again to determine the grammatical predictability of those sentences receiving consistently high scores (>90%). Highly predictable sentences were defined as those containing a straightforward syntactic structure of stated subject–verb–object. Sentences with low grammatical predictability included any other sentence structure, such as sentences with understood subjects, sentences with question transformations, and sentences that started with adverbial clauses. Fourteen sentences received average scores in excess of 90%. Of these, 71% (10 of 14) contained high grammatical predictability, while 29% (4 of 14) had low grammatical predictability. These findings must be interpreted with caution because the grammatical predictability was not controlled for equal distribution across speech samples, dysarthria severity, sentence length, or any other variable. However, this analysis does suggest that syntactic context might exert various degrees of influence over intelligibility depending on the predictability of the grammatical structures in a sentence. Further investigation is warranted.

Listener Evaluation Ability

Turning now to the listeners' evaluations of their own performance, the results of this study showed that listeners overestimated their transcription scores to a significant degree for all context conditions in both groups of speakers except for the no-context condition for the moderate speakers. Neither semantic nor syntactic context improved the accuracy of the evaluations, because the estimates were significantly higher than the actual scores in all context conditions.

This conclusion supports related literature that has demonstrated overconfidence in subjects on different memory and comprehension tasks (Glenberg et al., 1992; Koriat et al., 1992). This study demonstrates the potential for listeners to greatly influence their interactions with dysarthric speakers because they are assuming more successful comprehension than is actually occurring. It also signals the need for further investigation to determine why listeners are overconfident, how this affects their communication with dysarthric speakers in functional settings, and what variables might influence this phenomenon. There are other possible reasons for the disparity between the estimates and actual scores. For example, perhaps listeners relied on their own internal interpretations without comparing their judgments to the actual speech signal. Perhaps the task instructions and scoring format yielded inflated estimates by encouraging listeners to guess on the transcriptions (although they were instructed to not include guesses in the estimates). Although these are suggestions that warrant consideration, this discussion will remain focused on the first suggested variable of overconfidence.

The failure of context to affect listener evaluations might be attributed to several possible variables. One explanation might be that listeners relied on their own interpretations instead of attending to the information in the context. They may have estimated their transcriptions to be highly accurate according to what they thought they heard, instead of referring to the context for confirmation or correction. Another possible reason might be that the context does not provide the information needed by listeners even if they attend to the cue. Because of the vast number of sentences that might express concepts suggested by context, it is possible that listeners could write down sentences that agreed with both the context and their own perception of the speech signal but that were still incorrect transcriptions of the stimuli. The listeners would not be influenced by context to change their evaluations because their interpretations, however incorrect, were still in accord with the context. Other forms of input or feedback that would identify the disparity between the transcription and the stimuli are needed.

CLINICAL IMPLICATIONS

For clinical purposes, this study helps to define those dysarthric populations that might benefit most from context as a compensatory strategy for decreased speech intelligibility. According to the results of this study, context may prove to be helpful in improving communication effectiveness for severely dysarthric speakers, but context might not be highly beneficial for moderately dysarthric speakers.

It is also interesting to note that both semantic and syntactic context can be equally powerful in improving the sentence intelligibility of severely dysarthric persons. Semantic context was presented in a highly functional form in this study. Dysarthric persons and their communication partners could easily be instructed to use cue words to introduce semantic context during conversations. Unfortunately, in order to achieve the separation from semantic context, syntactic context was not presented in a highly functional form in this study. However, the principles of syntactic context can certainly be applied in daily communication. For example, dysarthric persons might be encouraged to use grammatically well-formed sentences to allow listeners to better interpret the message based on their knowledge of the structure of the language. Dysarthric speakers might also be instructed to use more common, simple, and predictable sentence structures, such as subject–verb–object structures, instead of more complex forms that are less predictable.

The results from the listener evaluations have clinical implications as well. The fact that listeners tended to overestimate their comprehension of the speakers suggests that listeners might assume they understand a speaker better than they actually did. The listeners may then forego the use of requests for clarification of the message, requests for repetitions, or other repair strategies that would ensure correct information transfer. Thus, in their overconfidence, listeners may reduce the success and efficiency of their interactions with dysarthric persons. Clinicians must educate communication partners and provide feedback to them regarding the accuracy with which they understand the dysarthric individual. Communication partners must be trained in the use of appropriate repair strategies to improve the quality of the interaction. In general, this study supports the view that therapy cannot be directed toward the dysarthric individual alone but must incorporate family and friends as well, because any communication partner has the potential to significantly impact the success of the interaction.

REFERENCES

Barefoot, S.M., Bochner, J.H., Johnson, B.A., & vom Eigen, B.A. (1993). Rating deaf speakers' comprehensibility: An exploratory investigation. *American Journal of Speech-Language Pathology, 2*, 31–35.

Dongilli, P.A. (1994). Semantic context and speech intelligibility. In J.A. Till, K.M. Yorkston, & D.R. Beukelman (Eds.), *Motor speech disorders: Advances in assessment and treatment* (pp. 175–191). Baltimore: Paul H. Brookes Publishing Company.

Dowden, P. (1992). *The effects of listener training on the speech intelligibility of severely dysarthric individuals.* Unpublished dissertation, University of Washington, Seattle.

Duffy, J.R., & Giolas, T.G. (1974). Sentence intelligibility as a function of key word selection. *Journal of Speech and Hearing Research, 17*, 631–637.

Ellis, L.W., & Fucci, D.J. (1991). Magnitude-estimation scaling of speech intelligibility: Effects of listeners' experience and semantic-syntactic context. *Perceptual and Motor Skills, 73*, 293–305.

Glenberg, A.M., Wilkenson, A.C., & Epstein, W. (1992). The illusion of knowing: Failure in the self-assessment of comprehension. In T.O. Nelson (Ed.), *Metacognition* (pp. 185–195). Boston: Allyn & Bacon.

Goodman, G.O., McClelland, J.L., & Gibbs, R.W., Jr. (1981). The role of syntactic context in word recognition. *Memory and Cognition, 9*, 580–586.

Hammen, V.L., Yorkston, K.M., & Dowden, P. (1991). Index of contextual intelligibility. In C.A. Moore, K.M. Yorkston, & D.R. Beukelman (Eds.), *Dysarthria and apraxia of speech* (pp. 43–53). Baltimore: Paul H. Brookes Publishing Company.

Kalikow, D.N., Stevens, K.N., & Elliot, L.L. (1977). Development of a test of speech intelligibility in noise using sentence materials with controlled word predictability. *Journal of the Acoustical Society of America, 61*, 1337–1351.

Koriat, A., Lichtenstein, S., & Fischhoff, B. (1992). Reasons for confidence. In T.O. Nelson (Ed.), *Metacognition* (pp. 171–184). Boston: Allyn & Bacon.

McAllister, J.M. (1988). The use of context in auditory word recognition. *Perception and Psychophysics, 44*, 94–97.

Miller, G.A., Heise, G.A., & Lichten, W. (1951). The intelligibility of speech as a function of the context of the test materials. *Journal of Experimental Psychology, 41*, 329–335.

Miller, G.A., & Isard, S. (1963). Some perceptual consequences of linguistic rules. *Journal of Verbal Learning and Verbal Behavior, 2*, 217–228.

Miller, G.A., & Selfridge, J.A. (1950). Verbal context and the recall of meaningful material. *American Journal of Psychology, 63*, 176–185.

Nelson, T.O., Gerler, D., & Narens, L. (1992). Accuracy of feeling-of-knowing judgments for predicting perceptual identification and relearning. In T.O. Nelson (Ed.), *Metacognition* (pp. 142–150). Boston: Allyn & Bacon.

O'Neill, J.J. (1957). Recognition of intelligibility test materials in context and isolation. *Journal of Speech and Hearing Disorders, 2*, 87–90.

Pierce, R.S., & Beekman, L.A. (1985). Effects of linguistic and extralinguistic context on semantic and syntactic processing in aphasia. *Journal of Speech and Hearing Research, 28*, 250–254.

Sitler, R.W., Schiavetti, N., & Metz, D.E. (1983). Contextual effects in the measurement of hearing-impaired speakers' intelligibility. *Journal of Speech and Hearing Research, 26*, 30–34.

Waller, M.R., & Darley, F.L. (1978). The influence of context on the auditory comprehension of paragraphs by aphasic subjects. *Journal of Speech and Hearing Research, 21*, 732–745.

Yorkston, K.M., & Beukelman, D.R. (1978). A comparison of techniques for measuring intelligibility of dysarthric speech. *Journal of Communication Disorders, 11*, 499–512.

Yorkston, K.M., & Beukelman, D.R. (1980). A clinician-judged technique for quantifying dysarthic speech based on single-word intelligibility. *Journal of Communication Disorders, 13*, 15–31.

Yorkston, K.M., Beukelman, D.R., & Traynor, C. (1984). *Computerized assessment of the intelligibility of dysarthric speakers (test manual)*. Austin, TX: PRO-ED.

Yorkston, K.M., Dowden, P.A., Honsinger, M.J., Marriner, N., & Smith, K. (1988). Comparison of standard and user vocabulary lists. *Augmentative and Alternative Communication, 4*(4), 189–210.

Zwitserlood, P. (1989). The locus of the effects of sentential-semantic context in spoken-word processing. *Cognition, 32*, 25–64.

Chapter 5

Top-Down Influences on the Intelligibility of a Dysarthric Speaker
Addition of Natural Gestures and Situational Context

Jane Mertz Garcia and Michael P. Cannito

VARIOUS TYPES OF intervention strategies are used in dysarthria management. Approaches such as behavioral exercises, use of prosthetic equipment, and pharmacologic or surgical intervention are applied with the ultimate goal of improving intelligibility of the patient's speech. Rosenbek and LaPointe (1985) acknowledged that "only if a dysarthric patient's nervous system returns to normal will speech return too" and, because this is an infrequent occurrence, the goal of treatment can best be described as "compensated intelligibility" (p. 104). Kent (1992) further described intelligibility as the "behavioral standard of communication," indicating that "an immediate principal criterion by which we judge a communicative attempt is the intelligibility of the talker" (p. 1). Overall, the vast majority of dysarthria treatment techniques have placed emphasis on improving the acoustic–phonetic information content intrinsic to the spoken signal. Although appropriate, these strategies are often inadequate in meeting the needs of the dysarthric speaker because the speech signal typically remains impaired to varying degrees. More recently, there has been increasing interest regarding information that is independent of the acoustic–phonetic content that may be utilized by listeners in the perception of degraded speech signals (Lindblom, 1990).

We gratefully acknowledge Celeste Kilpatrick for her assistance in this project.
Portions of this research were presented at the annual convention of the American Speech-Language-Hearing Association, Anaheim, CA, November 1993.

Numerous "top-down," or knowledge-driven, factors influence the perception of speech by human listeners (Marslen-Wilson & Tyler, 1980; Salasoo & Pisoni, 1985). Massaro (1987) identified top-down factors as contextual sources of information that influence speech perception. For example, Salasoo and Pisoni (1985) examined various knowledge sources (contextual and sensory information) applied by listeners in identifying missing content words from normally spoken sentences. One of their findings was that semantic and syntactic information provided by the sentence context aided normal word identification within meaningful sentences.

In addition to top-down influences, listeners perceive information employing bottom-up processes. Bottom-up processing is signal driven; the focus is on the different cues or specific features of the signal that contribute to discriminable contrasts (e.g., the visual features and letters comprising a word represent bottom-up perceptual influences). The combination of top-down and bottom-up processing is termed interactive processing. This is probably most representative of normal communication because listeners typically employ interactive processing to decode messages (Danks & Glucksberg, 1980; Massaro, 1987).

It has been recently suggested that intentional manipulation of top-down factors may provide a clinical strategy that can facilitate dysarthric speech intelligibility (Berry & Sanders, 1983; Vogel & Miller, 1991). A top-down approach to dysarthria treatment is knowledge driven, and the emphasis is on the communication interaction of the speaker and listener. Top-down influences, independent of the acoustic–phonetic information of the signal itself, are additional cues that listeners employ in an effort to process degraded speech signals. As a result of top-down information, the listener attempts to construct a "gestalt," or "whole," of the communication from all available sources of information (Vogel & Miller, 1991).

Bottom-up processing is more concerned with the speaker and quality of the dysarthric speech signal, in contrast to the focus on the listener and communication interaction described for top-down processing. With a bottom-up approach, the phonetic details are the salient features. As related to a dysarthric speaker, the specifics of the speech signal serve as the salient features from which a general pattern is constructed by the listener. In a bottom-up orientation to dysarthria treatment, the focus is on improving accurate production of the acoustic signal as the means to enhance listener perception.

Recent research studies have begun to focus on possible top-down influences on the intelligibility of dysarthric speech, especially those related to the benefit of semantic context cues. Hammen, Yorkston, and Dowden (1991) examined the effect of semantic context cues on single-word intelligibility of 21 dysarthric individuals. The dysarthric speakers were grouped according to level of impairment (i.e., profound, severe, or moderate) based on initial word intelligibility scores. When listeners were provided knowledge of the semantic context, word intelligibility scores improved for all speakers; however, the amount of gain was influenced by the severity of intelligibility impairment. The severe group demonstrated the greatest benefit, followed by the moderately impaired group. The dysarthric speakers classified as profoundly impaired in intelligibility had the least amount of gain in intelligibility when listeners were provided prior knowledge of the semantic context.

Dongilli (1994) extended this line of research by using semantic cues for stimulus words read in isolation and embedded within high-probability test sentences from the Speech Perception in Noise (SPIN) test (Kalikow, Stevens, & Elliott, 1977). Dongilli studied eight flaccid dysarthric speakers whose impairment of intelligibility ranged from mild to profound. His results also demonstrated the benefit of prior semantic context cues for single-word intelligibility. In addition, for all but his profoundly impaired speakers, findings showed that test words produced within sentences were more intelligible than when produced in isolation. This suggested that sentence context provided additional contextual information that aided listeners in perceiving the stimulus word. Of note, the effect of prior knowledge of the semantic context was found to be less beneficial for target words produced within sentences in comparison to isolated, single-word productions. Dongilli concluded that predictive information inherent within sentence utterances appeared to overpower the possible benefits of providing the listener an additional semantic context cue.

In these reported studies, listeners were provided additional contextualizing information in the form of a verbal cue; however, nonverbal cues may also enhance the speaker–listener interaction. Vogel and Miller (1991) described a case study in which a severely dysarthric speaker improved his communication by becoming more adept at employing top-down strategies. The speaker supplemented his residual speech with aspects of drawing, writing, and a communication board. In addition, gestures were incorporated to enhance pragmatic aspects of his communication. For other dysarthric speakers, gestures are sometimes recommended as an alternative communication modality or as a pacing strategy (Rosenbek, 1984; Yorkston, Beukelman, & Bell, 1988); however, the communicative effectiveness of using meaningful gestures during natural speech has not been well documented for dysarthric speakers. Within the latter treatment modality, gestures are used in conjunction with residual speech capabilities rather than as an alternative form of communication or deblocking strategy.

In the literature on normal interpersonal communication, gestures produced concurrently with speaking are termed *illustrators*. Ekman and Friesen (1969), in their classification of gestures, defined illustrators as movements that are directly tied to speech by serving to illustrate visually what is spoken verbally. McNeill (1985) further categorized concurrent gestures as those that spontaneously accompany speech, such as *referential* and *discourse-oriented* gestures. Popelka and Berger (1971) examined the use of appropriate or inappropriate gestures while speaking as possible influences on the speechreading skills of normal hearing listeners viewing a normal speaker. Using a visual-only presentation format for sentences of six words in length, their results demonstrated a significant increase in words understood when listeners viewed the speaker employing appropriate gestures while speaking, in contrast to a speechreading format only. Conversely, a significant decrease in communication was noted when inappropriate gestures accompanied speech.

Natural gestures used in conjunction with residual speech could potentially enhance the information exchanged between the dysarthric speaker and his or her listener(s). Gestures serve as a potential source of additional semantic information, which might aid the listener in decoding the distorted speech signal (i.e., top-down facilitation). In addition, it has been suggested that different types of gestures, such as simple, repetitive movements, may indirectly influence listener perception by reorganizing or modifying production aspects of the speaking process in some manner, resulting in an improvement in speaker intelligibility (i.e., bottom-up facilitation) (Rosenbek, 1984).

The purpose of this study was to determine how various sources of information, independent of acoustic–phonetic signal content, might contribute to listeners' understanding of sentences produced by a severely dysarthric speaker. Two separate experiments were conducted to determine if sentence intelligibility would be affected by manipulating sources of signal-independent information available to listeners. These factors included the speaker's use of illustrative gestures that accompanied the acoustic signal, the degree of predictiveness inherent to the gestured and spoken messages, and provision of prior knowledge of a situational theme to listeners. In Experiment 1, signal-independent factors were explored within an audio+video listening format. In Experiment 2, signal-dependent contributions to intelligibility were evaluated using an audio-only listening format. Results from the two experiments were compared in order to determine relative contributions of top-down and bottom-up sources of information influencing sentence intelligibility.

EXPERIMENT 1: AUDIO+VIDEO PRESENTATION FORMAT

The initial experiment was conducted to examine the facilitative influence of gestural information produced concurrently with speech, as well as the influence of predictiveness of the gestured information and spoken message. Because women are reportedly more accurate in interpreting nonverbal cues than men (Hickson & Stacks, 1989; Knapp & Hall, 1992), listener gender was included as a factor in order to determine if the speaker's use of gestures while speaking would differentially affect intelligibility scores of male and female listeners. Furthermore, the influence of situational context was studied, because listeners were provided prior knowledge regarding the situational theme of sentences. In Experiment 1, sentences were orthographically transcribed in response to an audio+video stimulus presentation format.

Methodology

Stimulus Material Development A pool of 60 sentences was developed, with each sentence 6–8 words in length. Sentences were classified as random (i.e., contextually unrelated) or related to situational contexts of "in the house" or "in the yard." For each sentence, two illustrative gestures were scripted to accompany the spoken sentence.

Nonverbal Predictiveness To determine the information value of the gestured message, the 60 sentences were pantomimed (without speaking) for a separate subject group of 10 normal undergraduate college students prior to this study. Subjects were asked to interpret the nonverbal communication by writing a complete sentence describing what was conveyed. This yielded a total of 10 written sentences for each of the 60 sentences pantomimed for the subjects. The 600 sentence responses (60 pantomimed sentences × 10 transcriptions per sentence) were scored separately by two different judges. Written responses were scored using a 4-point scale that combined dimensions related to accurate interpretation of the gestured content and semantic relatedness of the response to its target sentence (see Table 1). Scores were summed across all 10 subject responses for each sentence. The sentence total was then averaged across the two judges, resulting in a composite score for each of the 60 pantomimed sentences. Scores fell within a range of 0 (minimum predictability) to 40 (maximum predictability), reflecting the amount of predictable message information that was conveyed by gestures. From these scores, 16 test sentences were selected, equally divided between random (contextually unrelated) and situational (contextually related) themes. The selected test sen-

Table 1. Scoring criteria for nonverbal (gestural) predictability

Score	Gestural interpretation	Message similarity
0	None accurately interpreted	Unrelated
1	One gesture interpreted	Unrelated
2	One gesture interpreted	Related
3	Two gestures interpreted	Unrelated
4	Two gestures interpreted	Related

tences represented eight "high" and eight "low" predictives, based solely on the predictability of the gestured information. The eight high-predictive sentences had an overall mean score of 33.6 (four random sentences = 33.4; four context sentences = 33.8), and the overall mean score of the eight low predictives was 1.8 (four random sentences = 2.0; four context sentences = 1.6).

Verbal Predictiveness The 16 selected sentences were also examined with regard to verbal predictiveness. The verbal predictability of sentences was determined using a cloze testing procedure during a separate experiment involving 20 additional college students. For 10 of the subjects, the written sentence was provided with a blank in lieu of the word or words associated with the first gesture of the sentence. For the other 10 subjects, word(s) associated with the second gestured element were omitted within the printed sentence. Subjects were instructed to "fill in the blank" with the word(s) most likely to occur in each respective sentence. The percentage of words correctly predicted (from both halves) was computed for each sentence. The mean percent correct of high-predictive sentences was 57 (standard deviation [SD] = 21.08) and that of low-predictive sentences was 28 (SD = 22.51); this difference was statistically significant ($t14$ = 2.608, $p < .05$). In other words, in the absence of gestured information, the sentences could be differentiated as high or low predictive based only on their verbal content. In addition, gestural and verbal predictiveness measures were significantly correlated across sentences ($r16$ = .549, $p < .05$).

Speaker The speaker was a right-handed 62-year-old man who had suffered a stroke approximately 3 years earlier. As a result of his injury, his speech pattern was characteristic of a flaccid dysarthria, primarily related to his hypernasality, imprecise consonant productions, short phrases, and breathiness. Sentences of 5–15 words in length were observed to be 6% intelligible on the Assessment of Intelligibility of Dysarthric Speech (Yorkston & Beukelman, 1981a). The speaker demonstrated cognitive and linguistic abilities that allowed him to function independently within the community. The speaker used both upper extremities during gestural activities; he also demonstrated appropriate skills related to his production and recognition of gestures on the New England Pantomime Test (Duffy & Duffy, 1984).

Recording Procedure The audio–video recordings were made in a quiet room using a RCA (CCD) VHS camcorder, with a lapel-type 1/4″ condenser microphone positioned approximately 15 cm from the speaker's mouth. The speaker was seated during the videotaping, with a view range sufficient to include all hand gestures. Test sentences were printed on 3″ × 12″ cue cards for the speaker to orally read as a means to ensure the accurate production of sentences in each videotaped condition.

Speaking Conditions The dysarthric speaker was videotaped under two speaking conditions: 1) the 16 test sentences were orally read (no-gesture condition), and 2) the test sentences were orally read and accompanied by two scripted gestures (gestural condition). Sample sentences are given below, with italized words indicating the points at which gestures were performed. The gestural component is described in parentheses after each sentence.

Low-predictive test sentence:
The one in *front* went to the *back*.
(index finger pointing to front, then using thumb and motioning toward rear)

High-predictive test sentence:
Stop and *turn around* where you are.
(palm extended in a halting motion, then circular motion with index finger)

Listening Subjects The listening subjects included 16 normal adults, equally divided between men and women. Subjects were between 18 and 30 years of age and reported no history of psychological, neurologic, or hearing-related impairments. Listeners were naive with regard to the purpose of this study and also inexperienced in listening to disordered speech.

Listening Format and Procedures Half of the subjects were randomly assigned to the no-gesture condition and the remainder to the gestural condition. Each listening subject transcribed all 16 test sentences, which included eight high and eight low predictives. Within each level of predictiveness, half of the sentences were not related to each other and half were related by contextual themes of "in the house" or "in the yard." The tester stated the specific theme for the listener prior to each listening condition. All listening conditions were counterbalanced to reduce order effects. Listeners were tested individually or in pairs. Video presentation was on a standard commercial player and monitor, and audio signals were played in the sound field at a comfortable listening level approximating conversational speech.

Reliability Sentence transcriptions were scored with regard to exact word correctness. To determine interexaminer scoring reliability, 25% of the response sheets were randomly selected and rescored by a second judge; 98.5% exact interexaminer agreement was obtained.

Results and Discussion

Means and standard deviations for the audio–video listening format are presented in Table 2 and illustrated in Figures 1 and 2. To obtain the mean scores, the number of correct words were tabulated for each sentence, summed within the listening condition, and subsequently converted to a percent intelligibility score. The percentage of intelligible words within the no-gesture condition is illustrated in Figure 1. The mean percent intelligibility ranged from 13.9 to 63 in the no-gesture condition. Minimal change in intelligibility was apparent with regard to random versus context contrasts in the no-gesture condition. When averaged across the factor of context, high-predictive sentences were 60% intelligible and low predictives were 15% intelligible. In Figure 2, the results from the gestural condition are shown. The mean percent intelligibility varied from 38.9 to 88.5 when gestures accompanied residual speech. Within high-predictive sentences, 84% of the words were intelligible, as compared to 41% for low predictives. In comparing the no-gesture and gestural audio–video conditions, the overall percent intelligibility scores increased by approximately 25% when subjects were afforded the benefit of viewing gestures concurrently with speech. In both conditions, the high-predictive sentences were more intelligible than the low predictives.

To determine the statistical significance of these observed differences, the data were submitted to a four-way analysis of variance (Gestures × Predictiveness × Situational Context × Gender), with percentage of intelligible words as the dependent variable. Results indicated a main effect for gestures ($F_{1,12} = 42.277, p < .0001$) and a main effect for predictiveness ($F_{1,12} = 314.795, p < .0001$). These variables did not interact; that is, intelligibility scores of the gestural condition were significantly higher than those of the no-gesture condition, irrespective of predictiveness, and high predictives were significantly more intelligible than low predictives, regardless of the presence or absence of gestural information. In addition, there was a significant Predictiveness × Situational Context interaction ($F_{1,12} = 9.586, p < .01$). There was no significant effect of gender of the listening subjects ($F_{1,12} = .084, p > .50$), and no other interactions achieved statistical significance.

In Figure 3, the interaction of predictiveness with situational context is evident. Post hoc analysis (simple effects) demonstrated that high pre-

Table 2. Intelligibility means and standard deviations for low- and high-predictive sentences in the gestural and no-gesture listening conditions

	No gestures		Gestures	
	Mean	SD	Mean	SD
Low predictive				
Random	15.9%	(8.2)	44.4%	(11.1)
Context	13.9%	(7.3)	38.9%	(7.1)
High predictive				
Random	57.0%	(9.0)	79.5%	(15.9)
Context	63.0%	(14.8)	88.5%	(8.7)

Note: Data were collapsed across the factor of gender.

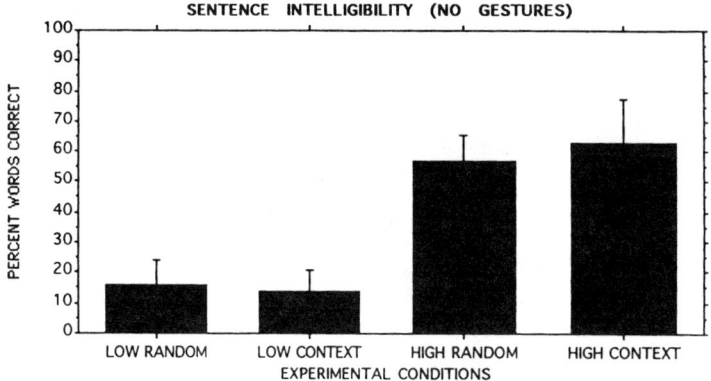

Figure 1. Mean percentages of intelligibility in the no-gesture listening conditions.

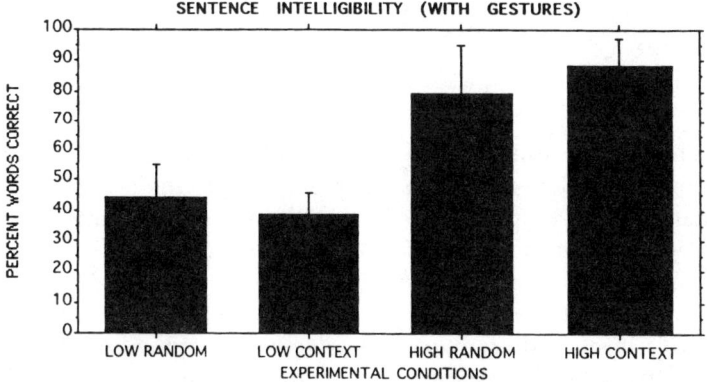

Figure 2. Mean percentages of intelligibility in the gestural listening conditions.

dictives differed from low predictives for both the random and context-related conditions ($p < .001$). In contrasting contextual conditions, contextually related and unrelated sentences did not differ for low-predictive sentences ($p > .20$); however, there was a significant difference between levels of situational context for high-predictive sentences ($p < .05$). High predictives with an identified situational context were 7.5% more intelligible than high predictives that were not situationally related.

Results from the first experiment, in which listeners were provided audio+video presentation, indicated there was an improvement in the speaker's intelligibility when natural gestures accompanied his speech. The use of naturalistic gestures enhanced this speaker's intelligibility by approximately 25%, and the benefit was constant for gestures of low- and high-predictive nonverbal information. Predictiveness was a facilitative cue with

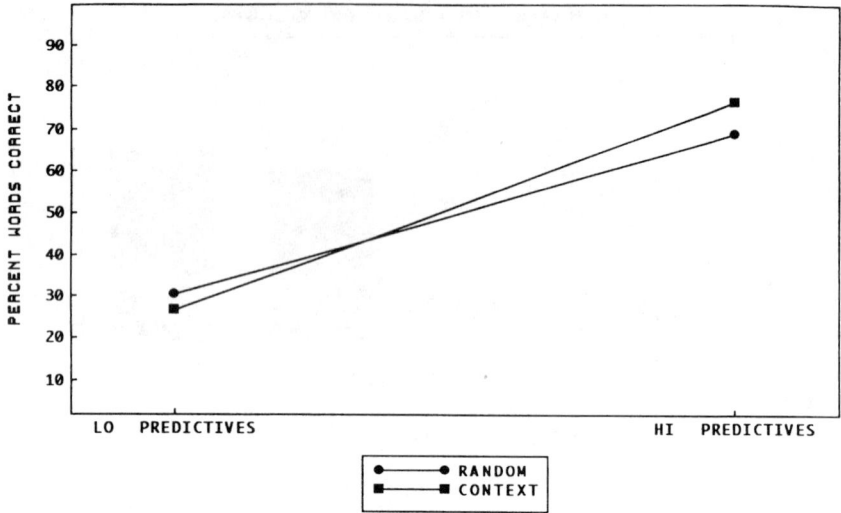

Figure 3. Plot of Predictiveness × Situational Context interaction, illustrating a selective benefit of context for highly predictive sentences.

gestures, but also proved to be a significant influence in the absence of gestured information. The overall mean intelligibility for high-predictive sentences was 72% in comparison to 28% for low-predictive sentences. This finding suggests that highly predictive sentences encode spoken messages containing greater "semantic cohesion," and this affords the listener additional information in perceiving the distorted speech signal.

For this speaker, there was also a selective benefit of context specific to the highly predictive sentences. Although the gain was statistically significant, the effect of context was less than either the benefit of gestures or predictiveness. This result appears consistent with the conclusion of Dongilli (1994), in that the benefit of semantic or situational context was overpowered by other factors aiding listener knowledge, such as predictive sentence context.

Although results from Experiment 1 indicated an improvement in the speaker's intelligibility when natural gestures accompanied speech, it was not certain whether the benefit of gestures was solely related to the additional visual source of information (top-down influence) or if the use of gestures positively influenced aspects of the dysarthric subject's speech pattern. For example, the use of simple, repetitive gestures may reduce articulatory distortion and slow speaking rate, resulting in improved speech intelligibility for some dysarthric speakers (Rosenbek, 1984). In order to address this issue, the experiment was replicated with listeners provided an audio-only format from which to orthographically transcribe test sentences.

EXPERIMENT 2: AUDIO PRESENTATION FORMAT

The purpose of the second experiment was to determine if the dysarthric speaker's use of gestures may have also provided a bottom-up influence on his speech. It was hypothesized that the speaker's intelligibility would be significantly greater in the gestural than in the no-gesture listening condition (audio-only listening format) if gestures influenced his speech production in a significant manner.

Methodology

Listening Subjects   For Experiment 2, 16 normal adult listeners who had not participated in Experiment 1 served as subjects. Again, subjects were equally divided between men and women. Listening subjects were native speakers of English ages 18–30. Subjects reported no significant history of hearing, psychological, or neurologic impairments. Listeners were unaware of the study's purpose and inexperienced with listening to disordered speech.

Procedure   The test sentences employed in Experiment 1 were used for Experiment 2. All procedures were identical to those of Experiment 1, with the exception that, in Experiment 2, the video monitor was concealed and sentences were orthographically transcribed solely on the basis of auditory information.

Results and Discussion

The mean scores, with standard deviations, comparing the no-gesture and gestural conditions with only the auditory signal available to the subjects were highly similar. For the no-gesture condition, the mean percent intelligibility was 39.3 ($SD = 6.3$), and that for the gestural condition was 35.4 ($SD = 10.5$). Results indicated no significant difference ($F_{1,14} = .824$, $p > .30$) in percent intelligibility contrasting the two listening conditions. The audio-only results demonstrated similar percentages of intelligibility for the no-gesture and gestural listening conditions, indicating that gestures did not influence the dysarthric subject's speech production in a manner sufficient to affect overall sentence intelligibility scores.

The absence of a discernible difference may have been influenced by a variety of factors. The speaker for this study had a stroke approximately 3 years earlier and presented a chronically dysarthric speech pattern that may have been less amenable to significant acoustic-phonetic alteration. Additionally, gestures that co-occur with speech vary in meaning and function (McNeill, 1992). Other gestural treatment approaches for dysarthria, such as combining speech with simple, repetitive hand gesturing (Rosenbek, 1984), are typically employed to facilitate rate control by imposing better phrasing or more appropriate pausing. The present study included a variety of gesture types; some gestures accentuated spoken content and others may have enhanced listener understanding by adding varying degrees of semantic content. As a consequence, the diversity of gesture types employed may have limited possible articulatory gain.

GENERAL DISCUSSION

These results support the position that various sources of information contribute to a listener's understanding of dysarthric speech. The findings of Experiment 1 clearly demonstrated that sentence intelligibility was significantly influenced by systematically manipulating the different sources of information available for listeners. For the low-predictive sentences, read orally without gestures, the speaker's average intelligibility was 16% for sentences without an identified context. In contrast, high-predictive sentences related to a situational theme were, on average, 88.5% intelligible in the gestural listening condition. The discrepancy within intelligibility scores resulted from the manipulation of factors that aided listener knowledge, because the same 16 test sentences were transcribed by all listeners. In other words, *intelligibility increased by approximately* 70% when listener knowledge was maximized through the speaker's use of gestures, messages of high predictiveness, and provision of prior knowledge of situational themes.

Experiment 2 demonstrated that use of gestures did not facilitate speech production to a degree sufficient to influence overall percent intelligibility. Although this finding seems at variance with prior literature utilizing pointing or pacing techniques to affect speech production (Crow & Enderby, 1989; Yorkston & Beukelman, 1981b), the absence of a difference in the present study may simply reflect the diversity (i.e., purpose and form) of natural gestures that accompany speech. Together, the findings of Experiments 1 and 2 suggest that naturalistic gestures while speaking served as a top-down influence for this particular speaker.

The results of this study showed that factors independent of the acoustic–phonetic signal itself (top-down influences) significantly contributed to listeners' understanding of sentences produced by a severely dysarthric speaker. Lindblom (1990) described the importance of signal-independent information in the presence of poor or degraded speech signals. Lindblom's mutuality model of communication describes a complementary relationship between the fidelity of a speech signal and signal–independent information, such as message and context information cues that influence what listeners hear. The mutuality model predicts that "rich" speech signal information can be easily understood by listeners provided minimal signal-independent information; however, when signal information is poor, the perception of speech is enhanced by maximizing listener knowledge through signal-independent information. In the present study, illustrative gestures, predictiveness of gestured and spoken (verbal) messages, and listener knowledge of a situational theme represented sources of signal-independent information that assisted listeners in decoding messages carried by a speech signal that was largely unintelligible.

The robust increase in the speaker's communicativeness associated with his use of gestures produced concurrently while speaking suggests an important relationship between spoken and gestured messages during natural speech. McNeill (1985) noted that "combining a spoken sentence and its concurrent gesture into a single observation gives two simultaneous views of the same process" (p. 350) and inferred that speech and gestures are overt manifestations of the same internal cognitive message. For the speaker in this study, gestures enhanced the amount of information understood by 25%. This preliminary finding raises the possibility of using naturalistic gestures as a therapeutic strategy to aid listener understanding of some dysarthric speakers.

In this study, sentences were differentiated as containing high or low predictiveness based on gestural and verbal content. Furthermore, test sentences were significantly correlated across gestural and verbal predictiveness measures. In other words, highly predictable gestured messages were associated with highly predictive spoken (verbal) sentences. The association of gestural and verbal sentence predictiveness is consistent with the "unity" of speech and gestures hypothesized by McNeill (1985), who noted that production of gestures and linguistic units are synchronized, with semantic and pragmatic functions completed in parallel. Although Experiment 1 demonstrated a similar communicative benefit of gestured information for both low- and high-predictive sentences, high-predictive sentences were more intelligible than low predictives in both the presence and absence of gestural information. This finding suggested that sentences of highly predictable message content greatly aided understanding of distorted (dysarthric) speech signals, even in the absence of corresponding gestural information.

CONCLUSION

Massaro (1987) noted that integration of information from multiple sources is a natural consequence of human behavior. Findings of this study indicate the importance of examining different sources of information in determining dysarthric speech intelligibility. For a severely dysarthric speaker, sentence intelligibility was significantly enhanced with top-down influences (i.e., factors independent of the acoustic information content of the spoken signal). It is hoped that future research will continue to examine the potential benefits of gestures produced concurrently with speech, especially related to the verbal predictiveness of its message content. Although gestures were limited to a top-down influence for this particular speaker, the potential benefit of spontaneous gesturing as a bottom-up influence needs further exploration with other similar dysarthric speakers. Expanding this research to include dysarthric patients of different diagnostic classifications and levels of severity may have important implications for both assessment and treatment of dysarthric speech.

REFERENCES

Berry, W., & Sanders, S. (1983). Environmental education: The universal management approach for adults with dysarthria. In W. Berry (Ed.), *Clinical dysarthria* (pp. 203–216). Boston: College-Hill Press.

Crow, E., & Enderby, P. (1989). The effects of an alphabet chart on the speaking rate and intelligibility of speakers with dysarthria. In K. Yorkston & D. Beukelman (Eds.), *Recent advances in clinical dysarthria* (pp. 99–108). Boston: College-Hill Press.

Danks, J.H., & Glucksberg, S. (1980). Experimental psycholinguistics. *Annual Review of Psychology, 31,* 391–417.

Dongilli, P. (1994). Semantic context and speech intelligibility. In J. Till, K. Yorkston, & D. Beukelman (Eds.), *Motor speech disorders: Advances in assessment and treatment* (pp. 175–191). Baltimore: Paul H. Brookes Publishing Co.

Duffy, R.J., & Duffy, J.R. (1984). *New England Pantomime Tests.* Tigard, OR: C.C. Publications.

Ekman, P., & Friesen, W.V. (1969). The repertoire of nonverbal behavior: Categories, origins, usage, and coding. *Semiotica, 1,* 49–98.

Hammen, V.L., Yorkston, K.M., & Dowden, P. (1991). Index of contextual intelligibility: Impact of semantic context in dysarthria. In C. Moore, K. Yorkston, & D. Beukelman (Eds.), *Dysarthria and apraxia of speech: Perspectives on management* (pp. 43–53). Baltimore: Paul H. Brookes Publishing Co.

Hickson, M.I., & Stacks, D.W. (1989). *Nonverbal communication: Studies and applications* (2nd ed.). Dubuque, IA: William C. Brown.

Kalikow, D.N., Stevens, K.N., & Elliott, L.L. (1977). Development of a test of speech intelligibility in noise using sentence materials with controlled word predictability. *Journal of the Acoustical Society of America, 61,* 1339–1351.

Kent, R.D. (1992). *Intelligibility in speech disorders: Theory, measurement, and management.* Philadelphia: John Benjamins.

Knapp, M.L., & Hall, J.A. (1992). *Nonverbal communication in human interaction* (3rd ed.). Orlando, FL: Harcourt Brace Jovanovich.

Lindblom, B. (1990). On the communication process: Speaker-listener interaction and the development of speech. *Augmentative and Alternative Communication, 6,* 220–230.

Marslen-Wilson, W., & Tyler, L. (1980). The temporal structure of spoken language understanding. *Cognition, 8,* 1–71.

Massaro, D.W. (1987). *Speech perception by ear and eye: A paradigm for psychological inquiry.* Hillsdale, NJ: Lawrence Erlbaum Associates.

McNeill, D. (1985). So you think gestures are nonverbal? *Psychological Review, 92,* 350–371.

McNeill, D. (1992). *Hand and mind.* Chicago: The University of Chicago Press.

Popelka, G.R., & Berger, K.W. (1971). Gestures and visual speech reception. *American Annals of the Deaf, 116,* 434–436.
Rosenbek, J.C. (1984). Selected alternatives to articulation training for the dysarthric adult. In H. Winitz (Ed.), *Treating articulation disorders: For clinicians by clinicians* (pp. 249–262). Austin, TX: PRO-ED.
Rosenbek, J.C., & LaPointe, L.L. (1985). The dysarthrias: Description, diagnosis, and treatment. In D. Johns (Ed.), *Clinical management of neurogenic disorders* (2nd ed., pp. 97–152). Boston: Little, Brown, & Co.
Salasoo, A., & Pisoni, D. (1985). Interaction of knowledge sources in spoken word identification. *Journal of Memory and Language, 24,* 210–231.
Vogel, D., & Miller, L. (1991). A top-down approach to treatment of dysarthric speech. In D. Vogel & M. Cannito (Eds.), *Treating disordered speech motor control* (pp. 87–109). Austin, TX: PRO-ED.
Yorkston, K.M., & Beukelman, D.R. (1981a). *Assessment of intelligibility of dysarthric speech.* Tigard, OR: C.C. Publications.
Yorkston, K.M., & Beukelman, D.R. (1981b). Ataxic dysarthria: Treatment sequences based on intelligibility and prosodic considerations. *Journal of Speech and Hearing Disorders, 46,* 398–404.
Yorkston, K.M., Beukelman, D.R., & Bell, K.R. (1988). *Clinical management of dysarthric speakers.* San Diego, CA: College-Hill Press.

Chapter 6

Effects of Insertion of Interword Pauses on the Intelligibility of Dysarthric Speech

Joanne M. Gutek and Anne Putnam Rochet

DECREASED INTELLIGIBILITY is a common characteristic of dysarthric speech. The reduction of speaking rate has been reported to be an effective mode of treatment to improve the intelligibility of dysarthric speakers (Yorkston & Beukelman, 1981a, 1981b; Yorkston, Hammen, Beukelman, & Traynor, 1990). Specific rate control techniques influence the pausal domain and the articulatory domain of speech differently (Crystal & House, 1982; Goldman-Eisler, 1961; Hammen, Yorkston, & Beukelman, 1989). Investigators remain uncertain about the components of rate (pausal, articulatory, or both) that may be responsible for the improved intelligibility. Preliminary research has suggested that rigid rate control techniques that promote a one-word-at-a-time speaking style by lengthening pause time and increasing the number of pauses may be especially beneficial for some dysarthric speakers (Crow & Enderby, 1989; Yorkston & Beukelman, 1981a; Yorkston, Beukelman, & Bell, 1988).

The effects of pausal manipulation on the intelligibility of speech samples have been examined for two groups of disordered speakers. Maassen (1986) and Maassen and Povel (1984, 1985) inserted interword pauses in samples of the speech of deaf persons. Hammen (1990) and Hammen, Yorkston, and Minifie (1994) inserted pauses at syntactically appropriate places in samples of dysarthric speech. Both investigations em-

---

This research was supported by the Province of Alberta Scholarship Fund.

ployed modern computer-processing techniques that enabled the relationship between pauses and intelligibility to be altered systematically.

To date, however, no computer alteration study that inserted *interword* pauses into dysarthric speech has been conducted. In addition, no studies have been reported that identify dysarthric speakers whose intelligibility is improved by a one-word-at-a-time style of speech. The present investigation experimentally manipulated the interword pause characteristics of 15 sentences of similar length spoken by three dysarthric speakers. Specifically, the following question was asked: Does the insertion of 160-ms interword pauses via a computer improve the intelligibility of sentences spoken by persons with dysarthric speech?

METHOD

Speech samples produced by 10 dysarthric speakers were recorded. The samples were transcribed, speech intelligibility was measured, and prosodic features were profiled. Then the samples of three speakers were digitally manipulated to create pause-altered versions of the samples. Two groups of listeners transcribed the altered and unaltered sentences. Intelligibility scores based on these transcriptions for unaltered and pause-altered sentences of dysarthric speakers were computed and compared statistically.

Acquisition of Experimental Samples of Dysarthric Speech

Ten adults with traumatic brain injury and dysarthria served as speakers. An 11-sentence version of the *Assessment of Intelligibility of Dysarthric Speech* (AIDS) (Yorkston & Beukelman, 1981a) was audiotaped for each speaker. Four additional 8-word sentences from the AIDS inventory were also recorded by each dysarthric speaker to provide an additional pool of experimental sentence material for later use. Sentence intelligibility recording procedures followed the protocol outlined in the AIDS manual (Yorkston & Beukelman, 1981a). Sentences were presented in a typed format, one sentence at a time. The investigator read the sentence aloud once, asking the dysarthric speaker to read along silently as the sentence was read. This procedure was used to ensure that intelligibility was not compromised by misreading and that speaking rate was not altered by reading difficulties (Yorkston & Beukelman, 1981a). As the speaker read the passage aloud, tape recordings were obtained using an audiocassette recorder (Marantz model PMD221) in a quiet room at the Alberta Hospital Ponoka during after-work hours. A close-talk, head-mounted, unidirectional microphone (Shure SM10A) was positioned 2.5 cm from the talker's lips at the left corner of the mouth, at an angle approximately 90 degrees to the direction of airflow from the mouth, throughout the recording session. Mouth-to-microphone distance and position were held constant within and across all 10 subjects. Recording sessions lasted approximately 30 minutes.

Intelligibility Transcriptions and Prosodic Ratings

Three listeners naive to the purposes of the experiment transcribed the sentences obtained from these 10 speakers according to the transcription standards for the AIDS. In preparation for this transcription task, the audio recordings of all the sentences were low-pass filtered at 8.6 kHz (Frequency Devices 901) and digitized at 22 kHz using a MacRecorder at 8-bit resolution on a Macintosh SE/30 microcomputer. The computer was programmed to replay the sentences to each listener in random order through a low-pass filter and loudspeaker by means of software written by the first author (Hypercard, version 2.0). Three listeners who had normal hearing, were native speakers of English, and were not speech-language pathologists transcribed the sentences. Results from the initial intelligibility transcriptions indicated that 5 of the 10 dysarthric speakers exhibited a moderate to severe impairment in sentence intelligibility; their scores ranged from 43% to 71% intelligibility (Table 1). These five speakers were selected for further study.

Ratings to profile the prosodic characteristics of the five dysarthric speakers were required to satisfy another potentially confounding variable in this research: homogeneity of subjects with respect to prosodic disturbance. In addition, it was hoped that specific profiles of the dysarthric speakers ultimately selected for the experimental speech sample might shed more light on the prosodic feature or constellation of prosodic features of dysarthric speech that could especially benefit from the addition of interword pauses in connected utterance. The abnormal prosodic char-

Table 1. Demographic information and intelligibility scores for the 10 dysarthric speakers

Speaker	Gender	Age	Primary etiology[a]	Years postinjury	Intelligibility (%)			
					Listener 1	Listener 2	Listener 3	Average
A	Male	37	TBI/fall	13	38	47	44	43%
B	Female	42	TBI/fall	3	87	89	93	90%
C	Male	47	TBI/fall	5	54	59	58	57%
D	Male	23	TBI/MVA	4	65	74	75	71%
E	Female	29	TBI/MVA	3	94	94	98	95%
F	Male	68	TBI/MVA	1	71	62	73	69%
G	Male	38	TBI/MVA	15	3	22	1	9%
H	Male	29	TBI/MVA	2	55	57	67	60%
I	Male	22	TBI/MVA	1	90	87	85	87%
J	Male	17	TBI/MVA	1	93	81	93	89%

[a] TBI, traumatic brain injury; MVA, motor vehicle accident.

acteristics of reduced stress, monopitch, monoloudness, and abnormal rate were considered to be the four most deviant features.

Three senior-level students in speech-language pathology with experience in the assessment and treatment of motor speech disorders participated in the perceptual judgment section of the study. Digital versions of 10 sentences (two 6- to 10-word sentences produced by each of the five dysarthric speakers who fit the speech intelligibility criteria) were played to the three judges by means of the same computer/loudspeaker system that had supported the intelligibility data collection. Each speech sample was rated on perceptual dimensions derived from those used in the Mayo Clinic Dysarthria Study (Darley, Aronson, & Brown, 1975) and modified by the investigator for this project. The series comprised 10 dimensions of prosody (Table 2). The speech samples were judged using a 7-point equal-interval scale. The 10 attributes were rated between 1 and 7, with 1 representing no abnormality, 2 representing mild and inconsistent (occurring less than 75% of the time) occurrence, 3 representing mild and consistent (occurring more than 75% of the time) occurrence, 4 representing moderate and inconsistent occurrence, 5 representing moderate and consistent occurrence, 6 representing severe and consistent occurrence, and 7 representing complete dysfunction.

The value of using perceptual rating scales in rating dysarthria depends on how well clinicians can agree on scale values and make reliable judgments (Kearns & Simmons, 1988; Sheard, Adams, & Davis, 1991). Therefore, the judges were trained by the first author to identify perceptual characteristics using samples of the Motor Speech Disorders tapes published by Darley et al. (1975). Following this training, judges were tested to determine their level of agreement on the various dimensions before judging of the experimental speech samples took place. Interrater agreement on two practice tests was calculated to be 90% (agreement within ±1 point on the rating scale).

The judges worked independently to produce the prosodic ratings for the 10 representative sentence samples from the five dysarthric speakers. They were allowed to listen to each sentence as many times as required to make their ratings.

After the judges completed the ratings of all 10 sentences, they were given a short break (30 minutes) and asked to re-rate 20% of the sample (2 sentences). Percentages of intrajudge agreement (agreement within ±1 point on the rating scale) were calculated for the repeated ratings. Judges demonstrated adequate intrarater agreement, which ranged from 80% to 100% (*mean* = 92%). Interjudge agreement (agreement within ±1 point on the rating scale) among the three judges was calculated for all 10 prosodic attributes for all the sentences they rated ($N = 20$). Interjudge agreement on the 7-point scale ranged from 65% to 85% (*mean* = 76%).

Table 2. Prosodic perceptual rating form

Rating	Characteristic	Description
1 2 3 4 5 6 7	Monoloudness	Voice shows monotony of loudness. It lacks normal variations in loudness.
1 2 3 4 5 6 7	Excessive loudness variation	Voice shows sudden, uncontrolled alterations in loudness, sometimes becoming too loud, sometimes too weak.
1 2 3 4 5 6 7	Loudness decay	There is progressive diminution or decay of loudness.
1 2 3 4 5 6 7	Monopitch	Voice lacks normal pitch and inflectional changes. It tends to stay at one pitch level.
1 2 3 4 5 6 7	Reduced stress	Speech shows reduction of proper stress or emphasis patterns.
1 2 3 4 5 6 7	Excess & equal stress	Excess stress on usually unstressed parts of speech.
1 2 3 4 5 6 7	Rate Slow Rapid	Rate of actual speech is abnormally slow or rapid.
1 2 3 4 5 6 7	Variable rate	Rate alternately changes from slow to fast.
1 2 3 4 5 6 7	Prolonged intervals	Prolongation of interword or intersyllable intervals.
1 2 3 4 5 6 7	Inappropriate silences	There are inappropriate silent intervals.

Prosodic attributes will be rated between 1 and 7, with

1. representing no abnormality
2. representing mild and inconsistent (occurring less than 75% of the time)
3. representing mild and consistent (occurring more than 75% of the time)
4. representing moderate and inconsistent
5. representing moderate and consistent
6. representing severe and consistent
7. representing complete dysfunction

The three dysarthric speakers on whom the best interjudge agreement for the prosodic features of interest occurred were chosen from those whose prosody rating profiles included high scores on the primary prosodic characteristics of reduced stress, monopitch, monoloudness, and abnormal rate. The final experimental material for pause alteration consisted of 15 sentences of similar length (6–10 words), five from each of these three speakers.

Digital Manipulation of Experimental Speech Samples

The digital recordings of the 15 sentences were pause-altered by the investigator using SoundEdit software (Figure 1). The following rules were employed in creating the pause-altered sentences:

- *All editing measurements were made by the investigator.*
- *Word boundaries were determined by alternately visually marking segment boundaries and listening to the enclosed fragments.* Osberger and Levitt (1979) established the majority (80%) of the phoneme boundaries in their experimental signals by ear, playing a digitized segment of speech repeatedly and systematically adjusting the start time until the last evidence of the phoneme of interest was heard. Twenty percent of the edits were determined by visual inspection of the waveform.
- *Pauses of 160 ms were inserted between all words.* Maassen (1986) found that pauses of 160 ms in length were just long enough to give the impression of a word boundary.
- *Pauses consisted of background tape noise.* Pure "silent" pauses that resulted in abrupt signal-to-silence and silence-to-signal transitions were found to introduce undesired audible clicks, onsets, and offsets. Therefore a 160-ms segment of silence between utterances on the audiotape for each speaker was digitized as the "pause" for insertion. It was less obtrusive as an insert because it contained the "background noise" that occurred naturally on the tape recordings between segments of speech.
- *When two words were already separated by a long pause (greater than 160 ms), that part of the signal was not altered by the addition of any more pause material.*
- *The accuracy of the pause adjustments was determined by remeasuring 30 randomly chosen pause placements and calculating the reliability of these measurements.* The values of the first pause placement and the second pause placement and the difference between the two measures were

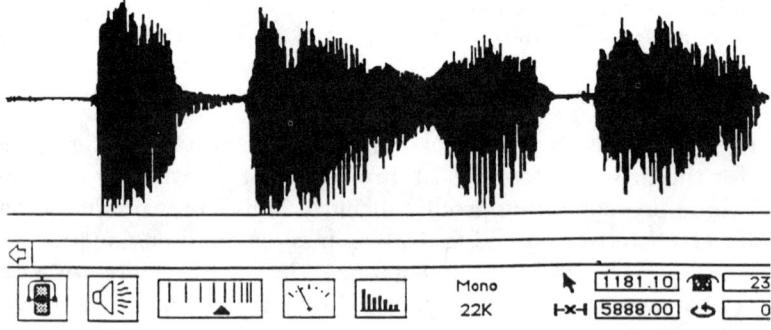

Figure 1. Example of SoundEdit waveform display.

obtained. Average measurement error was calculated to be 23.30 ms, with a range of 174.54 ms. Accurate and reliable determination of word boundaries for the insertion of pauses often was difficult because of the blurred word boundaries or the presence of continued voicing between words in the dysarthric speakers' utterances. For every measurement opportunity, the first author attempted to achieve pause insertions that were as valid and reliable as possible by utilizing both auditory and visual cues as often as necessary until the best possible pause placement was achieved.

Listener Judgments of Altered and Unaltered Speech Samples

Sixty students in rehabilitation medicine disciplines other than speech-language pathology served as listeners for the altered and unaltered speech samples; 30 transcribed the altered versions, and 30 transcribed the unaltered versions. All listeners had hearing perception within normal limits, similar language and educational backgrounds, and limited exposure to dysarthric speech. Listeners individually heard the audiosignal, which was low-pass filtered at 8.6 kHz (Frequency Devices 901), amplified (Realistic SA-150 stereo amplifier), and played through a loudspeaker (ProIII JBL) at a comfortable loudness level. A computer program (Hypercard, version 2.0) again was used to randomize the presentation of the unaltered or pause-altered sentences to each listener for verbatim transcription according to the AIDS protocol (Figures 2 and 3). An overall intelligibility score was derived from each listener's transcription of the 15 sentences he or she heard.

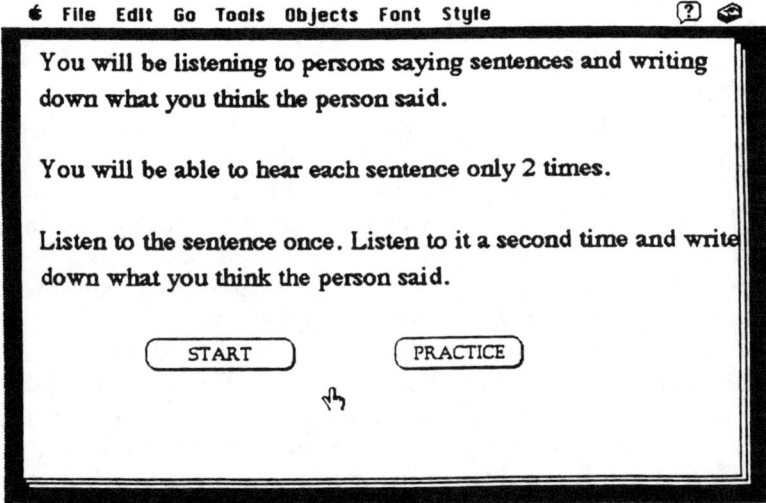

Figure 2. Instruction card of HyperCard stack for intelligibility listeners.

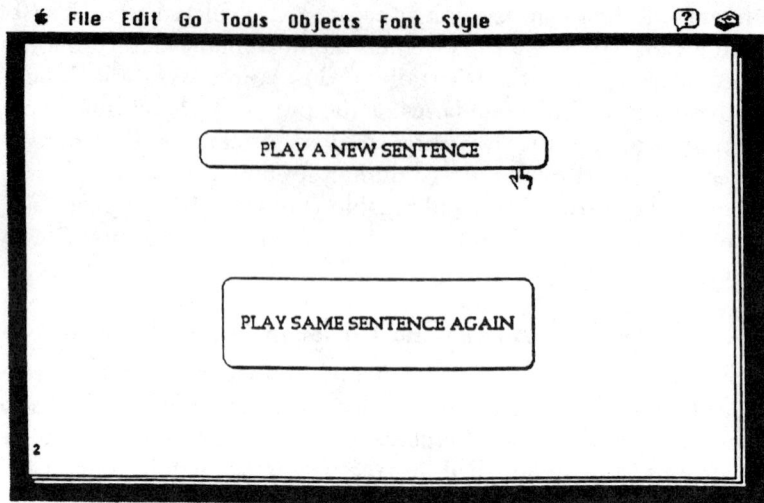

Figure 3. Trigger card of HyperCard stack for listeners.

STATISTICAL ANALYSIS

This study employed a between-group experimental design. The independent variable, within-sentence interword pause status, had two levels: unaltered and altered. The dependent variable consisted of mean intelligibility scores in the form of percentage values provided by an independent group of 30 listeners for each level of the independent variable. A one-tailed t-test for independent means was used to determine if a difference existed between the intelligibility scores obtained for the unaltered and pause-altered sentences. An alpha level of .01 and beta level of .60 were set for this test, with 58 degrees of freedom. The statistical analysis was run using Statview 512 software on a Macintosh SE/30 computer.

Yorkston and Beukelman (1981a) acknowledged the difference between clinical and statistical significance: "Important changes in speech performance may or may not be statistically significant; and vice versa, statistically significant differences may or may not be signaling functionally important changes in speech performance" (p. 21). Furthermore, they suggested that a clinically significant change includes an improvement in sentence intelligibility that is "beyond a speaker's day-to-day variability and beyond the range of difference that might be the result of sample selection (differences in word lists and sentence sets)" (Yorkston & Beukelman, 1981a, p. 21). Day-to-day variability must be considered because dysarthric speakers' recordings of different sentence sets on the same day have resulted in average differences of 8.6 percentage points for some speakers (Yorkston & Beukelman, 1981a). However, Yorkston and Beukelman noted that, although some dysarthric speakers may vary considerably from day to day, others may be exceptionally stable. Consequently, whereas a 10% difference in intelligibility might be clinically significant for one speaker, clinical significance might be decreased to 5% for a stable speaker or increased to 15% for a speaker whose intelligibility varies considerably. The final decision about the importance of any changes has been reported to be heavily based on clinical judgment (Yorkston & Beukelman, 1981a). For the purpose of this study, a clinically significant difference in intelligibility scores between the unaltered and pause-altered condition was set arbitrarily at 10% or higher.

RESULTS

An independent measures t-test calculated on the intelligibility scores for the control (unaltered) group and for the experimental (pause-altered) group revealed a significant difference ($p \leq .0001$). The insertion of interword pauses improved sentence intelligibility for the dysarthric speech samples used in this study by approximately 5%. Listeners transcribed unaltered sentences with an average of 50% accuracy (range = 41%–57%; standard deviation [SD] = 4.36%). Listeners transcribed pause-altered sentences with an average of 55% accuracy (range = 44%–67%; SD = 5.23%). The summary statistics are shown in Table 3. The clinical effect size of this statistical difference was small, however, at 0.35 (Ottenbacher & Barrett, 1989).

Intelligibility scores for the altered and unaltered versions were compared for individual speakers and revealed an overall increase in intelligibility for each speaker in the pause-altered sentences (Table 4). Speaker H

Table 3. Summary statistics for experimental hypothesis

	Count	Mean	SD	SE[a]
Experimental	30	54.893	5.23	.955
Control	30	49.972	4.36	.797

Degrees of freedom: 58
Unpaired t value: 3.957
Probability (1-tailed): .0001

[a]SE, standard error.

Table 4. Change in percent intelligibility for individual speakers averaged over 30 listeners

	Intelligibility (%)		
Speaker	Unaltered version (%)	Pause-altered version (%)	Difference (%)
C	59.92	65.37	+5.45
D	49.24	52.68	+3.44
H	39.50	46.42	+6.92

appeared to benefit most (7% improvement) from the addition of pauses, followed by speakers C (5% improvement) and D (3% improvement).

Intralistener agreement was calculated for six listeners (three in each condition) who agreed to transcribe the same sentences again after a minimum of 3 weeks had passed following the initial transcription. Although four of the six listeners (C-1, C-21, E-3, and E-17) did not differ in their two transcription scores by more than 5%, two others (C-4 and E-13) exhibited scores on their second transcription that were more than 10% higher than those obtained the first time (Table 5).

DISCUSSION

Clinical Versus Statistical Difference

The results of this investigation were associated with a statistically significant difference between intelligibility scores for sentences that were digitally altered by the addition of pauses (55%) and scores obtained for unaltered versions of those same sentences (50%). On the basis of these results, it can be concluded that interword pauses improved the sentence intelligibility of dysarthric speakers in this study by approximately 5%. Although this improvement in intelligibility was statistically significant, its clinical effect size was small (0.35), and it did not exceed the 10% criterion set arbitrarily by the investigator as a clinically significant change. The 5% change indicated that interword pauses may be only a part of improving intelligibility to a clinically significant level (10% improvement or greater, or an effect size of 0.80 or better).

Because none of the improvements in intelligibility produced by pause alteration resulted in a clinically significant change, it can be hypothesized that these improvements were not large enough to surpass the day-to-day variability of the speakers' performances and could not necessarily be expected to make a functional difference in their everyday attempts at successful, intelligible communication. However, to reach a

Table 5. Intralistener agreement

Listener[a]	Percent agreement		Percent difference
	1st listen	2nd listen	
C-1	47.46	52.54	+5.08
C-4	50.85	64.41	+13.56
C-21	52.54	56.78	+4.24
E-3	49.15	52.54	+3.39
E-13	50.85	61.86	+11.01
E-17	46.61	51.69	+5.08

[a] C, listeners who heard the control or unaltered sentences; E, listeners who heard the experimental or pause-altered sentences.

fully informed conclusion that the 5% improvement in intelligibility reported in this study did not surpass day-to-day fluctuations in intelligibility, an alternate methodology would have to have been implemented. Baseline measures of intelligibility of each of the three speakers would have to have been taken at several points during a single day. A measure of variance then could be obtained that could be compared with the intelligibility improvements derived from the pause-alteration process, and a less arbitrary and more subject-specific decision about the clinical significance of measurable improvements could be made.

Comparison of Results with Other Studies

The statistical results of this study can be compared and contrasted with the results of other pause alteration studies. The results reported here are similar to those reported by Maassen (1986), who artificially inserted silent pauses between words in sentences spoken by 10 deaf children. Maassen's (1986) procedure resulted in a small but statistically significant improvement in his subjects' speech intelligibility of 4% (27% unaltered, 31% pause-altered). In contrast, Hammen (1990) reported a 1% change (56% unaltered, 57% altered), and Hammen et al. (1994), using data from five of the six dysarthric speakers from the Hammen (1990) study, reported a 1.8% change (47.0% unaltered, 48.8% pause-altered). In both studies, changes in intelligibility following insertion of syntactically appropriate pauses (as opposed to interword pauses) in the sentences of speakers rendered dysarthric by parkinsonism were not significant.

Several explanations may be offered for the similarities and differences among the results obtained in each of the three studies. First, the place and length of pauses that were inserted differed in the investigations. Both these investigators and Maassen (1986) altered speech samples by adding 160-ms interword pauses; in contrast, Hammen (1990) and Hammen et al. (1994) added pauses of varying lengths only at syntactically appropriate locations. The decisions made regarding pause placement and distribution of pauses in the Hammen and Hammen et al. studies may have created samples that sounded unusual to their listeners and therefore interfered with improved transcriptions. Perhaps the interword pauses used in this study and in Maassen's were short enough (160 ms) to avoid creating altered sentences that sounded unusual. The rationale for pause placement in Hammen's study contrasts with the rationale for pause placement in this study and in Maassen's. Hammen's placement of pauses where syntactically appropriate was chosen to provide listeners with more processing time. Although the addition of brief interword pauses in this study and in Maassen's also increased processing time, the main purpose of the interword pauses was to create more well-defined word boundaries for the listener.

A second explanation for the differences obtained among the results of the studies may lie in the experimental materials used. In this study and in Maassen's (1986), short sentences were used as the experimental material; Hammen (1990) and Hammen et al. (1994) used longer sentences (20–26 words per sentence). The shorter sentences might have been easier for listeners to transcribe because they did not have to listen to and remember a great number of words. In contrast, listeners who participated in Hammen's study might have made transcription errors because of the large number of words they were required to remember and transcribe.

A third explanation for differences among the results of these studies involves the type of speech that was manipulated. Maassen (1986) manipulated speech of deaf persons that was characterized by continuous voicing and a slow rate. The dysarthric speech manipulated in this study was also slow in rate and was characterized by reduced stress, monoloudness, and monopitch. In contrast, Hammen (1990) and Hammen et al. (1994) manipulated parkinsonian dysarthric utterances, which were rapid in rate and often deficient in voicing. The perceptual characteristics of dysarthric speech in the present study are more similar to the characteristics of the speech of the deaf subjects in Maassen's study than to the characteristics of the parkinsonian dysarthric speech manipulated in Hammen's and Hammen et al.'s studies. Specific speech characteristics might therefore explain the statistically significant results that were obtained by Maassen (1986) and this study, yet not found by Hammen (1990) and Hammen et al. (1994).

A final important difference exists among the studies. Neither the Maassen (1986) study nor the Hammen (1990) study included a detailed perceptual profile of their speakers. Both studies manipulated the speech of what they thought were "homogeneous" groups (Maassen accessed "deaf speakers," Hammen accessed "parkinsonian speakers") without profiling the specific prosodic characteristics of each speaker. Both studies assumed that speakers with the same disease etiology would exhibit perceptual speech characteristics that would be similar. The development of perceptual profiles for speakers who might benefit from selective rate control techniques can be considered valuable and perhaps essential from both a clinical and a research perspective.

Implications for the Treatment of Dysarthric Speakers

The statistically significant results obtained from this study show that improvements in intelligibility can occur simply by the addition of short pauses between words, with no articulatory changes and no semantic or contextual cues. Thus, a measurable improvement in sentence intelligibility can be obtained by manipulating only the time between words—interword pauses. To the extent that the results of this study can be generalized to clinical settings, dysarthric speakers who present with moderate to severe intelligibility and prosodic characteristics of monopitch, monoloudness, reduced stress, and reduced rate should be encouraged to pause slightly between words. By inserting pauses between words, dysarthric speakers might enjoy the same small improvements (5%) in intelligibility that were documented in this study.

Dramatic improvements in the sentence intelligibility of dysarthric speakers reported in the literature (Crow & Enderby, 1989; Yorkston & Beukelman, 1981c; Yorkston et al. 1990) for word-by-word speech styles were not evident in this study. More remarkable improvements in intelligibility must therefore be attributed to something more than the achievement of well-marked word boundaries. Additional adjustments in speech articulation, loudness, and/or prosody may need to occur for more dramatic improvements in sentence intelligibility.

Although the addition of interword pauses might not create dramatic improvements in intelligibility it can be hypothesized that the elimination of certain pauses could be detrimental and could cause a decrease in intelligibility. The pauses already present in some types of dysarthric speech may actually be facilitating speech intelligibility. Deletion of those pauses may result in a decrease in intelligibility, as suggested by Maassen (1986), Hammen (1990), and Hammen et al. (1994). Research that involved the removal of pauses from speech samples of dysarthric speakers would provide information about the benefit of already existing pauses on the intelligibility of dysarthric speech.

Implications for the Training of Listeners

Listeners in the present study who had hearing perception within normal limits, similar language and educational backgrounds, and limited exposure to dysarthric speech differed substantially in their abilities to transcribe the same stimuli. The data in Table 5 for those six listeners who repeated the transcription task for the purpose of assessing intrajudge reliability illustrate a wide range of proficiency. In fact, the transcription scores across all the listeners in each group ranged from 41% to 57% for the 30 listeners who heard the unaltered sentences, and from 44% to 67% for the 30 who heard the pause-altered sentences. This observation has important clinical implications. It has been acknowledged that, when using intelligibility tests such as the AIDS to monitor the change in an individual dysarthric speaker over time, a "single judge is sufficient, providing that the judge is the same individual each time" (Yorkston & Beukelman, 1981a, p. 6). If different judges, who happen to differ substantially in natural listening abilities, were used to transcribe sentences spoken by a dysarthric speaker across a period of therapy, changes in intelligibility unrelated to treatment might be obtained.

Furthermore, if there are varying degrees of listener ability, perhaps listeners themselves can be trained to decode distorted speech with improved accuracy. Greenspan, Nusbaum, and Pisoni (1988) compared transcription accuracy before and after training with synthetic speech that included auditory–visual feedback about the identity of the stimuli. The training resulted in a substantial increase in intelligibility scores for both words and sentences that was not attributable merely to familiarity with the stimuli but was related to the listener's exposure to acoustic–phonetic information about the structural properties of the synthetic speech. Dysarthric speech can be compared to the synthetic speech reported by Greenspan et al. (1988). Both are degraded in quality. The signals synthesized by Greenspan et al. were "end-to-end concatenations of individual words with no pauses or coarticulation phenomena between words" (p. 422), not unlike the "blurred speech" of the dysarthric subjects in this study. Furthermore, just as synthetic speech has a limited repertoire of phonemes, dysarthric speakers tend to make general simplification errors that are highly consistent (Yorkston et al., 1988). Teaching a listener to attend to and learn the acoustic–phonetic information of a particular dysarthric speech pattern might be one effective way of achieving improved intelligibility and improved communication function for dysarthric speakers and their caregivers, especially when a dysarthric speaker's compensatory skills have plateaued or are declining. Further research on innate abilities among listeners or training programs in listeners' abilities would help determine if this is a productive clinical strategy to pursue.

Implications for Future Research

Continued research in the treatment of dysarthric speakers using various rate control techniques is needed. Future researchers in this area should be encouraged to identify groups of speakers by means of their intelligibility scores as well as by profiles of their prosodic features. Information about which dysarthric speech patterns respond to which types of speech rate intervention are needed for optimal treatment planning. Research involving intelligibility listening tasks should also use large samples of listeners for increased statistical power and external validity. This study revealed that individual listeners differed substantially in the ability to decode dysarthric speech. In order to offset the differences among listeners, large groups of listeners should be used.

Considering a clinical difference in addition to a statistical difference is an important step in the research process that forces a researcher to evaluate results on a functional level. In this study, the insertion of interword pauses was found to result in a statistically significant difference of approximately 5% ($p \leq .0001$). That same statistically significant difference was then considered on a functional level: Would the improvements in intelligibility produced by the insertion of interword pauses exhibited in this study make a functional difference in day-to-day intelligibility performance in the speech of someone with dysarthria? For this particular study, an arbitrary level of clinical significance was set at an average improvement in intelligibility of 10% or greater. Consequently, the results were not considered clinically significant. Furthermore, the statistical difference, although significant, was associated with only a small clinical effect size and may have been an artifact of the large number of listeners. Future studies may wish to consider the important distinction between a statistical and a clinical difference.

CONCLUSIONS

Results from the present study suggest that improvement in the sentence intelligibility of selected dysarthric speakers was exhibited after the insertion of interword pauses. Interpretation of these results must consider two major limiting variables: 1) the experimental design and methodology resulted in an artificial situation in which the speaker's task, the investigator's treatment, and the listener's environment were rigidly controlled, thus limiting their generalizability; and 2) the insertion of interword pauses did not result in a large effect size or improve intelligibility to a level considered to be clinically significant by the investigator.

Several valid conclusions can be drawn from this study: 1) the insertion of interword pauses improved intelligibility of selected dysarthric speech by a statistically significant, although small, percentage; 2) the insertion of interword pauses into dysarthric speech samples via a computer allowed for strong experimental control over the test stimuli and enhanced the internal validity of the study; 3) the large groups of listeners employed in generating the data that constituted the dependent variable in this study increased the statistical power of the results; and 4) the process of perceptually profiling the prosodic characteristics of reduced stress, monoloudness, monopitch, and reduced rate dysarthric speech, in addition to quantitative intelligibility measurements and knowledge of disease etiology, enhanced the homogeneity of the speaker group from which the experimental speech samples were obtained. Although the results of the present study may be somewhat limited with respect to internal and external validity, the method used and results obtained may be justified because those aspects of the research that are valid will provide essential information for further research in the area.

REFERENCES

Crow, E., & Enderby, P. (1989). The effects of an alphabet chart on the speaking rate and intelligibility of speakers with dysarthria. In K. Yorkston & D. Beukelman (Eds.), *Recent advances in clinical dysarthria* (pp. 99–108). Boston: College-Hill Press.

Crystal, T.H., & House, A.S. (1982). Segmental durations in connected speech signals: Preliminary results. *Journal of the Acoustical Society of America, 72,* 705–716.

Darley, F., Aronson, A., & Brown, J. (1975). *Motor speech disorders.* Philadelphia: W.B. Saunders.

Goldman-Eisler, R. (1961). The significance of changes in the rate of articulation. *Language and Speech, 4,* 171–174.

Greenspan, S.L., Nusbaum, H.C., & Pisoni, D.B. (1988). Perceptual learning of synthetic speech produced by rule. *Journal of Experimental Psychology, 14,* 421–433.

Hammen, V.L. (1990). *The effects of speech rate reduction in parkinsonian dysarthria.* Unpublished doctoral dissertation, University of Washington, Seattle.

Hammen, V.L., Yorkston, K.M., & Beukelman, D.R. (1989). Pausal and speech duration characteristics as a function of speaking rate in normal and dysarthric individuals. In K.M. Yorkston & D.R. Beukelman (Eds.), *Recent advances in clinical dysarthria* (pp. 213–224). Boston: College-Hill Press.

Hammen, V.L., Yorkston, K.M., & Minifie, F.D. (1994). Effects of temporal alterations on speech intelligibility in parkinsonian dysarthria. *Journal of Speech and Hearing Research, 37,* 244–253.

Kearns, K.P., & Simmons, N.N. (1988). Interobserver reliability and perceptual ratings: More than meets the ear. *Journal of Speech and Hearing Research, 31,* 131–136.

Maassen, B. (1986). Marking word boundaries to improve the intelligibility of the speech of the deaf. *Journal of Speech and Hearing Research, 29,* 227–230.

Maassen, B., & Povel, D.J. (1984). The effect of correcting temporal structure on the intelligibility of the deaf. *Speech and Communication, 3,* 123–135.

Maassen, B., & Povel, D.J. (1985). The effect of segmental and suprasegmental corrections on the intelligibility of deaf speech. *Journal of the Acoustical Society of America, 78,* 877–886.

Osberger, M.J., & Levitt, H. (1979). The effect of timing errors on the intelligibility of deaf children's speech. *Journal of the Acoustical Society of America, 66,* 1316–1324.

Ottenbacher, K.J., & Barrett, K.A. (1989). Measures of effect size in the reporting of rehabilitation research. *American Journal of Physical Medicine and Rehabilitation, 68,* 52–58.

Sheard, D., Adams, R.D., & Davis, P.J. (1991). Reliability and agreement of ratings of ataxic dysarthric speech samples with varying intelligibility. *Journal of Speech and Hearing Research, 34,* 285–293.

Yorkston, K.M., & Beukelman, D.R. (1981a). *Assessment of intelligibility of dysarthric speech.* Tigard, OR: C.C. Publications.

Yorkston, K.M., & Beukelman, D.R. (1981b). Ataxic dysarthria: Treatment sequences based on intelligibility and prosodic considerations. *Journal of Speech and Hearing Disorders, 46,* 398–404.

Yorkston, K.M., Beukelman, D.R., & Bell, K.R. (1988). *Clinical management of dysarthric speakers.* Austin, TX: PRO-ED.

Yorkston, K.M., Hammen, V.L., Beukelman, D.R., & Traynor, C. (1990). The effect of rate control on the intelligibility and naturalness of dysarthric speech. *Journal of Speech and Hearing Disorders, 55,* 550–560.

SECTION IV

RELIABILITY AND VALIDITY ISSUES IN ASSESSMENT

Chapter 7

The Multidimensional Nature of Pathologic Vocal Quality

Jody Kreiman, Bruce R. Gerratt, and Gerald S. Berke

"BREATHY" AND "ROUGH" are among the most familiar labels for pathologic voice qualities, and have been in common use since ancient times (see Laver, 1981, for review). Because of their importance for describing a wide variety of pathologies (e.g., Darley, Aronson, & Brown, 1969; Isshiki, Okamura, Tanabe, & Morimoto, 1969), these qualities are the subjects of frequent study in the literature on voice quality evaluation. For example, many papers have examined the correlation between acoustic and aerodynamic measures and rated breathiness and/or roughness (e.g., Arends, Povel, Os, & Speth, 1990; Arnold & Emanuel, 1979; Coleman, 1969; Fritzell, Hammarberg, Gauffin, Karlsson, & Sundberg, 1986).

However, despite a long history and extensive literature, the perceptual reality of breathiness, roughness, and related qualities (e.g., harshness, hoarseness) has never been systematically examined. In fact, these perceptual qualities have never received widely accepted definitions in the clinical literature, whether formal or informal. Thus, it is difficult to determine precisely what a particular author means by "hoarseness," "harshness," "breathiness," "roughness," or any other label for vocal quality. The general lack of research into the perceptual reality and meaning of important

---

Reprinted from the *Journal of the Acoustical Society of America*, 96, 1291–1302, 1994, by permission of the authors and the American Institute of Physics. © 1994 Acoustical Society of America.

This research was supported in part by National Institute on Deafness and Other Communication Disorders Grant No. DC 01797 and by Veterans Affairs Merit Review funds.

We thank Norma Antonanzas-Barroso for programming support, and Andrew Erman for his help in preparing the stimulus tapes.

descriptors of pathologic voices is a longstanding problem in voice research (Jensen, 1965; Reed, 1980).

Furthermore, listeners often disagree when they rate vocal qualities, suggesting that significant individual differences exist in the meaning assigned to such terms in practice. For example, Shipp and Huntington (1965) found interrater correlations (Pearson's r for pairs of raters) ranging from .33 to .78 for ratings of breathiness on an 8-point scale. Kreiman, Gerratt, Kempster, Erman, and Berke (1993) reported interrater correlations ranging from .55 to .92 for ratings of vocal roughness on a 7-point scale. Thus it appears that listeners may differ considerably from one another in the ratings assigned to any one voice, despite the fact that most individuals can rate voices consistently (see Kreiman et al., 1993, for review). Understanding the sources of this listener variability in voice quality ratings might lead to the development of more reliable rating protocols.

Perhaps because of the lack of systematic research in this area, authors also disagree about the relationships among breathiness, roughness, and other vocal qualities. Two implicit views are prominent in the literature on pathologic voices. In the first, different perceptual qualities are treated as independent features of voices that may reasonably be assessed individually. This view is implied by the many studies where ratings of a single quality are compared to objective measurements (e.g., Sansone & Emanuel, 1970; Wendahl, 1966; Yanagihara, 1967; Yumoto, Gould, & Baer, 1982; Yumoto, Sasaki, & Okamura, 1984), and occasionally is assumed explicitly (e.g., Whitehead & Emanuel, 1974). In the second, breathiness and roughness are both treated as subordinate aspects of some other quality (a hierarchical view). For example, Fairbanks (1960) argued that breathiness and harshness are both components of a superordinate "hoarse" quality. (See also Laver, 1980, for discussion of a descriptive phonetic approach to similar qualities in normal phonation.)

Very little experimental evidence is available regarding either of the traditional views of vocal quality. The "independent feature" view is supported by studies finding that raters agree highly when they rate individual qualities (e.g., Klich, 1982; Lively & Emanuel, 1970; Sapir & Aronson, 1985). However, many other studies have reported low or variable levels of interrater reliability (e.g., Cullinan, Prather, & Williams, 1963; Nieboer, De Graaf, & Schutte, 1988; Yumoto et al., 1984; see Kreiman et al., 1993, for review). Other studies provide limited support for a hierarchical view. Shipp and Huntington (1965) found ratings of breathiness and hoarseness were moderately correlated for three of four expert raters, suggesting that these qualities are related, but not in any simple way. One factor-analytic study also suggests that breathiness and roughness may be perceptually complex and interrelated: Hammarberg, Fritzell, Gauffin,

Sundberg, and Wedin (1980) found a "breathy–overtight" dimension (negatively associated with the scales "breathy," "wheezing," "lack of timbre," "moments of aphonia," and "husky," and positively associated with "creaky/vocal fry") and a "coarse–light" dimension (positively associated with the scales "coarse," "rough," and "harsh," and negatively associated with "high pitch," "middle register," and "restrained").

Other research has specifically addressed the perceptual structure of "hoarseness." Isshiki and Takeuchi (1970) used semantic differential techniques and factor analysis to examine subclassifications of hoarse voice quality. They found four factors, which they labeled "rough," "breathy," "asthenic" (lack of vocal strength), and "near-normal." The GRBAS protocol proposed by the Japanese Society of Logopedics (e.g., Hirano, 1981) maintained this distinction between rough, breathy, asthenic, and near-normal (the "grade" scale) aspects of hoarse voice, but added a scale for "strained" quality. Finally, Takahashi and Koike (1975) found that ratings of breathiness and roughness were moderately but significantly correlated ($r = .47$), and concluded that the two qualities are not independent factors in a perceptual space. They also described factor analyses that supported Isshiki and Takeuchi's (1970) breathy and rough factors for the description of hoarseness.

Previous studies using multidimensional scaling (MDS) suggest that breathiness and roughness are important perceptual features of pathologic voices, but that listeners differ from one another in how they judge these qualities. Kreiman, Gerratt, and Precoda (1990) found dimensions correlated with rated breathiness and roughness in a MDS study of 18 pathologic male voices. However, "rough" and "breathy" dimensions did not consistently emerge from a subsequent study examining individual differences in voice perception (Kreiman, Gerratt, Precoda, & Berke, 1992), suggesting these dimensions are not perceptually important for every listener, even in a fixed perceptual context. Other MDS studies have not consistently produced breathiness and roughness dimensions. Murry, Singh, and Sargent (1977) found dimensions associated with volume velocity (moderately correlated with breathiness ratings) and presence/absence of periodicity (related to rated hoarseness) in a study of pathologic male voices.[1] In contrast, Kempster, Kistler, and Hillenbrand (1991) found dimensions related to intensity, frequency, and perturbation in a MDS study of dysphonic female speakers. They did not speculate as to how these dimensions might relate to traditional labels for voice quality.

Thus, a number of issues remain unresolved, both with respect to the perceptual status of breathiness and roughness and to the perception of

---

[1]Three other dimensions were reported: ± tumor, F_0, and one uninterpreted dimension.

pathologic voices in general. In particular, the relationship among different labels for vocal quality has never been systematically investigated. Thus, it is unclear whether listeners can rate different (unidimensional) voice qualities independently or whether qualities are better viewed as multidimensional constructs whose dimensions may influence one another during the rating process. Such information is essential for designing valid and reliable protocols for clinically evaluating pathologic voice quality.

The present study combined MDS and unidimensional rating approaches to address these issues directly. MDS techniques have several advantages over more commonly used rating methods. They do not require a priori assumptions about the dimensionality of a quality, and thus allow unbiased investigation into the number of dimensions necessary to explain listeners' judgments, the nature of such dimensions, and the relationships among them. They also permit detailed examination of differences among listeners in the criteria used to rate a voice on some quality scale. The addition of unidimensional ratings of the same voices allowed us to relate multidimensional results to traditional impressionistic labels for voice quality, to determine how listeners may map multidimensional qualities onto unidimensional rating scales.

PERCEPTUAL SPACES FOR BREATHINESS AND ROUGHNESS

Method

Listeners (Group 1) Five native speakers of English participated in this study. None had participated in previous studies using these stimuli. Two were speech pathologists (Listeners 1 and 2), two were linguists specializing in voice research (Listeners 3 and 4), and one was trained in both linguistics and speech pathology (Listener 5). All were trained in the American tradition of voice quality description, and each had at least 3 years' postgraduate experience judging voices. Listeners worked with pathologic voices on a daily basis and regularly applied the terms studied here. Listeners reported no history of voice, speech, language, or hearing difficulties.

Stimuli The voices of 18 male speakers with voice disorders were selected at random from a library of audio recordings made as part of a phonatory function evaluation. During this evaluation, speakers sustained the vowel /ɑ/ at conversational levels of pitch and loudness. Speakers varied widely in the overall severity of their voice disorder. Mildly, moderately, and severely breathy and rough voices were all represented, as were a variety of diagnoses. A previous multidimensional scaling study using these voices (Kreiman et al., 1990) revealed breathiness and roughness dimensions that each accounted for more than 25% of the variance in listeners' dissimilarity judgments.[2]

Voice samples were low-pass filtered using two 4-pole Butterworth filters with cutoff frequencies of 6,300 Hz, and two with cutoff frequencies of 7,500 Hz, for a total reduction in amplitude of 3.2 dB at 5.6 kHz and 39.4 dB at 9 kHz. They were then sampled at 17,800 samples/second using a 16-bit A/D converter. A 1.7-s sample was taken from the middle portion of each speaker's /ɑ/. The digitized segments were normalized for peak voltage, and onsets and offsets were multiplied by 10-ms ramps to eliminate click artifacts. Stimuli were then output through a 16-bit D/A converter using the same filter settings.

Two experimental tapes were constructed. Each included both orders of all possible pairs of the 18 pathological voices (excluding pairs where voices were the same), for a total of 306 trials per tape. Stimuli were rerandomized for the second tape. For both tapes, voice samples within a pair were separated by 1 s, and pairs were separated by 6 s.

Procedure Each listener participated in two listening sessions separated by at least 1 week. Testing took place in a sound-treated booth. At one session, listeners judged the dissimilarity of each pair of voices with respect to levels of breathiness; at the other, they judged dissimilarity with respect to roughness. One experimental tape was used for the first session and the other for the second, so each listener made two judgments of each quality for each pair of voices. Order of task and tape presentation was randomized across listeners.

Listeners rated the dissimilarity of the pairs of voices on 7-point equal-appearing interval scales, where 1 represented identical levels of breathiness/roughness and 7 represented extreme difference in breathiness/roughness levels. Thus, a rating of 1 could mean voices were both very breathy, not breathy at all, and so on, while a rating of 7 meant that one voice was (near-) normal and one was severely breathy or rough. Formal definitions of breathiness and roughness were not offered. Instead, listeners were asked to use whatever standards they normally applied in their clinical practice or research. They were instructed to focus their attention on the quality being judged and to ignore any other qualities the voices might have. They were also asked to judge each pair of voices as independently as possible, and were discouraged from changing previous responses after hearing a new pair of voices.

Each test session lasted approximately 1.5 hr. Listeners were encouraged to take brief breaks during this period as needed.

---

[2]The only other dimension to emerge from this analysis accounted for 23% of the variance in dissimilarity judgments and was significantly correlated with F_0 for the voices.

Table 1. R^2 (variance accounted for) and stress for the group multidimensional scaling solutions

No. of dimensions in solution	Rating task			
	Breathiness judgments		Roughness judgments	
	R^2	Stress	R^2	Stress
6	.75	0.17	.81	0.19
5	.73	0.19	.81	0.20
4	.71	0.23	.80	0.23
3	.68	0.27	.76	0.26
2	.67	0.33	.75	0.30
1	.62	0.42	.70	0.36

Multidimensional Scaling Analyses Previous studies indicate that presentation order has a significant effect on listener judgments of vocal quality, because the first member of a pair of voices provides a context against which the second is judged, highlighting different facets of these complex stimuli (Gerratt, Kreiman, Antonanzas-Barroso, & Berke, 1993). To avoid losing such information, matrices of dissimilarity judgments were not symmetrized across the diagonal. Instead, each listener's judgments for each task were assembled into two half-matrices (upper and lower halves, minus the diagonal). Judgments from all listeners were combined and analyzed using the nonmetric individual differences model (INDSCAL) of SAS PROC MDS (Kruskal & Wish, 1978; SAS Institute, 1992; Schiffman, Reynolds, & Young, 1981). Separate analyses were undertaken for breathiness and roughness judgments. Each analysis included 10 half-matrices (two from each listener).

Scaling solutions were found in one to six dimensions for each rating task. Based on values of stress, on the amount of variance accounted for by each solution (R^2; Table 1), and on interpretability, two-dimensional solutions were selected for both the breathiness and roughness judgments.

Acoustic Analyses To assist in interpreting the scaling solutions, a number of time- and frequency-domain measurements were made on the test voices.[3] The fundamental frequency (F_0) and the frequencies of the first three formants (F_1, F_2, and F_3) were measured from spectrographic displays. F_0 was measured from narrow-band displays with a frequency range of 0–1 kHz; the center frequencies of the three clearest harmonics were measured to ensure accuracy. Formants were measured with reference to both narrow- and wide-band displays (with a frequency range of 0–4 kHz) and displays of line spectra of the vowels. Measurements were

---

[3] The voice of one pathologic speaker was clearly diplophonic. Thus, only formant measurements were available for him.

taken from sections of the display where the formants appeared most steady and level.

For jitter and shimmer measurements, a point on each waveform cycle that could be identified reliably from cycle to cycle was selected interactively. Measurements of mean jitter, standard deviation of jitter, and the coefficient of variation for jitter were then calculated using parabolic interpolation when the point marked was a peak and linear interpolation when a zero crossing was marked (Titze, Horii, & Scherer, 1987). Analogous shimmer measurements were also calculated, using the difference in decibels between the highest and lowest points in each marked cycle as the amplitude.

Several additional acoustic measures were also obtained. The natural logarithm of the standard deviation of the period lengths (LNSD; see Wolfe & Steinfatt, 1987) was calculated for each voice sample, as were the harmonics-to-noise ratio (HNR) (Yumoto et al., 1982) and the ratio of the amplitudes of the first to the second harmonic (H_1–H_2) (Bickley, 1982; Ladefoged, 1981). Finally, we calculated the "partial period comparison" (PPC), a time-domain comparison of the standard deviations of differences between moving vectors, each about 0.6 times the estimated period length (Ladefoged, Maddieson, & Jackson, 1988). To generalize this measure to long segments of speech, it was applied to a sample approximately three glottal cycles long; the next two cycles were skipped and the next three measured, continuing in this manner for the duration of the vowel sample. The mean of the indices generated for the entire voice sample was then calculated for use in this study. The PPC is moderately correlated with measures of jitter and shimmer and may measure variability within an utterance in levels of signal unsteadiness.

Unidimensional Perceptual Measures of Vocal Quality To assess the extent to which multidimensional spaces capture the information available from traditional unidimensional ratings of voice qualities, we gathered additional ratings of the stimulus voices using equal-appearing interval (EAI) scales for breathiness and roughness. A second group of eight expert listeners (four speech pathologists and four otolaryngologists) participated in this experiment. As above, listeners were trained in the American tradition of voice quality description, and each had a minimum of 3 years' experience evaluating pathologic voices. None had previous experience with these stimulus voices, and none participated in the study described above.

Judgments of breathiness and roughness were made at separate test sessions at least 1 week apart. Voices were rerandomized for each listener and rating task. Testing took place in a sound-treated booth. Stimulus digitization and playback were as described above. The rate of stimulus presentation was controlled by the listener.

At each listening session, listeners rated the voices using 7-point EAI scales. On these scales the value 1 represented minimum breathiness or roughness, and 7 represented severe breathiness or roughness. Scale end points were labeled accordingly. Listeners were asked to pay attention only to the quality being judged and to ignore any other qualities the voice might have. No formal definitions of breathiness or roughness were offered. Instead, listeners were asked to use whatever standards they usually applied in their clinical practices. Listeners were able to replay the voices if necessary before making their judgments.

Results

Independence of Breathiness and Roughness Ratings To determine if dissimilarity judgments of breathiness and roughness were independent, we examined the correlation between the two sets of unscaled ratings for each of the five listeners in Group 1. Values of Pearson's r averaged .25 (standard deviation [SD] = .10). Unidimensional (EAI) ratings of breathiness and roughness for Group 2 also were not highly correlated (mean Pearson's r = .27, SD = .17). These values are so low as to suggest that judgments of the two qualities were in fact independent, for both the dissimilarity ratings and the EAI task.

Rating Reliability Intrarater (test–retest) reliability for dissimilarity ratings of breathiness and roughness was assessed by calculating the correlation (Pearson's r) between the first and second rating of each pair of voices. Values for breathiness ratings ranged from .34 to .68, with a mean of .55. However, across listeners, 72.5% of repeated ratings differed by one scale value or less (range = 60.8%–90%; chance = 38.8%), suggesting the low correlation values reflect the limited range of the rating scale. Similarly, for the roughness ratings, repeated dissimilarity ratings were not particularly well correlated (mean r = .62; range = .37–.81), but the majority of repeated ratings were within one scale value (73.3%; range = 58.8%–85.6%). Note that these values also reflect the effects of the different presentation orders used for the first and second ratings of the voice pairs.

For the EAI ratings (listener Group 2), values of Pearson's r comparing a listener's first and second ratings of breathiness ranged from .63 to .93, with a mean of .81 (SD = .11). For roughness, intrarater correlations ranged from .66 to .91, with a mean of .78 (SD = .08). For interrater reliability, values of Pearson's r comparing all possible pairs of listeners indicated that individual listeners did not necessarily agree particularly well with one another. For breathiness, mean Pearson's r for pairs of raters was .69 (SD = .11, range = .44–.86). For roughness, mean Pearson's r = .54 (SD = .20, range = .05–.82). One listener in particular rated vocal roughness consistently (intrarater Pearson's r = .77) but differed considerably from the rest of the group (average r = .35; range = .05–.62). When that listener was excluded, the mean correlation among raters for roughness ratings increased to .60 (SD = .17, range = .22–.82).

However, average EAI ratings were sufficiently reliable for our purposes (e.g., Berk, 1979). For breathiness ratings, the intraclass correlation (ICC) = .93 [model (2,8); e.g., Ebel, 1951; Shrout & Fleiss, 1979]; for roughness, the ICC(2,8) = .86. Accordingly, average EAI ratings were used for interpreting group perceptual spaces. We will discuss issues surrounding the reliability of individual raters in more detail below.

Multidimensional Scaling Solutions As described above, two-dimensional solutions were selected for both the breathiness and roughness data. Stimuli were arranged roughly in a circle in both spaces (Figure 1). The breathiness space accounted for 67% of the variance in the underlying dissimilarity ratings of breathiness; the first dimension (D_1) accounted for 52% of the variance and the second dimension (D_2) for 15%.[4] The roughness solution accounted for 75% of the variance in the underlying dissimilarity ratings, with D_1 contributing 55% and D_2 contributing 20% to the explained variance.

Scaling solutions were interpreted by examining significant correlations between stimulus coordinates on each dimension and the acoustic parameters described above. In cases where dimensions were significantly correlated with more than one acoustic variable, multiple regression was used to determine whether the acoustic variables accounted for independent aspects of variance in stimulus coordinates.

Interpretations for the two spaces were similar. D_1 in the breathiness space was correlated with a weighted sum of H_1–H_2 and LNSD (R = .84); D_2 was correlated with a weighted sum of mean shimmer and F_0 (R = .82). In the roughness space, stimuli on D_1 were ordered according to a weighted sum of mean shimmer and H_1–H_2 (R = .91). D_2 correlated highly with a weighted sum of H_1–H_2 and F_0 (R = .81).

Stimulus coordinates in the two spaces were significantly correlated. Breathiness D_2 corresponded to roughness D_1 (r = .74, p < .01), and breathiness D_1 corresponded to roughness D_2 (r = .66, p < .01). These findings suggest that similar, multidimensional perceptual structures underlie ratings of vocal breathiness and roughness for our listeners.

Unidimensional Versus Multidimensional Ratings To examine how adequately unidimensional ratings capture this multidimensional information, multiple regression was used to compare stimulus coordinates on the dimensions derived above to average EAI ratings of breathiness and roughness for the same voices. Results are given in Table 2.

Unidimensional ratings did capture the majority of the information in both of the multidimensional spaces. Values of multiple R^2 ranged from

---

[4]The variance accounted for by each dimension is reported by the scaling program.

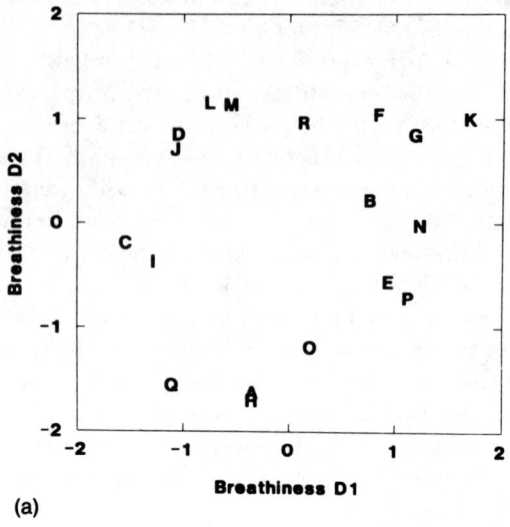

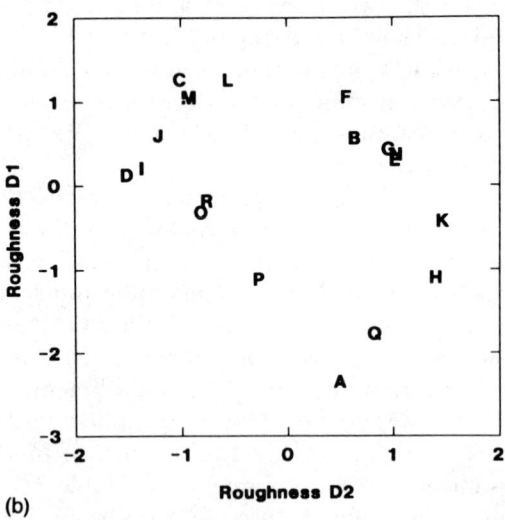

Figure 1. Multidimensional scaling solutions for the combined subject group. Letters indicate individual voices. *a*, space derived from dissimilarity ratings of breathiness. *b*, space derived from dissimilarity ratings of roughness.

Table 2. Results of multiple regressions comparing EAI ratings and stimulus coordinates in the group perceptual spaces

Dimension	Standardized regression coefficients		$F_{2,15}$[a]	Multiple R^2
	Breathiness ratings	Roughness ratings		
Breathy space D_1	1.03	−0.23	88.99	.92
Breathy space D_2	...	0.84	25.53	.77
Rough space D_1	−0.26	0.99	39.87	.84
Rough space D_2	−0.74	0.58	8.26	.52

[a]All F values are significant at $p < .01$.

.52 to .92 for the four dimensions. D_1 in the breathiness space was significantly related to unidimensional ratings of both breathiness and roughness; D_2 in the breathiness space was related only to rated roughness. Similarly, both dimensions in the roughness space were significantly related to both sets of unidimensional ratings. D_1 corresponded primarily to rated roughness, while D_2 was strongly related to both breathiness and roughness. Thus, EAI ratings of both breathiness and roughness were needed to describe each single perceptual space.

Individual Differences in Perceptual Strategy The R^2 values, squared subject weights, and weirdness values for individual subjects in the multidimensional scaling analyses are given in Table 3. Group values are included for comparison. The R^2 values in Table 3 represent the amount of

Table 3. R^2 values, squared subject weights, and weirdness values for individual listeners in the group scaling solutions

Listener/matrix	Breathiness space			Roughness space		
	R^2	Squared subject weights (D_1/D_2)	Weirdness	R^2	Squared subject weights (D_1/D_2)	Weirdness
1/1	.56	0.42/0.14	0.07	.59	0.29/0.30	0.34
1/2	.63	0.56/0.07	0.26	.68	0.38/0.30	0.27
2/1	.66	0.58/0.08	0.21	.71	0.53/0.18	0.00
2/2	.72	0.61/0.11	0.13	.72	0.59/0.13	0.14
3/1	.81	0.74/0.07	0.31	.80	0.52/0.28	0.16
3/2	.75	0.68/0.07	0.29	.85	0.45/0.40	0.31
4/1	.78	0.59/0.19	0.05	.78	0.58/0.20	0.02
4/2	.76	0.63/0.13	0.08	.83	0.72/0.11	0.24
5/1	.61	0.26/0.35	0.47	.80	0.78/0.02	0.66
5/2	.45	0.18/0.27	0.49	.71	0.64/0.07	0.34
Group	.67	0.53/0.16		.75	0.55/0.20	

Note: Each value represents the average of scores for the top and bottom half-matrix for that listener (see text for discussion).

variance in that subject's ratings that is accounted for by the group scaling solution. That is, they measure the overall fit of the group solution to an individual's data. Subject weights reflect the perceptual importance a given dimension has for an individual subject. The weights printed by the MDS procedure have been squared and sum to R^2 for a given subject. Weirdness reflects the extent to which an individual's weights on the dimensions are proportional to the group weights. A subject with weights proportional to the average weights has a weirdness of 0; a subject with one very large weight and one small weight has a weirdness near 1.

As Table 3 shows, subjects differed considerably in the extent to which the group solution reflected their perceptual strategies. For the breathiness space, weirdness values suggest that Listeners 3 and 5 differed substantially (and in different directions) from average in the relative importance given the two dimensions. Listener 3 relied relatively heavily on D_1 (which was correlated with a weighted sum of H_1–H_2 and LNSD). Because this dimension was much more important overall, this subject's R^2 value is high relative to the total group. In contrast, D_2 (correlated with a weighted sum of shimmer and F_0) was much more important for Listener 5 than for the group as a whole. Consequently, R^2 for this listener is lower than that for the group.

Listeners 1, 3, and 5 differed from the average in their dimension weights for the roughness space. D_2 (interpreted as a weighted sum of H_1–H_2 and F_0) was more important for Listeners 1 and 3 than for the group as a whole. D_1 (interpreted as a weighted sum of shimmer and H_1–H_2) was less important for Listener 1 than for the group and more important for Listeners 4 and 5. R^2 values are somewhat lower only for Listener 1, who differed from the group in the relative perceptual salience of both dimensions.

Discussion These data suggest that breathiness and roughness are not independent unidimensional aspects of vocal quality. Rather, they appear to be different aspects of a single multidimensional "quality." Rated breathiness and roughness were both needed to describe each of the MDS spaces. Thus, it appears that having listeners rate only breathiness or roughness is not adequate to assess the extent to which a voice possesses that individual quality. Our results indicate that information about both qualities is needed to measure either.

These data further suggest that consistent perceptual differences may underlie stable group scaling solutions. In particular, Listener 3 appears to have relied more heavily on dimensions correlated with H_1–H_2 than did the average listener; and Listener 5 apparently judged both breathiness and roughness in terms of acoustic signal perturbation.

To examine listener differences in more detail, we undertook a second set of multidimensional scaling analyses. Each new analysis included data from a single subject for a single vocal quality. We hoped such analyses would provide insight into the nature and extent of intersubject variability in perception of breathiness and roughness.

SCALING SOLUTIONS FOR INDIVIDUAL LISTENERS

Method

Separate breathiness and roughness spaces were calculated for each individual listener in Group 1 using the INDSCAL model of SAS PROC MDS, as above. Each analysis included the top and bottom half-matrices of dissimilarity judgments produced by that listener. This procedure was chosen over the traditional practice of symmetrizing matrices by averaging data points across the diagonal, because it preserves context-dependent information about vocal qualities, as argued above. Analyses of symmetrized data confirmed that one-dimensional solutions were appropriate for the symmetrized data, while solutions for the unsymmetrized data provided both higher overall R^2 values and more reasonable interpretations. Solutions were calculated in one to four dimensions. Based on values of stress, R^2, and interpretability, two-dimensional solutions were selected for all 10 analyses.

Results

Variance Accounted for by the Scaling Solutions R^2 values for the individual scaling solutions are given in Tables 4 and 5. In every case, scaling solutions accounted for the majority of the variance in an individual's dissimilarity ratings. For the breathiness spaces, R^2 values ranged from .66 to .87, with a mean of .80 ($SD = .09$). R^2 values for the roughness spaces ranged from .70 to .94, with a mean of .85 ($SD = .10$).

Interpretation of the Individual Spaces Individual perceptual spaces were interpreted using the methods described above. Results for the breathiness spaces are included in Table 4 and for the roughness spaces in Table 5. Stimulus configurations for individual breathiness spaces are shown in Figure 2 and for roughness spaces in Figure 3.

For breathiness, both dimension interpretations and stimulus configurations suggest that listeners are differentially weighing a fairly constant set of acoustic cues. There is little evidence of gross differences in perceptual strategy. Each listener's first dimension (which accounts for the majority of variance in the solutions) is significantly correlated with at least one dimension in the space for every other listener ($r = .64-.93$). Across solutions, only one dimension (D_2 for Listener 2) was not significantly related to any dimension in any other space.[5] All five spaces are interpretable

---
[5]Although this dimension shares acoustic correlates with D_1 for Listeners 3 and 5, stimuli are arranged differently. Listener 2 emphasized differences among mildly to moderately pathologic voices and compressed those between severely disordered voices, leading to low correlations with other listeners' perceptions.

Table 4. Interpretations for individual perceptual spaces: Breathiness ratings

Subject	R^2 for solution	Dimension	Weight	Interpretation	R for interpretation
1	.75	1	0.63	H_1-H_2+HNR	.83
		2	0.11	Shimmer SD	.59
2	.84	1	0.74	H_1-H_2+LNSD$+$PPC	.89
		2	0.10	Shimmer coefficient of variation$+$jitter SD	.73
3	.86	1	0.69	Shimmer coefficient of variation .	.62
		2	0.16	$F_0+H_1-H_2$	.71
4	.87	1	0.51	PPC$+H_1-H_2$	.78
		2	0.36	H_1-H_2+LNSD	.88
5	.66	1	0.39	Shimmer coefficient of variation $+F_0$	.70
		2	0.27	HNR$+H_1-H_2$	.76

in terms of H_1-H_2 and perturbation, and all contain two fairly continuous dimensions, with no obvious clusters of stimuli.

Listeners do differ in the relative weight given each dimension. For example, Listeners 3 and 5 relied more on shimmer and F_0, and less on H_1-H_2, than did Listeners 1, 2, and 4; and Listeners 1 and 5 attended to spectral noise (as measured by the harmonics-to-noise ratio) in addition to spectral slope (as measured by H_1-H_2). Overall, however, listeners seem to have used a fairly consistent set of perceptual parameters when judging the relative breathiness of the stimuli. This finding is consistent with the relatively high levels of interrater reliability for EAI ratings of breathiness reported above for these voices.

Listeners differed more in their roughness judgments. As Table 5 shows, only Listener 1's scaling solution matched the group solution. Lis-

Table 5. Interpretations for individual perceptual spaces: Roughness ratings

Subject	R^2 for solution	Dimension	Weight	Interpretation	R for interpretation
1	.70	1	0.42	Mean shimmer$+H_1-H_2$	.87
		2	0.28	$F_0+H_1-H_2+F3$	.91
2	.82	1	0.72	PPC$+H_1-H_2$	.93
		2	0.10	H_1-H_2	.58
3	.94	1	0.68	PPC$+H_1-H_2$	.90
		2	0.26	F_0	.62
4	.94	1	0.76	$F_0+H_1-H_2+$PPC	.86
		2	0.18	Jitter SD	.75
5	.86	1	0.53	PPC	.50
		2	0.33	PPC$+F_0$	.81

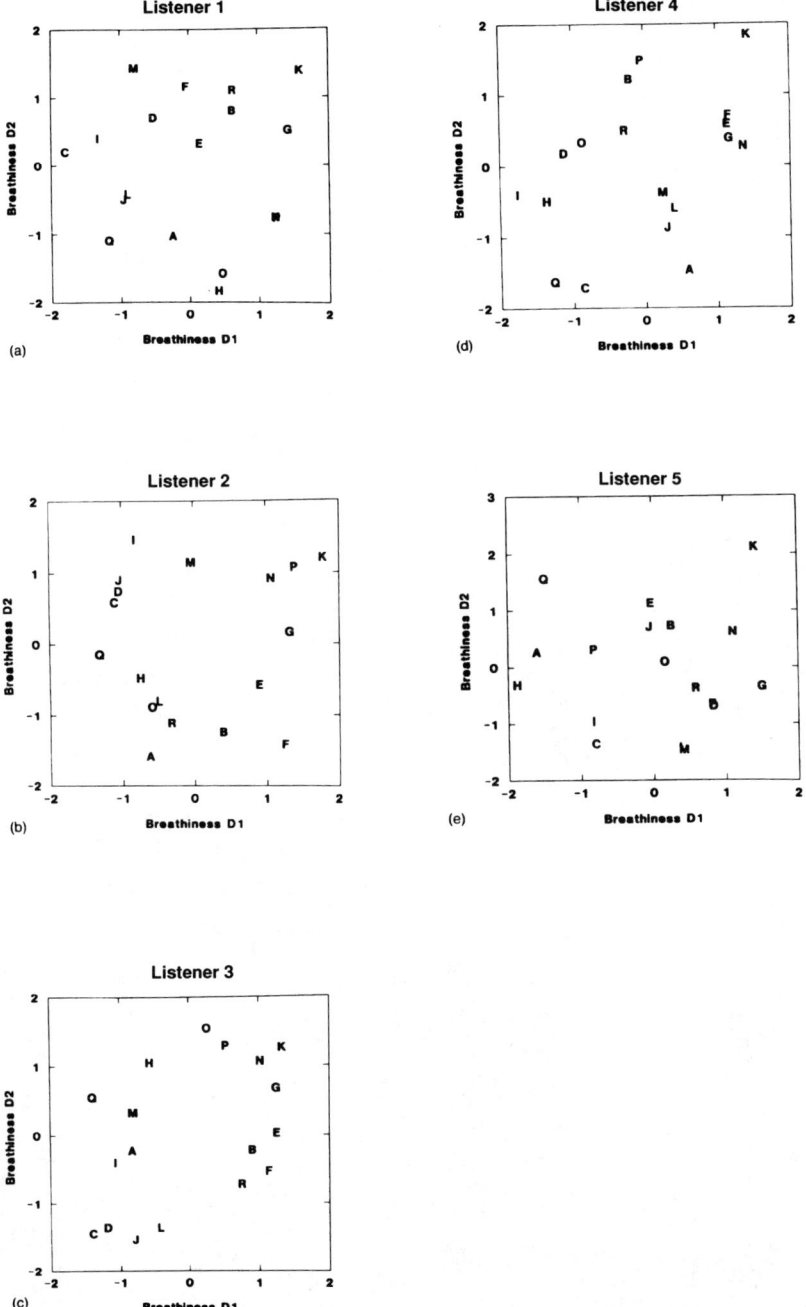

Figure 2. Multidimensional scaling solutions for individual listeners' dissimilarity ratings of breathiness.

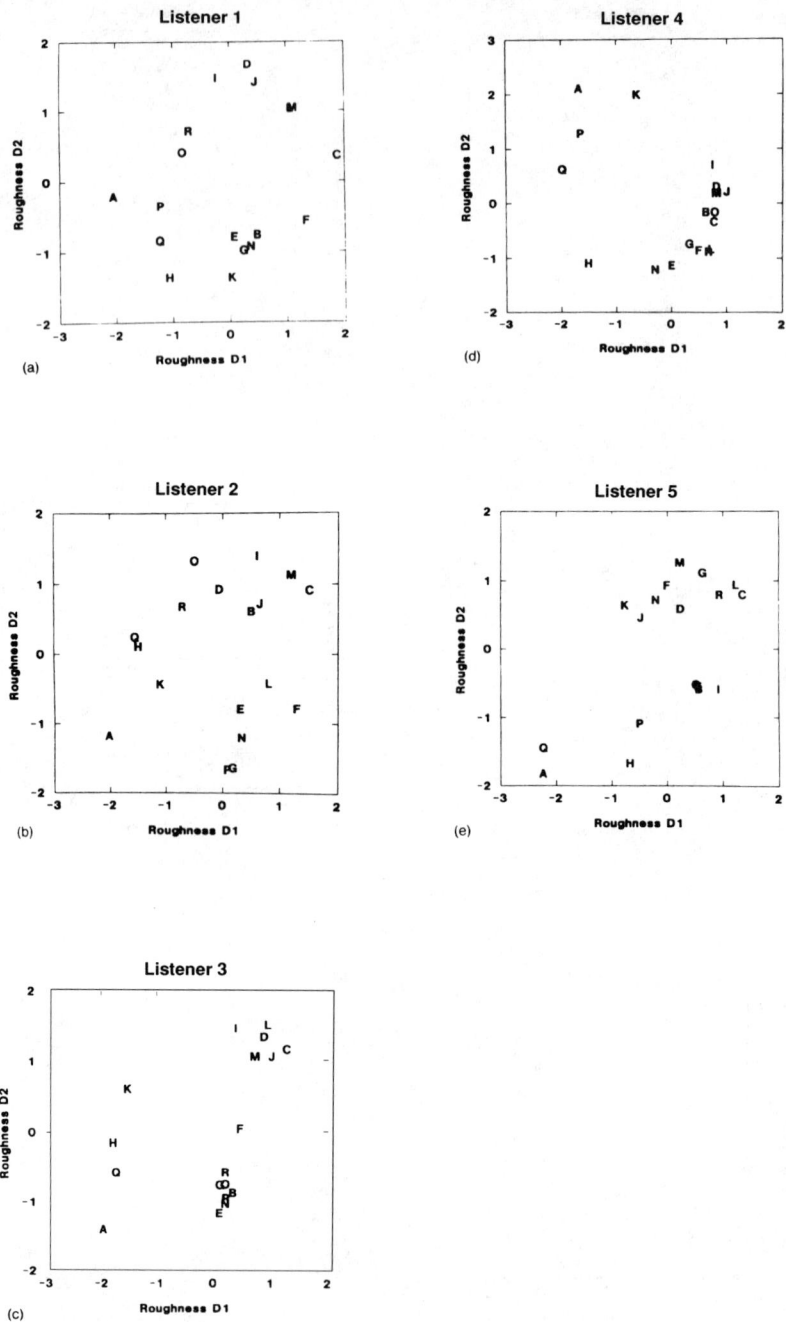

Figure 3. Multidimensional scaling solutions for individual listener's dissimilarity ratings of roughness.

tener 2 apparently did not use F_0 when judging roughness, while Listener 3 relied much more heavily on F_0 than the average listener. Listener 4 also relied heavily on F_0 but also apparently referred to levels of vocal jitter when judging roughness. Finally, neither dimension in the space for Listener 5 was significantly correlated with H_1–H_2, although that parameter was important for the other four listeners.

Figure 3 further suggests that some listeners judged roughness using continuous scales, while others seem to have used features that are dichotomous or trichotomous. The perceptual spaces for Listeners 1 and 2 suggest these subjects judged roughness using two features that varied continuously. However, Listener 3's perceptual space shows three tight clusters of stimuli. The first dimension divides the stimuli into those with fairly steady phonation and those with a tremulous or unsteady quality. The second dimension is well correlated with F_0; however, the upper cluster in this space includes voices that are simultaneously rough and breathy, while those in the lower cluster lack salient breathiness. Thus, the space for Listener 3 reflects a ternary division of voices into tremulous, breathy–rough, and other qualities. In contrast, the space for Listener 4 is divided along the major diagonal, with tremulous voices in quadrant IV and others in quadrant II. The space for Listener 5 also includes a cluster of tremulous voices, along with a small group of voices that seem to share a vowel quality nearer /æ/ than /ɑ/, and a cluster including the remainder of the voice set. Listeners 4 and 5 apparently treated roughness as a binary feature of voices (±tremulous), as compared to the ternary tremulous/breathy–rough/other distinction used by Listener 3.

PERCEPTUAL STRATEGIES AND INTERRATER RELIABILITY

As mentioned above, many researchers have reported low or variable levels of interrater reliability in studies of vocal quality, and reliability remains a serious problem in designing and using vocal quality rating systems in the clinic. The present findings suggest that one source of rating unreliability may be the tendency of different listeners to focus selectively on one or the other dimension of a given vocal quality. To test this hypothesis, we examined the correlations between the unidimensional (EAI) ratings of breathiness and roughness for listeners in Group 2 and the coordinates of the voice stimuli in the group multidimensional spaces. Significant correlations ($p < .01$, adjusted for multiple comparisons) are listed in Table 6.

This table suggests that listeners consistently focused their attention on a single dimension of breathiness when making EAI ratings. With the exception of Listener 5, whose perceptual strategy apparently deviated substantially from that of the other listeners, EAI ratings were well correlated

Table 6. Significant correlations between EAI ratings and perceptual dimensions in the group MDS spaces

Listener	EAI breathiness ratings correlated with:	EAI roughness ratings correlated with:
1	Breathiness: D_1 ($r = .78$)	Roughness: D_1 ($r = .88$)
	Roughness: . . .	Breathiness: D_2 ($r = .77$)
2	Breathiness: D_1 ($r = .80$)	Roughness: . . .
	Roughness: . . .	Breathiness: D_2 ($r = .75$)
3	Breathiness: D_1 ($r = .80$)	Roughness: . . .
	Roughness: . . .	Breathiness: . . .
4	Breathiness: D_1 ($r = .81$)	Roughness: D_1 ($r = .73$), D_2 ($r = .67$)
	Roughness: . . .	Breathiness: . . .
5	Breathiness: . . .	Roughness: . . .
	Roughness: . . .	Breathiness: D_2 ($r = .81$)
6	Breathiness: D_1 ($r = .94$)	Roughness: D_1 ($r = .80$)
	Roughness: . . .	Breathiness: . . .
7	Breathiness: D_1 ($r = .82$)	Roughness: D_1 ($r = .92$)
	Roughness: . . .	Breathiness: D_2 ($r = .69$)
8	Breathiness: D_1 ($r = .84$)	Roughness: D_1 ($r = .74$)
	Roughness: . . .	Breathiness: D_2 ($r = .83$)

with D_1 in the breathiness space and were not correlated with any dimensions in the roughness space. This finding is consistent with the relatively high levels of interrater reliability reported above for breathiness ratings.

In contrast, listeners differed considerably in the way they focused their attention while judging vocal roughness. As Table 6 shows, across listeners EAI ratings were correlated with a variety of perceptual dimensions, suggesting listeners varied considerably in the perceptual strategy they applied to the EAI task. Recall that D_1 in the roughness space and D_2 in the breathiness space were both correlated primarily with vocal shimmer; roughness D_1 was also correlated with H_1–H_2, and breathiness D_2 with F_0. Thus, listeners whose EAI ratings are correlated with D_1 in the roughness space apparently attended to simultaneous breathiness when judging roughness; those whose ratings correlated primarily with D_2 in the breathiness space attended to F_0 rather than to breathiness.

Interrater reliability for the roughness ratings varied significantly with apparent perceptual strategy. EAI ratings for listeners who apparently shared no inferred perceptual features (e.g., Listeners 1 and 3; Listeners 2 and 4) were poorly correlated (average Pearson's $r = .35$; $SD = .15$). Ratings for listeners whose inferred perceptual strategies had one feature in common (e.g., Listeners 1 and 4; Listeners 2 and 7) were better correlated (mean Pearson's $r = .64$; $SD = .12$). Listeners whose EAI ratings were correlated with two dimensions in the perceptual spaces (e.g.,

Listeners 1 and 7, Listeners 7 and 8) had the highest levels of interrater reliability (mean Pearson's $r = .73$; SD $= .08$). A one-way ANOVA comparing Pearson's r values for these three groups of subjects showed a significant effect of inferred perceptual strategy on interrater agreement [$F_{2,25} = 17.98$, $p < .01$]. Scheffé post hoc comparisons showed that listeners who shared one or two perceptual features agreed significantly better than those who shared no features. No difference was found between pairs of listeners sharing one or two features, possibly because of the small number of listeners in the latter group. These findings suggest that differences among listeners in how they focus attention on the different facets of vocal roughness are a significant cause of interrater unreliability.

GENERAL DISCUSSION

The limits of multidimensional scaling spaces as perceptual models are well known and have been discussed elsewhere (e.g., Yost, 1989). Furthermore, the present study used a relatively small set of male voices and a limited number of listeners. The perceptual features of female voices may differ significantly from those found for males, and interactions between listeners and speaker sex may occur (e.g., Batstone & Tuomi, 1981).

Nevertheless, our findings suggest that breathiness and roughness are related, multidimensional constructs. Most of the multidimensional information available from dissimilarity ratings was captured by the two sets of EAI ratings; however, EAI ratings of breathiness and roughness were both necessary to describe patterns of similarity with respect to either quality. Listeners differed in the relative importance given to different aspects of vocal quality, particularly when judging roughness. Simultaneous roughness did not appear to influence raters' judgments of breathiness; however, judgments of roughness were heavily influenced by degree of breathiness, the particular nature of the influence varying from listener to listener. Differential attention to different aspects of a quality is apparently a significant source of interrater unreliability in ratings of pathological voices.

This study indicates how traditional rating methods and scales may incorporate unsuspected sources of error. Problems of reliability have long plagued ratings of voice quality. We have previously argued that a significant portion of this unreliability in fact represents regular, predictable variability due to context effects, differences among listeners in background and perceptual strategy, characteristics of the task used to gather ratings, and interactions among these factors (Kreiman et al., 1993). The present results confirm the importance of differences among listeners in modeling voice perception. These differences range from dramatic (e.g., using unrelated perceptual strategies) to subtle (e.g., using continuous versus categorical dimensions for similar "features"). Listeners who differ more from one another agree less in their ratings; and listeners who differ less agree better.

Thus, it appears that the multidimensional nature of the acoustic voice signal greatly influences unidimensional ratings of voice quality. Our results strongly suggest that a given vocal quality cannot be evaluated reliably out of the context of other qualities a voice may possess. However, it may be possible to develop voice rating protocols that control this source of variability. A recent study (Gerratt et al., 1993) used an "anchored" EAI scale for vocal roughness, where each scale point was explicitly represented by a voice demonstrating that magnitude of vocal roughness. By fixing listener attention on a single dimension of roughness, this protocol produced significant improvements in interrater reliability relative to unanchored ratings. Such protocols may increase the likelihood that listeners will use similar perceptual strategies when judging a particular dimension.

The present study also highlights the need for more extensive, systematic investigation of the perceptual attributes of pathological voices and of the relationships among traditional terms for voice. The issues of what qualities are perceptually real and perceptually independent have been too long ignored in a field that is founded largely on perception (e.g., Jensen, 1965; Kreiman et al., 1993). Rating protocols that reflect the natural perceptual categories inherent in the population to be rated should be easier to use, more valid, and more reliable than those using arbitrary labels and categories whose meaning is questionable. Increased attention to these matters will benefit both research and clinical practice.

REFERENCES

Arends, N., Povel, D-J., Os, E. van, & Speth, L. (1990). Predicting voice quality of deaf speakers on the basis of glottal characteristics. *Journal of Speech and Hearing Research, 33,* 116–122.

Arnold, K.S., & Emanuel, F. (1979). Spectral noise levels and roughness severity ratings for vowels produced by male children. *Journal of Speech and Hearing Research, 22,* 613–626.

Batstone, S., & Tuomi, S.K. (1981). Perceptual characteristics of female voices. *Language and Speech, 24,* 111–123.

Berk, R. (1979). Generalizability of behavioral observations: A clarification of interobserver agreement and interobserver reliability. *American Journal of Mental Deficiency, 83,* 460–472.

Bickley, C. (1982). Acoustic analysis and perception of breathy vowels. *MIT., R.L.E. Speech Communications Group: Working Papers, 1,* 71–82.

Coleman, R.F. (1969). Effect of median frequency levels upon the roughness of jittered stimuli. *Journal of Speech and Hearing Research, 12,* 330–336.

Cullinan, W.L., Prather, E.M., & Williams, D.E. (1963). Comparison of procedures for scaling severity of stuttering. *Journal of Speech and Hearing Research, 6,* 187–194.
Darley, F., Aronson, A., & Brown, J. (1969). Differential diagnostic patterns of dysarthria. *Journal of Speech and Hearing Research, 12,* 246–269.
Ebel, R. (1951). Estimation of the reliability of ratings. *Psychometrica, 16,* 407–424.
Fairbanks, G. (1960). *Voice and articulation drillbook.* New York: Harper & Row.
Fritzell, B., Hammarberg, B., Gauffin, J., Karlsson, I., & Sundberg, J. (1986). Breathiness and insufficient vocal fold closure. *Journal of Phonetics, 14,* 549–553.
Gerratt, B.R., Kreiman, J., Antonanzas-Barroso, N., & Berke, G.S. (1993). Comparing internal and external standards in voice quality judgments. *Journal of Speech and Hearing Research, 36,* 14–20.
Hammarberg, B., Fritzell, B., Gauffin, J., Sundberg, J., & Wedin, L. (1980). Perceptual and acoustic correlates of abnormal voice qualities. *Acta Oto-laryngologica, 90,* 441–451.
Hirano, M. (1981). *Clinical examination of voice.* Vienna: Springer.
Isshiki, N., Okamura, H., Tanabe, M., & Morimoto, M. (1969). Differential diagnosis of hoarseness. *Folia Phoniatrica, 21,* 9–19.
Isshiki, N., & Takeuchi, Y. (1970). Factor analysis of hoarseness. *Studia Phonologica, 5,* 37–44.
Jensen, P.J. (1965, December). Adequacy of terminology for clinical judgment of voice quality deviation. *Eye, Ear, Nose and Throat Monthly, 44,* 77–82.
Kempster, G.B., Kistler, D.J., & Hillenbrand, J. (1991). Multidimensional scaling analysis of dysphonia in two speaker groups. *Journal of Speech and Hearing Research, 34,* 534–543.
Klich, R.J. (1982). Relationships of vowel characteristics to listener ratings of breathiness. *Journal of Speech and Hearing Research, 25,* 574–580.
Kreiman, J., Gerratt, B., Kempster, G., Erman, A., & Berke, G. (1993). Perceptual evaluation of voice quality: Review, tutorial, and a framework for future research. *Journal of Speech and Hearing Research, 36,* 21–40.
Kreiman, J., Gerratt, B.R., & Precoda, K. (1990). Listener experience and perception of voice quality. *Journal of Speech and Hearing Research, 33,* 103–115.
Kreiman, J., Gerratt, B.R., Precoda, K., & Berke, G.S. (1992). Individual differences in voice quality perception. *Journal of Speech and Hearing Research, 35,* 512–520.
Kruskal, J., & Wish, M. (1978). *Multidimensional scaling.* Sage University Series on Quantitative Applications in the Social Sciences No. 07-011. Beverly Hills, CA: Sage Publications.
Ladefoged, P. (1981). *The relative nature of voice quality.* Paper presented at the 101st Meeting of the Acoustical Society of America. Ottawa, Ontario.
Ladefoged, P., Maddieson, I., & Jackson, M. (1988). Investigating phonation types in different languages. In O. Fujimura (Ed.), *Vocal fold physiology: Voice production, mechanisms and functions* (pp. 297–317). New York: Raven Press.
Laver, J. (1980). *The phonetic description of voice quality.* Cambridge, England: Cambridge University Press.
Laver, J. (1981). The analysis of vocal quality: From the classical period to the 20th century. In R. Asher & E. Henderson (Eds.), *Toward a history of phonetics* (pp. 79–99). Edinburgh: University of Edinburgh Press.
Lively, M., & Emanuel, F. (1970). Spectral noise levels and roughness severity ratings for normal and simulated rough vowels produced by adult females. *Journal of Speech and Hearing Research, 13,* 503–517.

Murry, T., Singh, S., & Sargent, M. (1977). Multidimensional classification of abnormal voice qualities. *Journal of the Acoustical Society of America, 61*, 1630–1635.

Nieboer, G.L., De Graaf, T., & Schutte, H.K. (1988). Esophageal voice quality judgments by means of the semantic differential. *Journal of Phonetics, 16*, 417–436.

Reed, C.G. (1980). Voice therapy: A need for research. *Journal of Speech and Hearing Disorders, 45*, 157–189.

Sansone, F., Jr., & Emanuel, F. (1970). Spectral noise levels and roughness severity ratings for normal and simulated rough vowels produced by adult males. *Journal of Speech and Hearing Research, 13*, 489–502.

Sapir, S., & Aronson, A.E. (1985). Clinician reliability in rating voice improvement after laryngeal nerve section for spastic dysphonia. *Laryngoscope, 95*, 200–202.

SAS Institute, Inc. (1992). The MDS procedure. In SAS Tech. Rep. P-229, SAS/STAT Software: Changes and Enhancements, Release 6.07 (pp. 251–286). Cary, NC: SAS Institute, Inc.

Schiffman, S., Reynolds, M., & Young, F. (1981). *Introduction to multidimensional scaling: Theory, method, and applications.* New York: Academic Press.

Shipp, T., & Huntington, D. (1965). Some acoustic and perceptual factors in acute-laryngitic hoarseness. *Journal of Speech and Hearing Disorders, 30*, 350–359.

Shrout, P., & Fleiss, J. (1979). Intraclass correlations: Uses in assessing rater reliability. *Psychological Bulletin, 86*, 420–428.

Takahashi, H., & Koike, Y. (1975). Some perceptual dimensions and acoustic correlates of pathological voices. *Acta Oto-laryngologica, Supplement, 338*, 2–24.

Titze, I., Horii, Y., & Scherer, R.C. (1987). Some technical considerations in voice perturbation measurements. *Journal of Speech and Hearing Research, 30*, 252–260.

Wendahl, R. (1966). Some parameters of auditory roughness. *Folia Phoniatrica, 18*, 26–32.

Whitehead, R.L., & Emanuel, F.W. (1974). Some spectrographic and perceptual features of vocal fry, abnormally rough, and modal register vowel phonations. *Journal of Communication Disorders, 1*, 305–319.

Wolfe, V., & Steinfatt, T.M. (1987). Prediction of vocal severity within and across voice types. *Journal of Speech and Hearing Research, 30*, 230–240.

Yanagihara, N. (1967). Hoarseness: Investigation of the physiological mechanisms. *Annals of Otology, Rhinology and Laryngology, 76*, 472–488.

Yost, W.A. (Ed.). (1989). *Classification of complex nonspeech sounds.* Washington, DC: National Academy of Sciences Press.

Yumoto, E., Gould, W.J., & Baer, T. (1982). Harmonics-to-noise ratio as an index of the degree of hoarseness. *Journal of the Acoustical Society of America, 71*, 1544–1550.

Yumoto, E., Sasaki, Y., & Okamura, H. (1984). Harmonics-to-noise ratio and psychophysical measurement of the degree of hoarseness. *Journal of Speech and Hearing Research, 27*, 2–6.

Chapter 8

Reliability of Auditory–Perceptual Scaling of Dysarthria

Joslin Zeplin and Ray D. Kent

PERHAPS THE SINGLE most important contribution to the study of the dysarthrias was the identification of deviant perceptual dimensions by Darley, Aronson, and Brown (1969a, 1969b, 1975b). This work demonstrated that major forms of dysarthria could be distinguished by their auditory–perceptual characteristics and that, therefore, the nature of the speech disturbances could be used to infer site of lesion. The conclusions reached by Darley et al. are central to many contemporary descriptions of dysarthria and undergird one of the most comprehensive and popular systems of dysarthria classification. Moreover, the Darley et al. work has been cited as one of the most comprehensive systems of auditory–perceptual rating in the field of speech pathology (Gelfer, 1988).

In possibly the only published replication of the perceptual scaling studies of Darley et al., Zyski and Weisiger (1987) obtained ratings of dysarthric speech using recorded samples of dysarthria prepared by Darley et al. (1975a). The purpose of the replication was to determine the accuracy with which type of dysarthria could be classified by three groups of listeners who varied in experience. However, it should be noted that Zyski and Weisiger's procedures differed somewhat from those used by Darley et al. In the original study of Darley et al., the judges rated all perceptual dimensions, but, in the Zyski and Weisiger study, the judges rated only the most deviant dimensions. Zyski and Weisiger's results for the most clini-

---

This work was supported in part by National Institutes of Health research grant DC00319 from the National Institute on Deafness and Other Communication Disorders. It was also supported by a grant from the Trewartha Honors Undergraduate Research Fund, University of Wisconsin–Madison.

We thank the judges for their participation in the lengthy perceptual rating task.

cally experienced group are of special note. These individuals were 17 speech-language pathologists who had at least 5 years of clinical experience and who routinely diagnosed and treated persons with dysarthria. The accuracy of these 17 clinicians in identifying type of dysarthria from 28 recorded samples was 19% overall, ranging from a low of 1% for flaccid dysarthria to 55% for hypokinetic dysarthria. It is interesting that another group of subjects, graduate students who received 5 hours of classroom training on the perceptual evaluation of dysarthria, achieved an overall accuracy of 56%, or nearly three times better than the experienced clinicians. The superior performance of the graduate student group may have occurred because they were trained with the Audio Seminars materials used in the research study. Zyski and Weisiger concluded that the Mayo Clinic rating system was not sufficiently reliable for clinical purposes. This is a serious negative judgment for a classification system that is arguably the most widely used in the United States.

It appears that perceptual ratings continue to underlie the prevailing systems for clinical categorization and rating of severity of dysarthria (Collins, 1984; Enderby, 1980; Gerratt, Till, Rosenbek, Wertz, & Boysen, 1991). Perceptual ratings remain popular partly because alternative approaches, such as physiologic and acoustic methods, can be expensive, require specialized training, and may have limited application. In addition, the instrumental methods are themselves often validated against perceptual ratings of some kind. It is therefore difficult to avoid perceptual ratings of disordered speech as a primary, if not *the* primary, clinical evaluation. The importance of perceptual clinical evaluation does not necessarily rest on the need to infer site of lesion. In fact, rapid advances in brain imaging systems and other diagnostic tools may very well eclipse perceptual evaluation as a major source of information in this arena. However, perceptual evaluation continues to be essential to describe the nature of speech disorders and for the quantitation of change in speech performance as the result of management or altered status of the underlying disease. For both the layperson and the clinical specialist, the essence of speech is what we hear. If a person "sounds better" after therapeutic management, both client and clinician are likely to be satisfied, no matter what instrumental measures might reveal.

Given the continued importance of perceptual ratings, and given the discouraging replication reported by Zyski and Weisiger (1987), this study was designed to replicate some aspects of Darley et al.'s perceptual rating system for dysarthria. This study followed Zyski and Weisiger in using dysarthria samples from Darley et al. (1975a). However, unlike Zyski and Weisiger, the present investigation used a procedure more like that originally used by Darley et al.—the judges rated *all* perceptual dimensions, not just the most deviant, as done by the judges in the Zyski and Weisiger study. This report focuses on issues of reliability of perceptual scaling across six types of dysarthria.

METHODS

Recorded Samples of Dysarthric Speech

The dysarthric samples rated by the judges were obtained from the work of Darley et al. (1975a). These tapes contain samples of dysarthric speech selected from the original 212 speakers who were rated by Darley et al. (1969a, 1969b). The taped samples include 4–12 patients in each of seven categories: bulbar palsy (flaccid), pseudobulbar palsy (spastic), ataxic, hypokinetic, hyperkinetic chorea, hyperkinetic dystonia, and mixed (amyotrophic lateral sclerosis) [ALS]). The speaking tasks included syllable repetition, passage reading, and vowel prolongations. The passage reading ("Grandfather Passage") and syllable repetitions were selected for the present study because these tasks were present for most speakers on the tapes and because these tasks often are used in clinical assessment. The experimental tapes consisted of five dysarthric subjects in each category for a total of 35 speakers. The tape-recorded samples were digitized and then arranged on a stimulus tape in which speech samples were separated by a 7-second interval. Speakers were blindly numbered for identification and randomized in their order of appearance on both the reading passage and the syllable repetitions.

Subjects

The judges were selected from volunteers who responded to an announcement. Of the five judges, two were graduate students in the last year of a 2-year master's degree program who had taken a course in dysarthria. The three other judges were doctoral students, all of whom had had at least 1 year of clinical experience with dysarthric clients.

Rating Procedure

Judges were given a general description of the study, a copy of the definitions of the 38 dimensions used in the Darley et al. (1969a, 1969b) study, and an opportunity to ask questions about the procedure.

All perceptual dimensions but two were rated on a 7-point equal-appearing interval scale on which 1 represents normal speech and 7 represents a very severe deviation from normal speech. This rating scale replicates that used by Darley et al. The two dimensions of pitch and loudness level were scaled differently. For these two dimensions, speech could vary between bipolar extremes (low and high pitch; soft and loud level). Therefore, for ratings of these two dimensions, a value of 4 represented normal speech and the values of 1 and 7 represented deviations. The judges first heard the syllable repetition tape and later the reading passage. They were allowed as many replays as desired in performing their ratings.

RESULTS

Intrajudge and Interjudge Reliability

Intrajudge reliability was estimated by obtaining two sets of ratings for one speaker drawn by chance from each dysarthric category (a total of seven speakers). Discrepancy scores were determined for the replicate judgments (38 dimensions × 7 speakers × 5 judges × 2 speaking tasks). Table 1 summarizes the results for the passage-reading task. For each type of dysarthria, at least 33 of the rated dimensions had mean absolute discrepancy scores of 1 or less. A total of 24 Speaker × Dimension discrepancy scores were greater than 1. Of these, only eight exceeded a value of 2. Generally, then, the judges repeated their ratings reasonably well for the seven replicate speakers. The majority of dimensions were rescaled within 1 unit of the rating scale.

Interjudge reliability was estimated from standard deviations computed for the five judges's ratings of each dimension for each dysarthric speaker. A standard deviation of 1.0 was selected as a cutoff to distinguish the most reliable ratings, and a standard deviation of 2.0 was selected to distinguish the least reliable ratings. Table 2 summarizes the results for the passage-reading task. Across types of dysarthria, about half of the standard deviations were less than 1.0, and the great majority were less than 2.0. These results are interpreted to indicate a satisfactory interjudge reliability, especially given the large number of dimensions that were scaled. However, the interjudge reliability is not as high as might be desired for all dimensions. Among the dimensions that frequently appeared in the 10 most deviant, consistently small standard deviations were observed for imprecise consonants, pitch level, and fast rate.

Table 1. Summary of mean discrepancy scores used to estimate intrajudge reliability

	Discrepancy score	
Type of dysarthria	< 1	> 1
Flaccid	34	4
Spastic	38	0
Ataxic	37	1
Hypokinetic	34	4
Hyperkinetic (chorea)	33	5
Hyperkinetic (dystonia)	33	5
Mixed (ALS)	33	5

Table 2. Interjudge reliability: Percentages of standard deviations of judges' ratings that were less than 1.0 or greater than 2.0

Type of dysarthria	Standard deviation	
	< 1.0 (%)	> 2.0 (%)
Flaccid	44	8
Spastic	60	4
Ataxic	56	6
Hypokinetic	57	3
Hyperkinetic (chorea)	38	5
Hyperkinetic (dystonia)	42	8
Mixed (ALS)	32	19

Shared Deviant Dimensions Across Studies and Tasks

Two general comparisons are of primary interest. The first is a comparison of the ratings of the present study with those of Darley et al. (1969a, 1969b). For each type of dysarthria, a comparison was made of the 10 most deviant dimensions in the two studies, using the passage-reading task from the present investigation. Dimensions that appeared in the 10 most deviant dimensions listed in both studies are printed in bold in Table 3 (the dimensions listed for each type of dysarthria are ranked according to severity in the passage-reading task of the present study). These will be referred to as "shared deviant dimensions" (SDDs). The number of SDDs varied with type of dysarthria, ranging from four for ataxic dysarthria to seven for the mixed dysarthria in ALS. Across types of dysarthria, the dimensions most likely to be listed as SDDs are monopitch, monoloudness, imprecise consonants, breathy continuous voice, reduced (excess and equal) stress, and fast/slow rate. Some dimensions that tended to be rated highly deviant in the present study never appeared among the 10 most deviant dimensions listed in Darley et al. For example, *bizarreness* appeared in the 10 most deviant dimensions listed for all but one form of dysarthria in the present study but never appeared in Darley et al.'s study.

The second general comparison is between the two results for the two speaking tasks in the present study—syllable repetition versus passage reading. For this comparison, the SDDs are italicized in Table 3. The number of SDDs varied from five to seven across types of dysarthria. Of particular interest are the dysarthrias for which the top five ranked dimensions are the same for the contextual and syllable-repetition tasks. Only the two types of hyperkinetic dysarthria met this criterion.

DISCUSSION

A perceptual rating scale should, at the minimum, be characterized by 1) low intrajudge and interjudge variance and 2) high interspeaker vari-

Table 3. Shared deviant dimensions for seven types of dysarthria

FLACCID DYSARTHRIA
1. Pitch level
2. **Audible inspiration**
3. Bizarreness
4. **Imprecise consonants**
5. **Hypernasality**
6. **Breathy continuous voice**
7. **Phrases short**
8. Intelligibility overall
9. **Nasal emission**
10. Forced inspiration

SPASTIC DYSARTHRIA
1. **Monoloudness**
2. **Monopitch**
3. Loudness
4. **Pitch level**
5. Voice tremor
6. **Reduced stress (excess and equal)**
7. **Slow rate**
8. Strained–strangled
9. **Harsh voice**
10. Bizarreness

ATAXIC DYSARTHRIA
1. **Monoloudness**
2. **Monopitch**
3. Pitch level
4. **Imprecise consonants**
5. Loudness
6. **Reduced stress (excess and equal)**
7. Bizarreness
8. Intelligibility overall
9. Hypernasality
10. Fast rate

HYPOKINETIC DYSARTHRIA
1. **Monopitch**
2. **Monoloudness**
3. **Pitch level**
4. **Fast rate/short rushes**
5. Loudness
6. Increased rate in sequence
7. **Breathy continuous voice**
8. Audible inspiration
9. Phrases short
10. Excess/equal stress

HYPERKINETIC WITH CHOREA
1. Slow rate
2. **Imprecise consonants**
3. **Loudness**
4. Intelligibility overall
5. Bizarreness
6. Pitch level
7. **Intervals prolonged**
8. Reduced stress
9. **Inappropriate silences**
10. Voice tremor

HYPERKINETIC WITH DYSTONIA
1. Bizarreness
2. **Strained–strangled**
3. **Imprecise consonants**
4. Intelligibility overall
5. Loudness
6. Voice stoppages
7. Pitch level
8. Pitch breaks
9. **Irregular articulatory breakdown**
10. Voice tremor

MIXED (ALS)
1. **Imprecise consonants**
2. *Intelligibility overall*
3. Bizarreness
4. **Monopitch**
5. **Monoloudness**
6. **Hypernasality**
7. **Reduced stress (excess and equal)**
8. **Distorted vowels**
9. **Slow rate**
10. Loudness

Rank order reflects results for passage-reading task of present study. Dimensions printed in bold were common to the 10 most deviant dimensions in the present study (passage-reading task) and to those reported by Darley et al. (1969a, 1969b). Dimensions printed in italic were common to the 10 most deviant dimensions in the passage-reading task and syllable-repetition task in the present study.

ance for clinical samples (Dejonckere, Obbens, de Moor, & Wieneke, 1993). The perceptual dimensions proposed by Darley et al. appear to have the potential to meet these criteria, especially if the total set of dimensions is pruned to eliminate unreliable or undiscriminating dimensions. Unfortunately, very little is known about the pychometric properties of the various dimensions that constitute the Mayo Clinic rating system. An additional complication is that the dimensions are not uniformly applicable across types of dysarthria.

It is noteworthy that the five most deviant dimensions in the passage-reading task of the present study were almost entirely cross-listed with either the 10 most deviant dimensions in the syllable-repetition task of the present study or the 10 most deviant dimensions of the Darley et al. (1969a, 1969b) study. The shared appearance of these dimensions is one indication of validity. Those dimensions that appeared in the top 10 ranks for each form of dysarthria for both tasks of the present study and in the Darley et al. work may carry particular salience for perceptual classification across judges and speaking tasks. These features should define the perceptual essence of each dysarthric type (but they will not necessarily differentiate among types). The dimensions that held top-10 ranking in all three analyses are listed as the core features in Table 4.

The role of other perceptual dimensions could then be analyzed according to variables such as speaking task. Examples of the structure of perceptual features for the seven types of dysarthria are given in Table 4. These analyses are intended primarily to show the kind of analysis that could be undertaken. Confident identification of the features in each category awaits data from a larger sample of subjects and different speaking tasks.

A variety of factors could account for differences between the present results and those of Darley et al. (1969a, 1969b), and it is not possible to weigh their relative influence with the available information. First, the present results are based on only a subset of the subjects used by Darley et al. in their original ratings of dysarthria. Possibly, the speakers on the tapes, although selected by Darley et al., are not always representative of the larger subject groups from which they were derived. One example of this possibility is the rating of ataxic subjects as having fast rather than slow speech, contrary to the results reported by Darley et al. (1969a, 1969b). In fact, some of the ataxic speakers selected for the demonstration tape did have a rather fast speaking rate. Second, the judges in the present study had less experience with the scaling procedure than did Darley et al. Moreover, it is possible that the Mayo Clinic investigators consulted with one another in development of the rating scale dimensions and thereby achieved a degree of perceptual scaling uniformity that might not have been achieved by our listeners. Third, the judges in the present study may

Table 4. Structure of perceptual features for seven types of dysarthria

Dysarthria	Core features	Features for passage reading
Flaccid	Imprecise consonants Hypernasality Breathy continuous voice	Audible inspiration Short phrases Nasal emission
Spastic	Pitch level Reduced stress Slow rate	Monoloudness Monopitch Harsh voice
Ataxic	Imprecise consonants Reduced stress	Monoloudness Monopitch
Hypokinetic	Pitch level Fast rate/short rushes Breathy continuous voice	Monopitch Monoloudness
Hyperkinetic (chorea)	Imprecise consonants Loudness	Intervals prolonged Inappropriate silences
Hyperkinetic (dystonia)	Strained–strangled Imprecise consonants Irregular articulatory breakdown	
Mixed (ALS)	Imprecise consonants Reduced stress Distorted vowels Slow rate	Monopitch Monoloudness Hypernasality

Core features tend to occur across speaking tasks; features for passage reading are likely to occur in contextual speech, such as reading or conversation.

have interpreted some of the definitions of the dimensions differently from what was intended by Darley et al. One example may be the high ratings given by our judges to the dimension of bizarreness, which was seldom rated highly by Darley et al.

It is not surprising that some differences in the highest ranked dimensions should occur between the two tasks of passage reading and syllable repetition. For example, monopitch and monoloudness were the two most highly rated dimensions for passage reading by subjects with hypokinetic (parkinsonian) dysarthria, ataxic dysarthria, and spastic dysarthria, but neither dimension occurred in the 10 most severe dimensions for the syllable-repetition task by the same subjects. This result most likely is explained by the prosodic differences between the two tasks. Syllable repetition has little prosodic variation, so monoloudness and monopitch are not likely to be identified. Not so easily explained were the results for spastic dysarthria, in which intelligibility and imprecise consonants were the two most deviant dimensions for the syllable-repetition task, but neither was ranked in the 10 most deviant dimensions for passage reading. This result is particularly puzzling because imprecise consonants was a dimension with a high interjudge reliability and, for some other types of dysarthria, a good correspondence between the two tasks.

These results hold implications for the continued development of auditory–perceptual scaling of the dysarthrias. The challenge in perceptual ratings of dysarthria is very similar to that in perceptual ratings of voice disorder. A solution in the latter area was proposed by Kreiman, Gerratt, Kempster, Erman, & Berke (1993): "Variability in voice quality ratings might be reduced by replacing listeners' idiosyncratic, unstable, internal standards with fixed external standards for 'reference voices' for different vocal qualities" (p. 33). The tape by Darley et al. (1975a) and its successor (Aronson, 1993) give us "reference voices" for selected classifications of dysarthria. Because speech-language clinicians assess motor speech disorders primarily—and often exclusively—by perceptual methods, audiotaped and videotaped references are needed to standardize the rating and classification of the dysarthrias. In addition, attempts to correlate acoustic or physiologic measures of dysarthric speech with perceptual ratings assume that the latter are valid and reliable. It does not appear that this assumption can be safely made in all situations. Therefore, studies that compare perceptual ratings with other kinds of measures should demonstrate that the perceptual values have adequate reliability.

CONCLUSIONS

This study demonstrated that, for most of the perceptual dimensions evaluated, listeners were able to assign ratings to samples of dysarthric speech that were fairly repeatable. However, the dimensions differed in the degree of both intrarater and interrater agreement. These differences warrant careful study in future research to determine if some dimensions are preferable to others by a reliability criterion. In a comparison of the 10 most deviant dimensions for each type of dysarthria, there were only general similarities between the present results and those of Darley et al. (1969a, 1969b). Although some dimensions were shared, notable differences also were observed. It is not possible to determine the source of differences in the two sets of data, but both speaker and rater variables likely were primary factors.

REFERENCES

Aronson, A.E. (1993). *Dysarthria: Differential diagnosis* [audiotape]. Rochester, MN: Mentor Seminars.

Collins, M. (1984). Integrating perceptual and instrumental procedures in dysarthria assessment. *Communicative Disorders, 9,* 159–170.

Darley, F.L., Aronson, A.E., & Brown, J.R. (1969a). Clusters of deviant speech dimensions in the dysarthrias. *Journal of Speech and Hearing Research, 12,* 462–496.
Darley, F.L., Aronson, A.E., & Brown, J.R. (1969b). Differential diagnostic patterns of dysarthria. *Journal of Speech and Hearing Research, 12,* 246–269.
Darley, F.L., Aronson, A.E., & Brown, J.R. (1975a). *Audio seminars in speech pathology: Motor speech disorders.* Philadelphia: W.B. Saunders.
Darley, F.L., Aronson, A.E., & Brown, J.R. (1975b). *Motor speech disorders.* Philadelphia: W.B. Saunders.
Dejonckere, P.H., Obbens, C., de Moor, G.M., & Wieneke, G.H. (1993). Perceptual evaluation of dysphonia: Reliability and relevance. *Folia Phoniatrica, 45,* 76–83.
Enderby, P. (1980). Frenchay dysarthria assessment. *British Journal of Disorders of Communication, 15,* 165–173.
Gelfer, M.P. (1988). Perceptual attributes of voice: Development and use of rating scales. *Journal of Voice, 2,* 320–326.
Gerratt, B.R., Till, J.A., Rosenbek, J.C., Wertz, R.T., & Boysen, A.E. (1991). Use and perceived value of perceptual and instrumental measures in dysarthria management. In C.A. Moore, K.M. Yorkston & D.R. Beukelman (Eds.), *Dysarthria and apraxia of speech: Perspectives on management* (pp. 77–93). Baltimore: Paul H. Brookes Publishing Co.
Kreiman, J., Gerratt, B.R., Kempster, G.B., Erman, A., & Berke, G.S. (1993). Perceptual evaluation of voice quality: Review, tutorial, and a framework for future research. *Journal of Speech and Hearing Research, 36,* 21–40.
Zyski, B.J., & Weisiger, B.E. (1987). Identification of dysarthria types based on perceptual analysis. *Journal of Communication Disorders, 20,* 367–378.

Chapter 9

Prosodic Assessment of Dysarthria
Effects of Sampling Task and Issues of Variability

Anja Leuschel and Gerard J. Docherty

THE LITERATURE ADDRESSING the role of prosody in speech intelligibility has gradually increased over the years, but much remains to be investigated. In arguing for an increased focus on this aspect of dysarthric speech, Weismer and Martin (1992) provided an overview of this area, discussing relevant studies from the literature on synthetic speech, speech perception, and deaf speech. Huggins (1977), for example, found that the intelligibility of synthesized sentences decreases when they are produced with abnormal timing or pitch contours or both. Similar findings are discussed by Silverman (1987), who concluded that differences in intelligibility between natural and synthetic speech "can be largely accounted for by synthetic speech exhibiting inadequate prosody rather than just poor segmental quality" (p. 1.11). Research on speech perception has suggested that prosodic features are particularly important for word recognition by giving prominence to the key words in an utterance, helping to identify word boundaries, and distinguishing between new and given information (Cutler, 1994; Cutler & Foss, 1977; Cutler & Norris, 1988; Nooteboom, Brokx, & de Rooij, 1978). Any deviation from the normal prosodic pattern may have implications for this recognition process and potentially render

---

The first author has been supported by a research studentship awarded by the University of Newcastle-upon-Tyne Research Committee.

We would like to thank Nick Miller, Anne Whitworth, and participants at the Sedona Motor Speech Conference for comments on earlier versions of this chapter. Responsibility for remaining blemishes is our own.

speech less intelligible. This view is supported by the results of studies on hearing-impaired speakers. Several researchers have investigated the relationship between intelligibility and prosodic impairment in the speech of deaf persons by carrying out correlational studies to determine if the subjects' intelligibility scores could be successfully predicted by their suprasegmental characteristics (e.g., Osberger & Levitt, 1979; Parkhurst & Levitt, 1978; Smith, 1975). Although the results are not entirely consistent, the majority of the studies have found strong relationships between these two factors.

This previous literature suggests that prosody can have substantial effects on intelligibility. However, in the treatment of dysarthria, the value of adequate prosody for intelligibility has not been widely recognized. Some researchers have stressed the importance of treating prosody along with or even before articulatory impairments (Hargrove & McGarr, 1994; Robin, Klouda, & Hug, 1991; Rosenbek & LaPointe, 1985), and a small number of studies have tried to support this notion empirically by manipulating aspects of prosody in order to improve intelligibility (Berry & Goshorn, 1983; Yorkston, Hammen, Beukelman, & Traynor, 1990). However, these have focused chiefly on the reduction of speech rate using pacing techniques or pause insertion. No studies have yet investigated the effects of other prosodic factors, such as adequate stress and pause placement. The lack of research exemplifying the importance of prosody for intelligibility is somewhat reflected in those treatment materials (e.g., Robertson & Thomson, 1986) that advocate initial treatment of segmental impairments, such as vowel inaccuracy or restricted phonologic contrasts, as a means of improving intelligibility, and only address prosodic problems toward the end of the therapy program in order to increase the naturalness of speech. However, given that prosody may have substantial effects on intelligibility, it is important that prosodic aspects of speech are not neglected in the remediation of both types of deficit, segmental and suprasegmental, in dysarthria.

In order to treat prosodic impairment in dysarthria in the most effective way, it is important to have an account of the nature of the impairment. Recent years have seen an increase in the number of studies designed to investigate the prosodic characteristics of dysarthric speakers (Darkins, Fromkin, & Benson, 1988; Hertrich & Ackermann, 1993a, 1993b; Illes, Metter, Hanson, & Iritani, 1988; Kent & Rosenbek, 1982; Liss & Weismer, 1994; Ludlow & Bassich, 1983, 1984; Ludlow, Connor, & Bassick, 1987; Murry, 1983; Schlenck, Bettrich, & Willmes, 1993; Yorkston, Beukelman, Minifie, & Sapir, 1984). These studies have concentrated mainly on those types of dysarthria identified by Darley, Aronson, and Brown (1975) as being particularly prone to prosodic impairment (ataxic and hypokinetic dysarthria) in order to contrast them with each other (e.g., Ludlow & Bassich, 1983, 1984; Ludlow et al., 1987) or with other neurologic diseases that cause prosodic impairments, such as apraxia (e.g., Kent & Rosenbek, 1982). Research on the prosodic characteristics of dysarthria has primarily investigated the speakers' performance in various forms of contrastive stress drills, looking predominantly at their ability to modulate syllable or vowel duration, intensity, and fundamental frequency (F_0) between stressed and unstressed syllables. The main finding of this work is that the majority of dysarthric speakers are less efficient than normal speakers in modulating the acoustic parameters of prominence in order to achieve stress contrasts. Furthermore, it has been found that the different phonetic parameters implicated in producing stress contrasts can be affected to different degrees and that there is not necessarily any consistency across the subjects regarding which parameter is most impaired.

Although these studies provide much valuable information on certain aspects of the prosodic abilities of dysarthric speakers of different etiologies and severities, they are, in some respects, somewhat limited. First, they have investigated a restricted number of parameters. Most studies have focused on subjects' abilities to differentiate between stressed and unstressed syllables by looking at syllable duration, intensity, and F_0. There is therefore relatively little information on other prosodic parameters, such as pausing, speech rate and intensity, and F_0 modulation across whole utterances. This reflects the limited data that can be obtained from the tasks predominately used in such research (i.e., contrastive stress tasks). Some researchers have widened the scope of analysis by including other tasks, such as prolonged vowel production or response latency tasks, in the design (Ludlow & Bassich, 1983, 1984; Ludlow, Bassich, & Connor, 1985; Ludlow et al., 1987). However, except for studies by Kent and Rosenbek (1982), Schlenck et al. (1993), and Illes et al. (1988), researchers have almost exclusively investigated structured speech data, such as contrastive stress drills. This emphasis represents a second significant limitation of the research on prosodic aspects of dysarthria, in that there has been increasing evidence that it may not be possible to generalize the speech behavior in such highly structured tasks to that in more naturalistic speech situations.

Differences between various speech tasks in normal subjects have been documented as early as the 1960s, and recently researchers have started to find these differences in impaired speakers as well. Read and spontaneous speech material of normal speakers appears to differ in various prosodic aspects, such as speech rate; placement and duration of pauses (Barik, 1979; Goldman-Eisler, 1968; Grosjean & Deschamps, 1973; Levin, Schaffer, & Snow, 1982); intonation patterns; tone unit boundaries (Crystal & Davy, 1969; Howell & Kadi-Hanifi, 1991); mean F_0 and degree of F_0 variation (Graddol, 1986; Johns-Lewis, 1986); and segmental characteristics (Farnetani & Faber, 1992; Harmegnies & Poch-Olivé, 1992). In the context of impaired speech, Morrison and Shriberg (1992) argued that standard articulation test scores are not representative of the intelligibility in natural discourse of speech-delayed children. Frearson (1985) showed that the same is true for dysarthric speakers' sentence intelligibility scores, such as those from the Assessment of Intelligibility of Dysarthric Speech (AIDS) of Yorkston and Beukelman (1981). Recently, Brown and Docherty (1995) have reported differences in various prosodic features of dysarthric and normal speech depending on whether speech is sampled from a read passage or from a naturalistic conversation. A considerable amount of research has thus shown that differences exist between structured tasks such as reading aloud and more naturalistic tasks such as conversation. This means that the results gained from structured tasks might be unrepresentative of natural speech behavior and cannot be generalized without caution. The choice of sampling task therefore seems an important factor in the study of prosody in the dysarthric or any other speaker population.

The current study sets out to address some of the shortcomings of this previous research. Its aims were to investigate dysarthric and normal speakers' prosodic characteristics by measuring in naturalistic speech situations a wider range of prosodic parameters than is typically found in the literature and to compare this performance with that in the more structured tasks most commonly used in this area of research (i.e., contrastive stress drills and passage reading). Furthermore, the study compared the performance of two types of dysarthria, a hypokinetic and a mixed group of speakers as defined by Darley et al. (1975). Studies of the validity of Darley et al.'s typology have produced conflicting results. Acoustic as well as perceptual studies either confirm their categorization (Ludlow & Bassich, 1983) or find sufficient overlap in speech characteristics between different groups or differences within groups to justify questioning the utility of the etiologically based distinctions (Metter & Hanson, 1986; Portnoy & Aronson, 1982; Yorkston et al., 1984; Zyski & Weisiger, 1987). A further aim of the present study was to investigate whether two types of dysarthric speakers who, according to Darley et al.'s (1975) findings, would be predicted to have distinct prosodic profiles could be distinguished on the basis of their performance on a range of prosodic parameters.

METHODOLOGY

Subjects

Ten dysarthric and 10 control subjects were analyzed for this research. The two groups were matched for age, sex, and accent. All speakers were age 50 years or older. To ensure the absence of aphasia, apraxia, and other factors that might affect speech and language, only subjects with degenerative diseases were admitted to the research. The dysarthric group consisted of four subjects with idiopathic Parkinson's disease, three with motor neuron disease (of an amyotrophic lateral sclerosis type), and three with multiple sclerosis. Table 1 provides information on subjects' sex, age, medical diagnosis, intelligibility score, and, in the case of the parkinsonian speakers, the medication and dosage taken. Because the investigated disorders are often associated with dementia, depression, and cognitive difficulties, all subjects were screened for these problems by means of their medical notes and language testing. The parkinsonian speakers were all

Table 1. Description of subjects by clinical diagnosis, sex, age, medication for the parkinsonian speakers, and severity of dysarthria expressed in single-word intelligibility scores

Subject	Diagnosis	Sex	Age	Medication[a]	Intelligibility score (%)
PF1	Parksinson's disease	F	82	Gaviscon 10 ml tid, Madopar 125 mg 6 × day, Temazepam 10 mg nocte, Terguride 0.5 mg tid	81
PF2	Parkinson's disease	F	66	Adalat Retarde 10 mg/day, selegiline 10 mg/day, Sinemet Plus 1 qid, bromocriptine 2.5 mg bid, Dothiapen 75 mg nocte, Co-Proxamol 2 tablets nocte	56
PM1	Parkinson's disease	M	60	Sinemet Plus 8 × day, bromocriptine 10 mg bid, selegiline 5 mg bid, benzhexol hydrochloride 1 mg tid	95
PM2	Parkinson's disease	M	56	Sinemet CR 1 tablet/day, selegiline 10 mg/day, bromocriptine 2 mg nocte, 2.5 mg bid	87
MF1	Motor neuron disease	F	68		82
MF2	Motor neuron disease	F	70		79
MF3	Motor neuron disease	F	74		20
MSF1	Multiple sclerosis	F	57		71
MSM1	Multiple sclerosis	M	58		88
MSM2	Multiple sclerosis	M	65		62
			Mean: 65.5		Range: 56–95
Control subjects			Mean: 65.7		Range: 93–100

[a] bid, twice a day; tid, three times a day; qid, four times a day; nocte, at night.

recorded early in the afternoon at a time when their medication had taken its optimum effect. If the speakers experienced any "off periods" during the recording, the session was repeated at a later date. The exclusion criteria for the dysarthric group were 1) the presence of any speech and language problems other than their dysarthria, 2) the presence of any neurologic problems other than those causing the dysarthria, 3) hearing loss, 4) inadequate vision, 5) inadequate reading skills, and 6) a previous history of speech or language problems. This information was extracted from the medical notes, the notes of the speech and language therapists, and a personal interview with the subjects. All subjects were further screened for language and hearing problems during the recording session by means of a naming task and an informal hearing assessment. Only subjects with a mild to moderate dysarthria were admitted to the study, because the more severe cases were not able to perform the connected speech tasks aimed at investigating their prosodic abilities. The same exclusion criteria were applied to the nondysarthric control group.

Design

The data for analysis were obtained from four elicitation tasks: a word list, a contrastive stress task, a reading passage, and some conversation. The word list had the purpose of establishing a single-word intelligibility score that was used as a severity measure. The score was established by two listeners who were unfamiliar with the words and subjects and had no linguistic training. The word list was scored in an open response mode, following the instructions given to listeners in the AIDS (Yorkston & Beukelman, 1981). The words also provided a basis for a detailed segmental analysis of the subjects. The list was an adaptation of Kent, Netsell, and Abbs's (1989) word list. Minimal pairs for two additional phonetic contrasts were added to the list together with 14 words designed to provide a larger sample of voice onset time measurements (not reported in this paper).

The remaining tasks elicited data for the elaboration of subjects' prosodic profiles. The contrastive stress drills consisted of two subtasks, a sentence stress task and a lexical stress task (noun–verb distinctions). The latter was presented as a reading task including sentences with the target words and distracter sentences matched for length. The sentence stress task consisted of one sentence that was produced in four different versions (each word appeared once in a stressed and three times in an unstressed position). The lexical stress task included four word pairs with stress on either the first or second syllable, generating eight sentences. Both the sentence and the word pairs were adapted from the prosody section of Robertson and Thomson's (1986) dysarthria workbook and are comparable to those used in previous studies on dysarthria.

The reading passage was adapted from Beresford (1986). It consisted of a dialogue that was designed to elicit a greater variety of intonation patterns than the prose found in the "Grandfather Passage" (Darley et al., 1975). The passage was 172 syllables long and phonetically balanced by including all sounds of English: consonants, vowels, diphthongs, and various consonant clusters. All consonants occurred in initial position where appropriate, with the majority also occurring in medial and final positions.

In the conversational task, the subjects were asked to describe a recent vacation. The experimenter then started a conversation continuing on this topic. This elicited more natural data than the immediately preceding monologue task (in most cases, the subjects showed no awareness that they were still being recorded). Approximately 15 minutes of conversation were recorded for each subject. However, a section of approximately 170 syllables, comparable to the reading passage, was taken from the middle part of the conversation for the purposes of the analysis.

This paper reports the results obtained from the reading and conversation tasks.

Apparatus

The recordings were made with a Technics Portable Digital Audio Tape Recorder (model SV-260An) on Ampex 467 R-46 digital audiotapes, using a Panasonic Ramsa Condenser Microphone (model P 50). The microphone was placed on a table approximately 30 cm away from the subject. Acoustic analysis of the recordings was performed on a Kay Elemetrics Computerized Speech Laboratory (CSL) 4300, version 4.01. The signal was digitized at a sampling rate of 20 kHz (with anti-aliasing filtering), and wide-band spectrograms of the data were displayed on the monitor screen. The analysis bandwidth was varied in order to provide the clearest wide-band display for each individual subject. This had no implications for the measurements taken because they were all in the time domain. Intensity and F_0 analysis was performed with a frame length of 20 and 15 ms for male and female speakers, respectively.

Measurement Criteria

Weismer and Liss (1991) have discussed the limitations of using normal speech behavior as a basis for comparison with disordered speech—namely, that a great deal of information can be lost by restricting the analysis to features that are important for speech production in normal speakers. The following measures were devised in order to capture salient aspects of the dysarthric speakers' prosodic capabilities.

- *Articulation rate*—This measure indicated the rate of speech excluding pauses, and was calculated in syllables per minute.

- *Mean pause duration*—No minimum duration threshold was applied for pause identification, because criteria suggested by the literature have been established on the basis of normal speech data and might therefore not apply to dysarthric speech. Instead, a period of silence in the acoustic signal that was not associated with a stop closure was taken as an indicator for a pause. The data included all types of pauses, not only breath pauses. Although no threshold was applied to the data, the pause durations were comparable to the values given in the literature (Arlington, Brenninkmeyer, Arn, Grundhauser, & O'Connel, 1992; Brubaker, 1972), with a minimum value of approximately 100 ms.
- *Number of pauses*—The total number of pauses in the reading passage.
- *Articulation/pause time ratio*—This measure was obtained by calculating the percentage of the total speech time occupied by articulation and pause time.
- *Mean length of utterance*—An utterance was defined as a stretch of speech delimited by pauses. The mean length was expressed in syllables rather than words. This was necessary to be able to include unintelligible utterances into the calculation where the word boundaries could not be defined reliably.
- *Mean utterance duration*—Expressed in seconds.
- *Unstressed vowel duration*—Unstressed vowels were defined as those that had been reduced to /ə/ and /ɪ/, such as in *the* [ðə] or *because* [bɪkɔz]. No durational criteria were applied regarding their maximum length because they have been found to be prolonged in dysarthric speech in various studies (e.g., Kent & Rosenbek, 1982; Kent et al., 1979).
- *Percentage of unstressed vowel time*—This measure expresses the percentage of the whole articulation time represented by the sum of all unstressed vowel durations.
- *Intensity range*—To measure intensity, the peak intensity values were taken from each vowel. Reduced vowels were excluded from the analysis. The intensity values were normalized with a procedure adapted from Kent and Rosenbek (1983). Each utterance was treated as an entity, and all values within this utterance were normalized against the highest value on a scale of 0.5 dB. The highest value was assigned the rank 0, and all subsequent values 1 to n. The greater n was, the wider the range of intensity values in the utterance. To arrive at the range of variation for the whole passage, the mean of the highest normalized values of each utterance was calculated. Again, a greater value in this measure represented a wider range of variation in the signal.
- *Intensity envelope*—This measure was applied to investigate the amount of variation between vowels within utterances. The difference between the ranks of neighboring vowels was calculated and averaged across the

whole signal. A higher result represents a greater difference between vowels (i.e., a higher degree of intensity variation).
- F_0 *range*—Because a significant amount of F_0 modulation can take place within one vowel, it was considered unrepresentative to measure a single F_0 value. The maximum and minimum values were therefore chosen to represent the F_0 of each vowel. Although this is still not an ideal technique to measure F_0, it was considered to be the most suitable for the present analysis because it captured more information on F_0 modulation than the more commonly applied method of taking the F_0 value at the midpoint of the vowel. The data were normalized with the same procedure as for the intensity analysis but on a scale of 5 Hz.
- F_0 *envelope*—To calculate this measure, it was impractical to work with two F_0 values per vowel, and the midpoint between the minimum and maximum was used instead. The calculation of the envelope value was comparable to that for the intensity measure.
- F_0 *intravowel variation*—As mentioned above, a great deal of F_0 variation took place within one vowel. To capture this phenomenon, the intravowel variation of F_0 was additionally investigated by calculating the difference between the minimum and maximum rank values of each vowel. These differences were then averaged across the whole signal. As for the other measures, a higher value expressed a wider range of F_0 variation.
- *Mean* F_0—The mean F_0 was calculated by averaging all F_0 values measured in the signal (i.e., using both the maximum and minimum values of each vowel).

The pause measurements as well as mean length of utterance and mean utterance duration have been omitted from the analysis of the conversation data because most pauses occurred between the turns of the two speakers or when the speaker thought about the next utterance. They were therefore not comparable to those between the phrases in the reading passage.

RESULTS

The control subjects' performance was comparable to other published research findings on normal speakers of that age (Amerman & Parnell, 1990, 1992; Ramig, 1983), and their results were therefore taken as a reasonable baseline measure against which to compare the dysarthric group.

Reading Versus Conversation
First, the results are considered with respect to whether there were differences between sampling tasks and whether the dysarthric speakers showed

the same differences as the control subjects. As mentioned above, only 9 of the 14 parameters were investigated in both reading and conversation and are therefore used in the comparison.

The statistical results of the Wilcoxon test for the control group (see Table 2) show that these subjects had significantly different patterns of performance across the two sampling tasks in five out of the nine parameters measured (percentage of unstressed vowels, intensity envelope, and three F_0 measures: range, envelope, and intravowel variation). In contrast, the dysarthric group showed no significant differences in any of the parameters (see Table 2). However, differences were observed in the performance of some subjects on some parameters, although there was no consistency regarding which subjects showed differences between the tasks or which parameters were involved.

Comparison of the performance of the dysarthric and control subjects in each separate parameter also generated some interesting results (see Table 3). The differences between the two groups were of the same significance level in reading and conversation for only two parameters, articulation rate and intensity range, with all other parameters showing differences in significance level between the tasks. For two parameters (percentage of unstressed vowels and intensity envelope), the differences between the groups were significant in one task but not the other. For one parameter (mean unstressed vowel duration), on which the groups differed significantly in both tasks, the differences were significant at a higher level in one of the tasks. For the remaining five parameters, which showed no significant differences between the groups in any of the two tasks, the p values were nearer to the 5% significance level in one of the tasks. These findings suggest that the two groups differed to a greater extent from each other in one task than the other, and inspection of the results indicates that, in five of the nine parameters measured, greater differences between

Table 2. Statistical results (Wilcoxon test) for the comparison of the reading and conversation data

Parameters	p Values[a]	
	Control subjects	Dysarthric subjects
Articulation rate	.683	.683
Unstressed vowel duration	.813	.053
Unstressed vowel percentage	**.009**	.959
Intensity range	.083	.262
Intensity envelope	**.009**	.683
Mean F_0	.163	.359
F_0 range	**.014**	.477
F_0 envelope	**.033**	.093
F_0 intravowel variation	**.042**	1.000

[a]Significant results ($p < .05$) are indicated by bold type.

Table 3. Statistical results (Mann–Whitney test) for the comparison of the dysarthric and control groups for reading and conversation

Parameters	p Values[a]	
	Reading	Conversation
Articulation rate	.10	.10
Mean pause duration	.20	NA
Number of pauses	**.02**	NA
Articulation/pause time ratio	**.04**	NA
Mean length of utterance	**.007**	NA
Mean utterance duration	.55	NA
Mean unstressed vowel duration	**.009**	**.002**
Percentage of unstressed vowels	.406	**.007**
Intensity range	**.023**	**.023**
Intensity envelope	.820	**.034**
Mean F_0	.97	.39
F_0 range	.212	.678
F_0 envelope	.326	.706
F_0 intravowel variation	.850	.096

[a] Significant results ($p < .05$) are indicated by bold type.

the two groups were found in the conversational task. Only F_0 range and envelope showed greater differences in the reading task.

These results support the findings of previous studies on normal and impaired speech production (Barik, 1979; Brown & Docherty, 1995; Frearson, 1985; Goldman-Eisler, 1968; Grosjean & Deschamps, 1973; Howell & Kadi-Hanifi, 1991; Johns-Lewis, 1986; Levin et al., 1982; Morrison & Shriberg, 1992) and suggest that speech performance in a structured task such as reading, as measured by a range of prosodic parameters, may not be wholly representative of performance in a more naturalistic task such as conversation. This became evident from the fact that the control speakers exhibited differences in their speech behavior between the two tasks. This differentiation was not consistently observed in the dysarthric group. Additionally, differences were found between the performance of the two groups in each task, suggesting that the dysarthric speakers generally differ more from the control subjects in conversation than in reading. It is therefore likely that the performance of dysarthric subjects, especially those of milder severity, will fall within the normal limits in a reading assessment, and that impairments will only become evident in a conversational situation. For speakers with dysarthria of greater severity, who are different from normal subjects on both tasks, it will also be important to conduct a comparative assessment to see whether differences are present in the two tasks, and in which parameters. Results from both the present and the previous studies have therefore shown that it is important to investigate the performance of dysarthric speakers in different sorts of elicitation tasks, structured and unstructured, in order to arrive at a complete evaluation of individual patients' abilities.

Prosodic Impairment

The next results to be reported relate to the question of which prosodic parameters were impaired in the dysarthric group, and whether the two etiologically defined groups of dysarthric speakers showed different patterns of impairment. For this analysis, the dysarthric group was compared with the control group (see Table 3). In the reading task, only 5 of 14 parameters, and in conversation, only 4 of 9 parameters, showed significant differences between the two groups (i.e., less than 50% of the measures showed differences in each of the tasks). These results contradict previous research findings in which significant differences between dysarthric and control speakers have been observed in many of the param-eters investigated in this study (Illes et al., 1988; Ludlow et al., 1987; Murry, 1983; Schlenck et al., 1993). They are also not in keeping with the perceptual impression of the dysarthric group, which suggested impairments in a larger number of prosodic factors.

Visual inspection of the data revealed that, in most cases, high intersubject variability in the dysarthric group seemed to be the reason for the nonsignificant statistical results. This high amount of variability has been a common finding in the field of motor speech disorders, although it has not always been the main focus of discussion. Interspeaker variability is manifested in a high standard deviation of the group data and can account for the fact that the findings of one study differ from those of other studies, even though all other conditions, such as sampling task, measurement criteria, and severity and etiology of the subjects, are equal. Various explanations have been provided for the presence of interspeaker variability in the literature. Some investigators (Weismer & Liss, 1991; Yorkston et al., 1984) have discussed the fact that inter- and intraspeaker variability are often inherent characteristics of disordered speech and prevent any generalization being made from the results. They therefore argue against the quantification of dysarthric speech in terms of group performance. Most other researchers, however, have tried to provide explanations for the high amount of variability within their subject groups or the discrepancy of their results with other studies (Hertrich & Ackermann, 1993a; Ludlow & Bassich, 1983; Portnoy & Aronson, 1982). Etiology and severity of the subjects are commonly invoked in order to account for variability. These factors are difficult to control and are therefore likely to have affected subjects' performance. Severity, for example, can be quantified in a number of different ways, either by measuring the performance on certain speech characteristics (intelligibility score, speech rate, etc.) or by describing the clinical symptoms (e.g., degree of spasticity, tremor in Parkinson's disease). Etiology is an even more difficult factor to control. Although one clinical feature, such as spasticity, might prevail, the subjects could have another hidden component that could also affect their speech. This is especially the case with subjects who have diffuse lesions, such as a cerebrovascular accident, a head injury, or a degenerative disorder that can affect the whole nervous system (e.g., motor neuron disease or multiple sclerosis). With regard to the present subject group, differences in severity and etiology seem to be an appropriate explanation for the high degree of variability in the data. Subjects with three different kinds of etiology had been admitted to the study, and speakers with the same type of dysarthria had different single-word intelligibility scores, which were used as an index of severity. One might therefore expect every dysarthric subject to behave differently from the others as a result of differing in either the etiology or the severity of the dysarthria. However, as the following data will exemplify, neither of the two factors can fully account for the variability found in the data.

Etiology For this analysis, the dysarthric speakers were classified into two groups. In Darley et al.'s (1975) terms, they can be referred to as a hypokinetic group and a group of speakers with mixed dysarthria. The multiple sclerosis and motor neuron disease subjects were grouped together for statistical reasons. It was possible to do this because all of these speakers exhibited mainly spastic features of dysarthria, and statistical tests comparing the two groups showed no significant differences in any of the prosodic parameters investigated. According to Darley et al.'s (1975) description of the three etiologies (Parkinson's disease, amyotrophic lateral sclerosis, and multiple sclerosis), differences could be expected between the two groups in the measures of articulation rate, F_0 and intensity range, and F_0 and intensity envelope. These measures are most closely related to Darley et al.'s dimensions of rate, monopitch and loudness, and impaired pitch and loudness control. However, these differences were largely not found, with the exception of the articulation rate measure and mean unstressed vowel duration, the latter being unrelated to Darley et al.'s (1975) findings. This finding is clearly shown on the graphic representation of the data (see Figures 1–4). Figure 1 shows a clear division between the two groups. The parkinsonian speakers had significantly higher articulation rates than the speakers with a mixed type of dysarthria (reading, $p = .014$; conversation, $p = .043$). However, no division was evident in the other parameters mentioned above. The group mean and range are nearly equal for the intensity range and envelope, and only the conversational data of the F_0 envelope show small but statistically insignificant differences between the two groups. The data therefore suggest that etiologic differences cannot account entirely for the high degree of variability that has been observed within the dysarthric group.

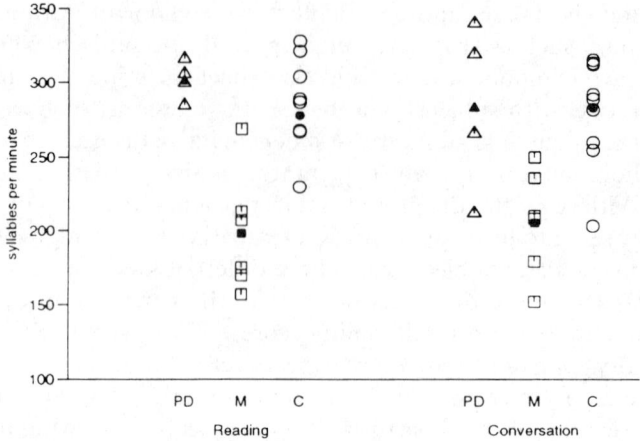

Figure 1. Articulation rate (in syllables per minute) for the parkinsonian (PD), mixed (M), and control (C) subjects in reading and conversation. Each subject is represented by one symbol; the solid symbol indicates the group mean. If fewer symbols than group members are shown, two or more subjects had the same score.

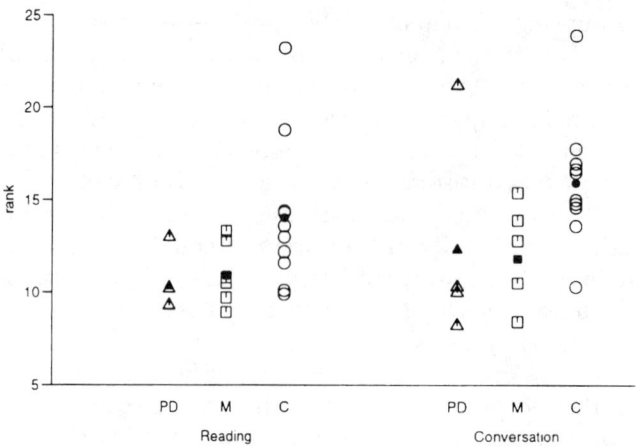

Figure 2. Range of intensity variation in ranks for the parkinsonian (PD), mixed (M), and control (C) subjects in reading and conversation. Each subject is represented by one symbol; the solid symbol indicates the group mean. If fewer symbols than group members are shown, two or more subjects had the same score.

Severity Another plausible explanatory factor for the variability in the study data is that the dysarthric speakers analyzed were impaired to different degrees of severity, as indicated by the subjects' single-word intelligibility scores. To address this point (and to avoid an interaction of etiology and severity), only the data from the parkinsonian subjects will be discussed. For the purpose of this discussion, the parameters have been grouped into four categories: speech timing (rate, pausing behavior, mean

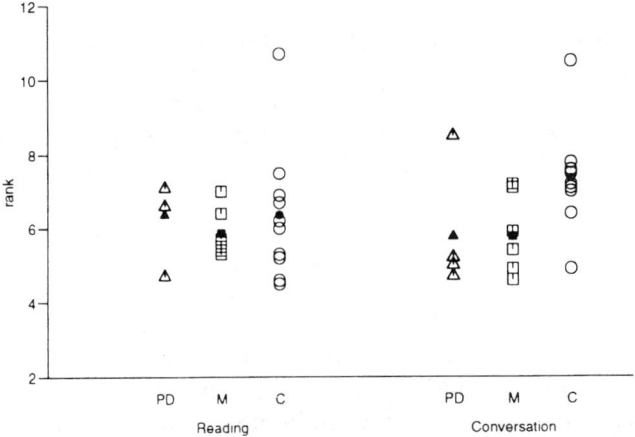

Figure 3. Intensity envelope in ranks for the parkinsonian (PD), mixed (M), and control (C) subjects in reading and conversation. Each subject is represented by one symbol; the solid symbol indicates the group mean. If fewer symbols than group members are shown, two or more subjects had the same score.

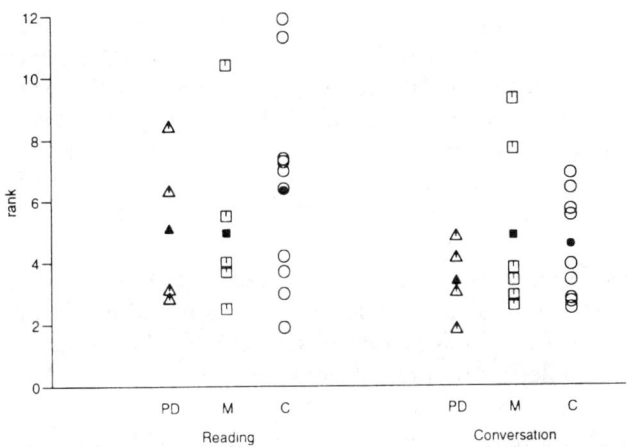

Figure 4. F_0 envelope in ranks for the parkinsonian (PD), mixed (M), and control (C) subjects in reading and conversation. Each subject is represented by one symbol; the solid symbol indicates the group mean. If fewer symbols than group members are shown, two or more subjects had the same score.

length of utterance, and mean utterance duration); segmental timing (unstressed vowel measures); intensity (range and envelope); and F_0 (mean, range, envelope, and intravowel variation). The individual results have been normalized by rank ordering the control and dysarthric subjects, in order to allow for a comparison of the parameters with one another. A rank value between 1 and 10 designates a performance within, and a value between 11 and 20 one outside, the normal range.

Table 4 shows, from left to right, the score for each category (i.e., the mean rank of all parameters subsumed within each category); the mean of all four categories; and the normalized scores for the intelligibility measure established from the word list, which has been used as a severity measure. The intelligibility scores suggest that PM1 is the least impaired subject, followed by PM2, PF1, and then PF2. If these scores are compared with the mean performance for the four categories, it is evident that the two measures are closely related to each other and consequently that overall performance on the prosodic parameters is in fact related to severity. However, the individual scores show variations in the degree of impairment of each category. This means that one cannot predict from the severity measure how much each category, and consequently each individual speech parameter, will be affected. Furthermore, the data show that there is no uniform pattern of prosodic impairment in the hypokinetic group. Not all subjects, for example, had increased speech rates or monopitch. Indeed, each of the four subjects had an individual profile of prosodic performance.

These data therefore suggest that, although severity seems to be reflected in the overall prosodic performance of subjects, no statements can be made about the degree to which different prosodic characteristics are affected. Furthermore, the data do not highlight any particular patterns of impairment for the hypokinetic group. The same would appear to be true for the other two etiologies, although no reliable statements can be made about these speakers because of the small sample size.

Summary

Although a relatively small number of subjects has been investigated, the results suggest that subjects are differentially affected in each parameter, independent of their etiology or the severity of other parameters. This generates a high degree of intersubject variability, which, perhaps not sur-

Table 4. Individual performances (expressed in ranks) of Parkinson's disease subjects on parameter groups plus mean and severity scores[a]

Subjects	Parameter groups				Mean	Severity
	Speech timing	Segmental timing	Intensity	F_0		
PF1	5	15	16	11	11.8	15
PF2	15	8	15	11	12.3	19
PM1	10	14	11	5	10.0	8.5
PM2	16	7	14	6	10.8	13

[a] Scores are rank ordering as noted in text.

[b] Parameters are grouped as follows: speech timing (articulation rate, number of pauses, mean length of utterance, mean utterance duration); segmental timing (mean unstressed vowel duration, percentage of unstressed vowels); intensity (range, envelope); and F_0 (mean, range, envelope, and intravowel variation).

prisingly, renders the statistical tests for group comparisons nonsignificant. As a result, there is no consistency regarding which parameters are affected most in the various types of dysarthria, which means that no distinctions in etiology are possible on the basis of the speakers' prosodic profiles.

DISCUSSION

As mentioned above, the issue of variability in the speech data is not often the major focus of discussion in the literature. This might seem surprising considering that, to judge from the means and standard deviations provided by most researchers, considerable interspeaker variability is always present in the data. One of the earliest investigators to discuss variability was Canter (1961). He investigated various speech characteristics of parkinsonian speakers and observed that "there was no single speech characteristic which was consistently deviant in the Parkinsonian patients" (p. 157). He therefore concluded that parkinsonian speakers did not necessarily have the same profiles and furthermore claimed that the fact that he did not observe an impairment in certain speech parameters did not mean that these parameters would never be impaired in a parkinsonian speaker. Although he did not describe his subjects individually, Canter (1961) still recognized the need to discuss the data in more detail than simply by looking at pooled group results in order to account for the variability found in the data. Lehiste (1965) also followed this approach, providing a detailed acoustic analysis of each individual investigated.

Following Darley, Aronson, and Brown's (1969a, 1969b) research, however, the study of dysarthric subjects underwent a change of focus. They proposed a list of speech characteristics that were observed to be frequently impaired in each of seven etiologic groups of dysarthric speakers and that could be used diagnostically to identify the clinical type of dysarthria. They found that "each of the seven neurologic disorders is characterized by its unique set of clusters, no two disorders having the same set" (Darley et al., 1969a, p. 465). Intersubject variability was not a major focus of their discussion, despite the fact that not every subject belonging to a particular group showed an impairment in the same dimensions and, conversely, that many speech dimensions and clusters of dimensions were found to occur across different types of dysarthria. Although a few studies provided detailed accounts of various types of dysarthria without particularly attempting to contrast the groups with each other (e.g., Kent & Rosenbek, 1982), most subsequent studies took up Darley et al.'s (1969a, 1969b) strand of investigation, and experiments were designed to empirically test their typology or to find additional characteristics of certain types of dysarthria. If the results did not confirm Darley et al.'s

(1969a, 1969b) findings, the reason was often thought to be differences in etiology or severity, as discussed above. Portnoy and Aronson (1982), for example, found considerable overlap between ataxic and spastic speakers in certain characteristics that were previously thought to appear exclusively in one or the other type. Rather than suggesting that speakers could be affected in different ways by their disorder and might show speech abnormalities mainly associated with another type of dysarthria, they tried to explain the problem by proposing that the ataxic subjects might not have been pure ataxics but may also have had a hidden spastic feature in their pathology, and vice versa.

One of the reasons that the issue of intersubject variability has been neglected in the research literature would appear to be the number of subjects included in many previous studies. Darley et al.'s (1969a, 1969b) research included approximately 30 subjects per type, and Portnoy and Aronson (1982) used a similar number for each group. With such high subject numbers, it is more likely that statistical tests will identify certain trends that characterize the different groups of dysarthric speakers and that intersubject variability will be effectively relegated to a secondary issue. Studies of smaller groups of subjects have tended to give greater attention to interspeaker variability. Yorkston et al. (1984), for example, looked at the stress production of three ataxic speakers of similar severity and found no commonalities in their patterns of production. Metter and Hanson (1986) investigated some prosodic aspects of the speech of 10 subjects with Parkinson's disease and progressive supranuclear palsy. They observed that the performance of the subjects on seven speech parameters was highly variable, noting that the performance on one parameter could not predict that on the others. Furthermore, the speech performance on individual parameters was unrelated to the severity of the dysarthria or to the other clinical symptoms. Subjects with different etiologies could show speech impairments similar to those of parkinsonian speakers, and subjects with the same type of dysarthria could exhibit different patterns of impairment. Like Yorkston et al. (1984), Metter and Hanson (1986) advocated an individual detailed assessment of each speaker and stressed the importance of using a multivariate approach as opposed to one that merely considers the speech variables that have previously been identified as prone to impairment in a particular type of dysarthria. Ludlow and Bassich (1983) also argued for this approach as a result of their investigation of the speech characteristics of subjects with Parkinson's disease and Shy-Drager syndrome. They found that no single speech characteristic could distinguish between the two etiologies, but that successful differentiation was possible using a multivariate approach. Weismer and Liss (1991; Liss & Weismer, 1992) also supported the need to assess each subject individually across a number of parameters, although they offered a rather different perspective. They were alert to the problems created by group studies of impaired speech and by approaching the analysis with preset ideas from the literature on normal speech behavior and previous findings from the motor speech disorders literature about what factors are responsible for the speech impairment. Instead, they advocated letting the data guide the analysis of the speaker, investigating each subject individually.

CONCLUSIONS

The findings summarized above and those reported in this paper have implications for assessment procedures investigating dysarthric speech. Because a great deal of variability between different subjects has been found, and each dysarthric speaker seems to behave differently from the others in some respect, assessments must consider as many speech parameters as possible in order to obtain a full picture of an individual's impairment. These parameters must be investigated thoroughly in order to provide the clinician with sufficient information on how to treat the patient in the most effective way. Furthermore, because previous and the present results suggest that differences exist between speech behavior in structured and unstructured tasks, it is important to include both types of task in an assessment protocol.

The dysarthria assessments that are most commonly used in the United Kingdom only partly fulfill these criteria. The Frenchay Dysarthria Assessment (Enderby, 1983) and the Robertson Dysarthria Profile (Robertson, 1982) provide a detailed description of the speakers' breathing, phonatory, and oromotor skills, but give little indication of their performance on the segmental and prosodic aspects of speech. The AIDS (Yorkston & Beukelman, 1981) provides the clinician with reliable single-word and sentence intelligibility scores for both baseline measures and retests, but gives no guidance regarding which segmental aspects are particularly impaired in a speaker. Kent, Weismer, Kent, and Rosenbek (1989) recognized this problem and designed a word list containing minimal pairs for the phonetic contrasts that are most likely to be impaired in dysarthria. This gives the clinician a detailed analysis from which to plan treatment effectively, but does not look at performance in connected speech.

The assessment of oromotor functions and the segmental aspects of speech can thus be carried out in sufficient detail with a combination of tests already available. However, none of these tests provides an in-depth analysis of the patients' performance on naturalistic speech tasks or compares this performance with that in more structured tasks. Furthermore, none of the tests investigates the prosodic aspects of speech in sufficient detail to identify the pattern and the severity of the impairment and to provide a baseline measure for monitoring change. Present assessments only indicate the presence or absence of a problem, and the scores obtained give little indication regarding which prosodic aspects are specifically impaired, to what degree each aspect is impaired, and which should be treated.

Yorkston et al. (1984) have suggested a more detailed analysis procedure that looks at a variety of prosodic features with acoustic and perceptual means. However, their analysis is based largely on contrastive stress data. Considering the results described above on the differences between reading and a more naturalistic type of discourse, there is still the need for a procedure that can be applied to both structured and naturalistic speech data.

A more comprehensive prosodic profile would incorporate both structured and naturalistic speech tasks, such as contrastive stress drills, reading, and conversation. It would include analysis of a variety of prosodic features and investigate these in as much detail as possible. Rather than looking at monopitch, for example, F_0 range, envelope, and intravowel variation could be considered separately, as has been done in the present research. This would allow for a more detailed account of the factors that give rise to the auditory impression of impaired prosody and would give more directions for therapy planning. If, in addition, the data could be analyzed acoustically, the profile would enable the clinician to provide a detailed quantification of the degree of impairment of different aspects of prosody, a feature that is crucial for the identification of improvement or deterioration in speech performance.

For the assessment to be clinically viable, there must be a balance between the need to arrive at a detailed account of the speaker's abilities and the time constraints of the clinician. As discussed above, the currently available procedures do not provide sufficient detail to indicate the precise areas of prosodic impairment to the clinician. In contrast, the approach advocated by Weismer and Liss (1991), investigating speech in a data-driven fashion, may provide a more detailed account of a speaker's impairment but is also potentially very time consuming. This may not, therefore, be the most practical approach for the clinician. Although the present study looked at a restricted number of prosodic dimensions, a certain amount of detail was provided by considering a range of acoustic parameters associated with each dimension. The approach taken in this study may therefore represent a compromise between the need for detailed analysis and the time constraints of the clinician. A prosodic profile is currently being developed incorporating the above-mentioned tasks and parameters (Leuschel & Docherty, 1994) that is intended to provide an in-depth, quantitative account of a dysarthric speaker's prosodic impairment while still being concise enough to be applied in a clinical setting.

REFERENCES

Amerman, J.D., & Parnell, M.M. (1990). Auditory impressions of the speech of normal elderly adults. *British Journal of Disorders of Communication, 25*, 35–43.
Amerman, J.D., & Parnell, M.M. (1992). Speech timing strategies in elderly adults. *Journal of Phonetics, 20*, 65–76.
Arlington, J., Brenninkmeyer, S.M., Arn, D., Grundhauser, R., & O'Connell, D.C. (1992). A usual extreme case—pause reports of informal spontaneous dialogue. *Bulletin of the Psychonomic Society, 30*, 161–163.
Barik, H.C. (1979). Crosslinguistic study of temporal characteristics of different types of speech materials. *Language and Speech, 20*, 116–126.
Beresford, R. (1986). *Unpublished reading passage.* Newcastle-upon-Tyne, England: University of Newcastle-upon-Tyne.
Berry, W.R., & Goshorn, E.L. (1983). Immediate visual feedback in the treatment of ataxic dysarthria: A case study. In W.R. Berry (Ed.), *Clinical dysarthria* (pp. 253–265). San Diego: College-Hill Press.
Brown, A., & Docherty, G.J. (1995). Phonetic variation in dysarthric speech as a function of sampling task. *European Journal of Disorders of Communication, 30*, 17–35.
Brubaker, R.S. (1972). Rate and pause characteristics of oral reading. *Journal of Psycholinguistic Research, 1*, 141–147.
Canter, J.G. (1961). *An investigation of speech characteristics of a group of patients with Parkinson's disease.* Unpublished doctoral thesis, Northwestern University, Evanston, IL.
Crystal, D., & Davy, D. (1969). *Investigating English style.* Hong Kong: Longman.
Cutler, A. (1994). Segmentation problems, rhythmic solutions. *Lingua, 92*, 81–104.
Cutler, A., & Foss, D.J. (1977). On the role of sentence stress in sentence processing. *Language and Speech, 20*, 1–10.
Cutler, A., & Norris, D. (1988). The role of strong syllables in segmentation for lexical access. *Journal of Experimental Psychology: Human Perception and Performance, 14*, 113–121.
Darkins, A.W., Fromkin, V.A., & Benson, D.F. (1988). A characterisation of the prosodic loss in Parkinson's disease. *Brain and Language, 34*, 315–327.
Darley, F.L., Aronson, A.E., & Brown, J.R. (1969a). Clusters of deviant speech dimensions in the dysarthrias. *Journal of Speech and Hearing Research, 12*, 462–496.
Darley, F.L., Aronson, A.E., & Brown, J.R. (1969b). Differential diagnostic patterns of dysarthria. *Journal of Speech and Hearing Research, 12*, 246–269.
Darley, F.L., Aronson, A.E., & Brown, J.R. (1975). *Motor speech disorders.* Philadelphia: W.B. Saunders.
Enderby, P.M. (1983). *Frenchay Dysarthria Assessment.* San Diego: College-Hill Press.
Farnetani, E., & Faber, A. (1992). Tongue-jaw coordination in vowel production: Isolated words versus connected speech. *Speech Communication, 11*, 401–410.
Frearson, B. (1985). A comparison of the AIDS sentence list and spontaneous speech intelligibility scores for dysarthric speech. *Australian Journal of Human Communication Disorders, 13*, 5–21.
Goldman-Eisler, F. (1968). *Psycholinguistics: Experiments in spontaneous speech.* London: Academic Press.
Graddol, D. (1986). Discourse specific pitch behaviour. In C. Johns-Lewis (Ed.), *Intonation in discourse* (pp. 221–237). San Diego: College-Hill Press.

Grosjean, F., & Deschamps, A. (1973). Analyse des variables temporelles du français spontané. II: Comparaison du français oral dans la description avec l'anglais (description) et avec le français (interview radiophonique). *Phonetica, 28,* 191–226.

Hargrove, P.M., & McGarr, N.S. (1994). *Prosody management of communication disorders.* London: Whurr Publishers.

Harmegnies, B., & Poch-Olivé, D. (1992). A study of style-induced variability: Laboratory versus spontaneous speech in Spanish. *Speech Communication, 11,* 429–437.

Hertrich, I., & Ackermann, H. (1993a). Acoustic analysis of speech prosody in Huntington's and Parkinson's disease—a preliminary report. *Clinical Linguistics and Phonetics, 7,* 285–297.

Hertrich, I., & Ackermann, H. (1993b). Dysarthria in Friedreich's ataxia: Syllable intensity and fundamental frequency patterns. *Clinical Linguistics and Phonetics, 7,* 177–190.

Howell, P., & Kadi-Hanifi, K. (1991). Comparison of prosodic properties between read and spontaneous speech material. *Speech Communication, 10,* 163–169.

Huggins, A.W.F. (1977). Speech timing and intelligibility. *Attention and Performance, VII,* 279–298.

Illes, J., Metter, E.J., Hanson, W.R., & Iritani, S. (1988). Language production in Parkinson's disease: Acoustic and linguistic considerations. *Brain and Language, 33,* 146–160.

Johns-Lewis, C. (1986). Prosodic differentiation of discourse modes. In C. Johns-Lewis (Ed.), *Intonation in discourse* (pp. 199–219). San Diego: College-Hill Press.

Kent, R.D., Netsell, R., & Abbs, J.H. (1979). Acoustic characteristics of dysarthria associated with cerebellar disease. *Journal of Speech and Hearing Research, 22,* 627–648.

Kent, R.D., & Rosenbek, J.C. (1982). Prosodic disturbances and neurologic lesion. *Brain and Language, 15,* 259–291.

Kent, R.D., & Rosenbek, J.C. (1983). Acoustic patterns of apraxia of speech. *Journal of Speech and Hearing Research, 26,* 231–249.

Kent, R.D., Weismer, G., Kent, J.F., & Rosenbek, J.C. (1989). Towards phonetic intelligibility testing in dysarthria. *Journal of Speech and Hearing Disorders, 54,* 482–499.

Lehiste, I. (1965). *Some acoustic characteristics of dysarthric speech.* Bibliotheca Phonetica, Fasc. 2. Basel: Karger.

Leuschel, A., & Docherty, G.J. (1994, November). *An assessment tool for prosody in dysarthric speech.* Paper presented at the 4th Symposium of the International Clinical Phonetics and Linguistics Association, New Orleans.

Levin, H., Schaffer, C.A., & Snow, C. (1982). The prosodic and paralinguistic features of reading and telling stories. *Language and Speech, 25,* 43–54.

Liss, J., & Weismer, G. (1992). Qualitative acoustic analysis in the study of motor speech disorders. *Journal of the Acoustical Society of America, 92,* 2984–2987.

Liss, J., & Weismer, G. (1994). Selected acoustic characteristics of contrastive stress production in control geriatric, apraxic, and ataxic dysarthric speakers. *Clinical Linguistics and Phonetics, 8,* 45–66.

Ludlow, C.L., & Bassich, C.J. (1983). The result of acoustic and perceptual assessment of two types of dysarthria. In W.R. Berry (Ed.), *Clinical dysarthria* (pp. 121–153). San Diego: College-Hill Press.

Ludlow, C.L., & Bassich, C.J. (1984). Relationships between perceptual ratings and acoustic measures of hypokinetic speech. In M.R. McNeil, J.C. Rosenbek,

& A.E. Aronson (Eds.), *The dysarthrias: Physiology, acoustics, perception, management* (pp. 163–195). San Diego: College-Hill Press.

Ludlow, C.L., Bassich, C.J., & Connor, N.P. (1985). An objective system for assessment and analysis of dysarthric speech. In J. Darby (Ed.), *Speech and language evaluation in neurology: Adult disorders* (pp. 393–425). New York: Grune & Stratton.

Ludlow, C.L., Connor, N.P., & Bassich, C.J. (1987). Speech timing in Parkinson's and Huntington's disease. *Brain and Language, 32,* 195–214.

Metter, E.J., & Hanson, W.R. (1986). Clinical and acoustical variability in hypokinetic dysarthria. *Journal of Communication Disorders, 19,* 347–366.

Morrison, J.A., & Shriberg, L.D. (1992). Articulation testing versus conversational speech sampling. *Journal of Speech and Hearing Research, 35,* 259–273.

Murry, T. (1983). The production of stress in three types of dysarthric speech. In W.R. Berry (Ed.), *Clinical dysarthria* (pp. 69–83). San Diego: College-Hill Press.

Nooteboom, S.G., Brokx, J.P.L., & de Rooij, J.J. (1978). Contributions of prosody to speech perception. in W.J.M. Levelt & G.B. Flores d'Arcais (Eds.), *Studies in the perception of language* (pp. 75–107). New York: John Wiley & Sons.

Osberger, M.J., & Levitt, H. (1979). The effect of timing errors on the intelligibility of deaf children's speech. *Journal of the Acoustical Society of America, 66,* 1316–1324.

Parkhurst, B.G., & Levitt, H. (1978). The effect of selected prosodic errors on the intelligibility of deaf children's speech. *Journal of Communication Disorders, 11,* 249–256.

Portnoy, R.A., & Aronson, A.E. (1982). Diadochokinetic syllable rate and regularity in normal and in spastic and ataxic dysarthric speakers. *Journal of Speech and Hearing Disorders, 47,* 324–328.

Ramig, L.A. (1983). Effects of physiological aging on speaking and reading rates. *Journal of Communication Disorders, 16,* 217–226.

Robertson, S. (1982). *Dysarthria profile.* San Diego: College-Hill Press.

Robertson, S., & Thomson, F. (1986). *Working with dysarthric clients: A practical guide to therapy for dysarthria.* Bicester, England: Winslow Press.

Robin, D.A., Klouda, G.V., & Hug, L.N. (1991). Neurogenic disorders of prosody. In D. Vogel & M.P. Cannito (Eds.), *Treating disordered speech motor control: For clinicians by clinicians* (pp. 241–271). Austin, TX: PRO-ED.

Rosenbek, J.C., & LaPointe, L. (1985). The dysarthrias: Description, diagnosis, and treatment. In D. Johns (Ed.), *Clinical management of neurogenic communicative disorders* (2nd ed.) (pp. 97–152). Boston: Little, Brown.

Schlenck, K.-J., Bettrich, R., & Willmes, K. (1993). Aspects of disturbed prosody in dysarthria. *Clinical Linguistics and Phonetics, 7,* 119–128.

Silverman, K.E.A. (1987). *Structure of fundamental frequency contours.* Unpublished doctoral thesis, University of Cambridge, England.

Smith, C.R. (1975). Residual hearing and speech production in deaf children. *Journal of Speech and Hearing Research, 18,* 795–811.

Weismer, G., & Liss, J.M. (1991). Acoustic/perceptual taxonomies of speech production in motor speech disorders. In C.A. Moore, K.M. Yorkston, & D.R. Beukelman (Eds.), *Dysarthria and apraxia of speech: Perspectives on management* (pp. 245–270). Baltimore: Paul H. Brookes Publishing Co.

Weismer, G., & Martin, R.E. (1992). Acoustic and perceptual approaches to the study of intelligibility. In R.D. Kent (Ed.), *Intelligibility in speech disorders: Theory, measurement and management* (pp. 67–118). Amsterdam: John Benjamins Publishing Company.

Yorkston, K.M., & Beukelman, D.R. (1981). *Assessment of intelligibility of dysarthric speech*. Tigard, OR: C.C. Publications.

Yorkston, K.M., Beukelman, D.R., Minifie, F.D., & Sapir, S. (1984). Assessment of stress patterning. In M.R. McNeil, J.C. Rosenbek, & A.E. Aronson (Eds.), *The dysarthrias: Physiology, acoustics, perception, management* (pp. 130–162). San Diego: College-Hill Press.

Yorkston, K.M., Hammen, V.L., Beukelman, D.R., & Traynor, C.D. (1990). The effect of rate control on the intelligibility and naturalness of dysarthric speech. *Journal of Speech and Hearing Disorders, 55*, 550–560.

Zyski, B.J., & Weisiger, B.E. (1987). Identification of dysarthria types based on perceptual analysis. *Journal of Communication Disorders, 20*, 367–378.

SECTION V

RESPIRATORY INVOLVEMENT IN DYSARTHRIA

Chapter 10

Respiratory Patterning and Variability in Dysarthric Speech

Vicki L. Hammen and Kathryn M. Yorkston

ADEQUATE RESPIRATORY SUPPORT is important not only for the production of intelligible speech, but for its potential impact on prosodic characteristics and therefore speech naturalness. Determination of the adequacy of respiratory support must go beyond measures of vital capacity to include measures of speech breathing. The work of Hixon and colleagues (Hixon, Goldman, & Mead, 1973; Hoit & Hixon, 1986, 1987; Hoit, Hixon, Altman, & Morgan, 1989; Hoit, Hixon, Watson, & Morgan, 1990) has provided a rich normative data base of speech breathing characteristics. Recently, the types of respiratory problems occurring with neurologic disease have been documented (Annoni, Chevrolet, & Kesselring, 1993). Additionally, the speech breathing literature has been expanded to include investigations of the effects of neurologic impairment on speech breathing (Hixon, 1982, 1987; Murdoch, Chenery, Bowler, & Ingram, 1989; Putnam & Hixon, 1984; Solomon & Hixon, 1993). The study of speech breathing in neurologically impaired populations has focused primarily on the relative contributions of the rib cage and abdomen to changes in lung volume level during conversation and reading. Although

---

Reprinted from the *Journal of Medical Speech-Language Pathology*, 2(4), 253–261, 1994, by permission of the authors and Singular Publishing Group, Inc.

This work was supported in part by Grant No. H133B80081 from the National Institute on Disability and Rehabilitation Research, Department of Education, Washington, DC. Portions of this work were presented at the 1993 American Speech-Language-Hearing Association convention in Anaheim, CA, and the 1994 Conference on Motor Speech, Sedona, AZ.

Many thanks to Mary Towne, who assisted in collecting data for this project.

the number of syllables per breath group have been reported in a number of these studies (Hoit & Hixon, 1987; Hoit et al., 1989, 1990; Solomon & Hixon, 1993), other more global aspects of speech breathing, such as location of breaths and consistency of breath group length, have received much less research attention. These aspects of speech breathing (i.e., breath group length, location of breaths, and consistency of breaths) may be best defined as respiratory patterning. In particular, the location of breaths has rarely been investigated (Beukelman, Yorkston, Dowden, & Minifie, 1986; Winkworth, Davis, Ellis, & Adams, 1994).

The study of breath group location has important implications for speech intelligibility as well as naturalness. Breath group units serve to partition speech into meaningful units. Grosjean and Collins (1979) showed that most speakers breathe at major syntactic boundaries (e.g., end of sentences, clause boundaries). These findings were replicated by Winkworth and colleagues (1994) in a study of speech breathing during reading for a group of healthy young women. The authors found that breaths occurred at major syntactic boundaries and that there was high intra- and intersubject agreement for location of breaths. If the location of a breath is not tied to appropriate syntactic boundaries, the listener may become "lost" and intelligibility can be reduced. Huggins (1978), in his work on the importance of timing in the intelligibility of deaf speech, referred to this phenomenon as the "garden path" effect. The incidence of breath group location abnormalities in individuals with dysarthria has not been well documented.

In addition to speech intelligibility, the length of breath groups can affect speech naturalness. Bellaire, Yorkston, and Beukelman (1986) related decreased naturalness of speech in a young head-injured subject to the presence of short, uniform breath groups, as well as reduced fundamental frequency range. The dysarthric speaker produced fewer words per breath group when reading a standard passage than a control speaker. It seems reasonable to expect that it would be more difficult to produce natural fundamental frequency contours in a substantially shortened breath group.

As the above discussion suggests, our knowledge of breath group lengths and the location of breaths for dysarthric speakers is quite limited. Therefore, this investigation into the more global aspects of respiratory control was conducted with the following questions as its focus:

1. Do mean breath group length and range differ between dysarthric and control speakers?
2. Does the location of breaths differ for the two groups of speakers?
3. Do the subject groups differ in trial-to-trial variability for breath group location?

METHODS

Subjects

Twenty-two individuals with dysarthria identified from the Speech Pathology Service in the Department of Rehabilitation Medicine, University of Washington, served as experimental subjects. Demographic information for the dysarthric subjects is presented in Table 1. Severity levels were established based on the judgment of a certified speech-language pathologist at the time of the experimental session. All subjects were medically stable; none had a history of pulmonary disease; all had adequate vision (with correction) to read printed material, had no history of hearing loss, and had adequate respiratory abilities to read sentence-level material. The age range of the dysarthric subjects was 21–81 years. Twenty-two nonneurologically impaired individuals were recruited as control subjects. The control group consisted of 20 females and 2 males. Although this gender distribution is different from that of the dysarthric subject group, gender does not appear to be a significant factor when speech breathing is examined (Hoit et al., 1989). The age range for the control group was 23–73 years.

Experimental Task

The subjects read a standard paragraph-length passage (Hammen, Yorkston, & Minifie, 1994) while the Respitrace system (Respiratory Monitoring, Inc.) was used to transduce changes in the circumference of the rib cage and abdomen. The rib cage, abdomen, and sum signals from the Respitrace were FM recorded (Hewlett-Packard 3964A) onto high-quality tape. The audio signal obtained from a microphone positioned approximately 10 inches from the subject also was FM recorded.

The subjects were provided a large-print copy of the paragraph and asked to read the paragraph silently to familiarize themselves with the text. They were then instructed to read the paragraph in their typical style at a comfortable loudness level. If numerous reading errors occurred, the trial was discontinued and the paragraph was reviewed again. Subjects read the

Table 1. Severity information for the dysarthric subjects ($n = 22$)

Medical diagnosis	Dysarthria severity level			Total
	Mild	Moderate	Moderate–severe	
Traumatic brain injury	4	5	1	10
Parkinson's disease	4	2	1	7
Cerebrovascular accident	2	1	1	4
Amyotrophic lateral sclerosis			1	1
Total	10	8	4	22

passage two times. Because this task was part of a larger data collection effort, several other tasks were completed during an experimental session. All experimental tasks were randomly ordered. Usually a number of other speech samples were recorded prior to the second trial of paragraph reading.

Data Analysis

The rib cage, abdomen, and sum signals from the Respitrace unit were displayed on the face of an oscilloscope, and the audio signal was monitored via headphones. Transcripts of the reading passage were marked for occurrence of breaths based on a combined judgment of both the Respitrace and audio signals. Interrater agreement calculated on 20% of the data was 100%. The following measures were obtained from the marked transcripts: breath group length, frequency of occurrence, location of breath, and concurrence. Operational definitions for each of the measures were as follows:

Breath Group Length: The number of words per breath group served as the measure of breath group length. Mean, maximum, and minimum words per breath group length were determined for each reading of the passage for each subject.

Frequency of Occurrence: The number of times a given breath group length was observed during the reading passage.

Location of Breath: The location of breaths was coded into the following three categories:

1 = Primary Syntactic Boundary: Breaths that occurred at sentence boundaries.
2 = Secondary Syntactic Boundary: Breaths that occurred at phrase and/or subordinate clause boundaries.
3 = Other: Breaths occurring within a phrase or clause.

Concurrence: As an initial attempt at quantifying trial-to-trial variability, a measure of concurrence was developed. For the purposes of this experiment, concurrence was defined as the percentage of total breaths (Trial 1 + Trial 2) occurring at the same location across both trials. Concurrence was calculated for each syntactic boundary. An example of the manner by which concurrence was determined is presented in Figure 1. This dysarthric subject had five breaths in Trial 1 and five breaths in Trial 2, for a total of 10 breaths across the two paragraph readings. Those breaths occurred at exactly the same location four times; thus, there were four instances of concurrence. Because two breaths must occur in the same location to be considered concurrent, this corresponds to 8 breaths. The percentage of concurrence for this subject was calculated as 80% (8/10).

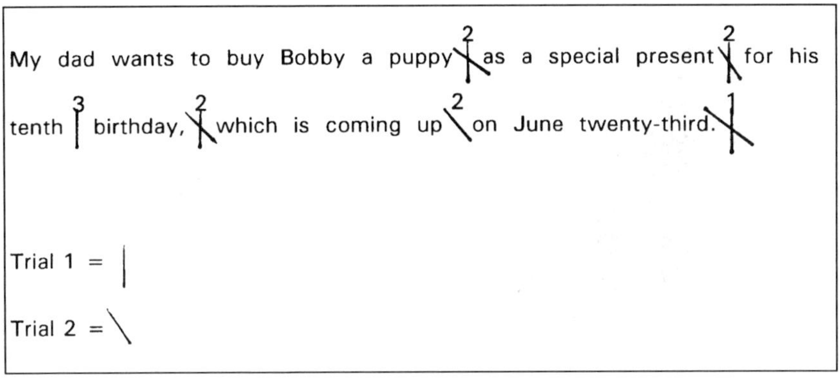

```
                                    2                    2
My  dad  wants  to  buy  Bobby  a  puppy\ as  a  special  present\ for  his
       3           2                       2
tenth | birthday, \which  is  coming  up \on  June  twenty-third.\
```

Trial 1 = |

Trial 2 = \

Figure 1. An example of the method used to determine concurrence from a dysarthric subject. The vertical and backward slashes indicate a breath taken at that location during Trial 1 and Trial 2, respectively. The numbers above the slashes indicate the assigned syntactic boundary code.

RESULTS AND DISCUSSION

Breath Group Length

The first question of interest was: Do mean breath group length and range differ between dysarthric and control speakers? Table 2 presents the results for the number of words per breath group (WPBG). Mean WPBG was significantly shorter for the subjects with dysarthria (9.3) than for the control subjects (16.9) ($F_{1,42} = 15.18, p < .001$). Mean maximum WPBG was also significantly shorter for the subjects with dysarthria (17.5) than for the control subjects (27.6) ($F_{1,42} = 15.45, p < .001$). Finally, a significant difference between groups was found for minimum WPBG: 3.5 for the subjects with dysarthria versus 8.5 for the control subjects ($F_{1,42} = 14.39, p < .001$).

Frequency of Occurrence

Another method of examining the range of breath group lengths is through the use of frequency of occurrence. This allows the pattern of group performance on this task to be observed in a way not possible with overall mean data. Frequency of occurrence for breath group length plotted for the two groups to examine the patterns appears in Figures 2 and 3.

Table 2. Mean, maximum, and minimum words per breath group (WPBG) for the dysarthric and control subjects

Group	Mean WPBG	Maximum WPBG	Minimum WPBG
Dysarthria	9.3 (7.4)	17.5 (10.3)	3.5 (4.1)
Control	16.9 (5.3)	27.6 (6.1)	8.5 (4.7)

Data have been averaged across subjects ($n = 22$) and trials (2) within each group. Standard deviations are shown in parentheses.

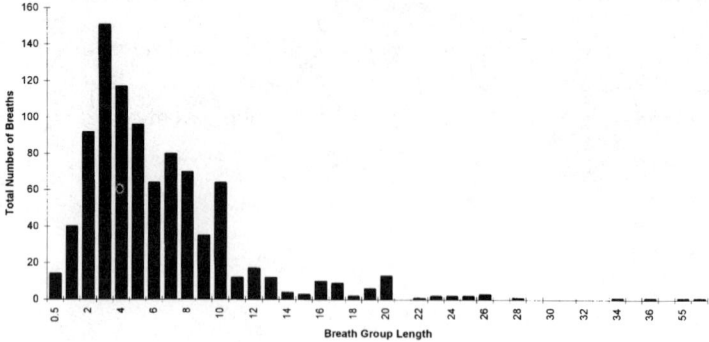

Figure 2. Frequency of occurrence of breath group lengths (in words) for the dysarthria group speakers.

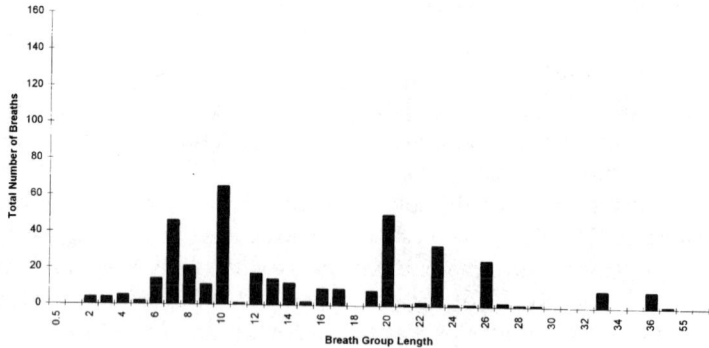

Figure 3. Frequency of occurrence of breath group lengths (in words) for the control group speakers.

These graphs were created by pooling the breath group lengths for all 22 speakers in each group across both reading trials and determining the overall frequency of occurrence for each length. The 0.5 length indicates that the individual took a breath between syllables of multisyllabic words.

Note that for the dysarthric speakers the distribution is skewed to the right, toward shorter breath group lengths (Figure 2). Some subjects took a breath within a word, although the frequency is fairly small. Also, the subjects with dysarthria have a number of breath group lengths that occur more than 80 times. The shape of the distribution is more difficult to discern for the control speakers (Figure 3), but it is certainly different from that of the dysarthric speakers. No within-word breaths occurred, and none of the breath group lengths occurred more than 80 times for this group. Overall, it is clear that the control subjects did not breathe as frequently as the dysarthric subjects. Finally, the distributions for both groups contain some outliers of extremely long breath group lengths, a finding not readily apparent in the mean data.

Breath Location

The next research question was: Does the location of breaths differ for the two groups of speakers? Figure 4 represents the percentage of breaths occurring at each syntactic boundary for the two groups. The number of breaths occurring at the syntactic locations coded as 1s, 2s, or 3s across both reading trials were divided by the total number of breaths occurring in both samples to determine the percentage of breaths taken at each type of syntactic boundary. These percentages were then averaged across the 22 subjects for each group. Figure 4 shows that the control subjects took a greater proportion of their breaths at primary syntactic boundaries than

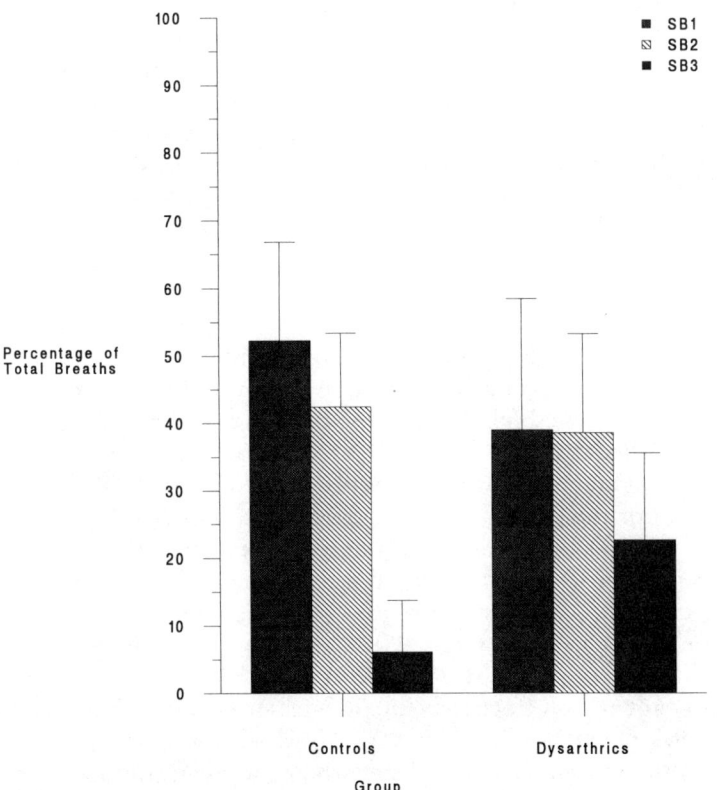

Figure 4. Mean percentage of breaths occurring at syntactic boundaries (SB) (1 = primary, 2 = secondary, 3 = other) for dysarthria and control group subjects. Error bars represent the standard deviation from the mean.

did the dysarthric group. The control subjects had 73.71% of their breaths at locations coded as 1s versus 38.89% for the dysarthric subjects. The dysarthric speakers had a greater proportion of their breaths occur within a phrase or clause (22.58%) than did the control group, which averaged only 2.08% at this location.

Following arcsin transformation of the percentages, a 2 × 3 (Group × Syntactic Boundary) repeated-measures ANOVA was performed on the data. A significant between-subjects effect for group ($F_{1,42} = 11.79, p = .001$) was found. A significant interaction for Group × Syntactic Boundary ($F_{2,84} = 25.55, p < .001$) was also found during statistical analysis.

To aid in the interpretation of these results, it was important to determine the likelihood of taking a breath at syntactic boundary "3." That is, what breath group lengths were required for subjects to breathe at all primary and secondary boundaries? The number of words between locations coded as "1" or "2" were calculated and the mean and mode determined. The mean breath group length if breaths occurred at primary and secondary locations was 3.67 words, and the mode was 4. Therefore, if a subject could produce four words per breath group, he or she would have been able to avoid taking a breath within a phrase. All subjects had maximum breath group lengths that were greater than four words, indicating that this subject group demonstrated adequate respiratory capacity to breath at only primary or secondary locations. Their failure to do so, as indicated by breaths at syntactic boundary "3," may be indicative of an inability to adequately plan the pattern of respiratory use in speech tasks.

Concurrence

The final research question was: Do the subjects differ in trial-to-trial variability for breath group location? Mean percentages of concurrence for each syntactic boundary for the two speaker groups are presented in Figure 5. Both groups had a high percentage of concurrence for breaths at primary syntactic boundaries, 90.18% for the dysarthric speakers and 92.36% for the control speakers. Separation between the groups appears in the data for concurrence for the secondary syntactic boundaries. Control subjects had 28.59% concurrence at this location, while the dysarthric subjects had 50.77% concurrence. These percentages were arcsin transformed prior to entry into a 2 × 3 (Group × Concurrence at Syntactic Boundary) repeated-measures ANOVA. Results of this analysis showed a significant main effect for concurrence at syntactic boundary ($F_{2,84} = 122.19; p < .001$).

Although the Group × Concurrence at Syntactic Boundary interaction approached, but failed to reach, statistical significance, it was interesting that none of the control subjects demonstrated concurrence for syn-

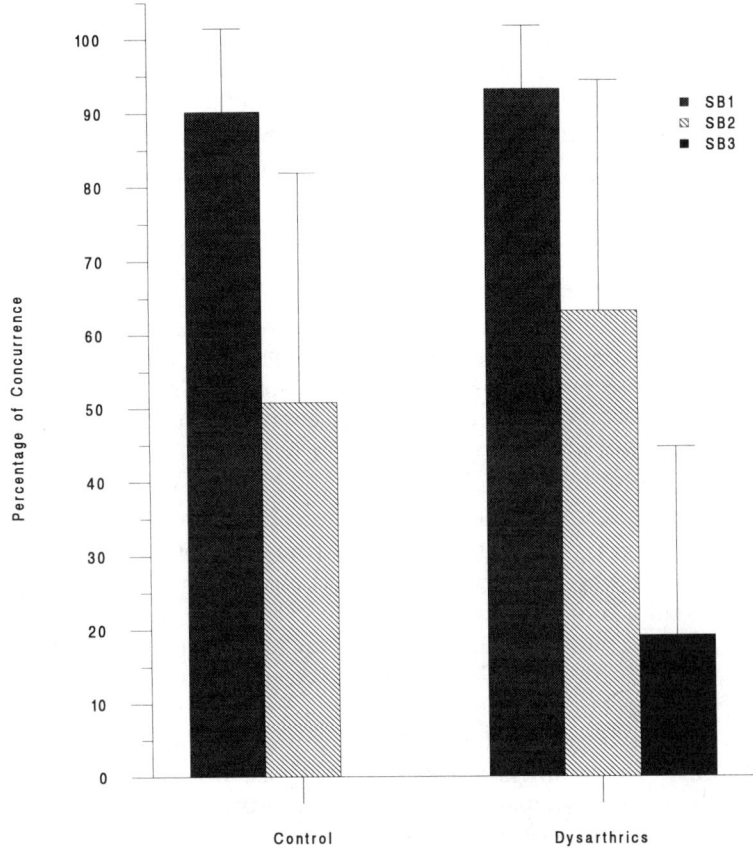

Figure 5. Mean percentage of concurrent breaths occurring at syntactic boundaries (SB) (1 = primary, 2 = secondary, 3 = other) for dysarthria and control group subjects. Error bars represent the standard deviation from the mean.

tactic boundaries coded as "3" (i.e., occurring at boundaries other than primary or secondary). Although some control subjects took a breath at a syntactic boundary "3" location during the first reading of the paragraph, they did not do so during the second reading. The dysarthric subjects, in contrast, had 19.09% concurrence for "other" locations. It should be noted that there was a large amount of variability in these data. The standard deviation for the data was actually greater than the mean. This can be attributed in part to the complete lack of concurrence at syntactic boundary "3" for some dysarthric subjects. Twelve out of 22 (54%) dysarthric subjects had some concurrence for this location. Among those 12 subjects, the percentage of concurrence ranged from 9% to 100%.

It was also of interest to determine if the 12 subjects who exhibited concurrence at syntactic boundary "3" were similar with respect to dysarthria severity level. Forty percent (4/10) of the mildly dysarthric subjects, 62% (5/8) of the moderately dysarthric subjects, and 75% (3/4) of the moderately severe dysarthric subjects showed concurrence for syntactic boundary "3."

CONCLUSIONS

The results of this investigation indicated that the dysarthric and control groups differed for the mean number of words that occur during a breath group. This is consistent with other reports in the literature on breath group length for both normally aging and neurologically impaired individuals. For example, Solomon and Hixon (1993) found that individuals with Parkinson's disease produced fewer words per breath group than their group of healthy adults.

Not only were there significant differences in mean, maximum, and minimum breath group length, the distributions, or pattern, of breath group lengths were quite different for the two groups. The dysarthric subjects had a more skewed distribution, favoring quite short breath group lengths, whereas the control group subjects showed much more variation in breath group length. These results from a larger, more diverse group of dysarthric subjects are in agreement with Bellaire et al.'s (1986) study of a single subject with unnatural speech following a closed head injury. The findings in this study suggest that the high number of shorter breath groups may contribute to the alterations in naturalness observed in many types of dysarthric speakers. Clearly, the relationship between speech naturalness and breath group length and/or location needs further investigation.

The greater proportion of breaths occurring within phrases/clauses in the dysarthric group may suggest inappropriate respiratory support; however, it also may indicate poor planning. In an attempt to exclude individuals with more severe respiratory compromise, the subjects recruited for this study did not exhibit substantial respiratory deficits. However, some subjects may have had difficulty planning how to utilize their respiratory support for speech. There were not sufficient numbers of subjects within each severity or medical diagnosis category to do correlation analyses between breath group length or location and these factors. An inspection of the data suggested that subjects with traumatic brain injuries were more likely to take a breath at a nonsyntactic boundary than were subjects who had had a cerebrovascular accident. Differences in breath group location for different etiologies or dysarthria severity levels might be interesting to pursue in future studies.

The most obvious difference between the groups was that the dysarthric subjects showed concurrence for breaths taken within phrases and clauses (i.e., syntactic boundary "3"). Not only do some dysarthric speakers pause to breathe at ungrammatical locations, they also do so at the same location in a second trial. This finding has important implications for speech intelligibility. A listener may be more likely to rely on the location of a breath as marking the boundary of a meaningful unit if it occurs consistently. As mentioned earlier, Huggins (1978) has suggested that these errors can create a "garden path" effect. That is, the listener makes some assumptions regarding the message based on the chunking of the utterance into units. If the breath occurs at a location that is not syntactically correct, a wrong decision is made and the listener may be misled in subsequent attempts to understand the speaker. It is likely that this would have a negative impact on speech intelligibility, especially of the more severely dysarthric speakers.

Speech naturalness may also be affected when the speaker interrupts the speech stream at an ungrammatical location to breathe. Lieberman (1967) suggested that the breath group defined a prosodic pattern that is used to mark the boundaries of declarative sentences. This definition was subsequently extended to include smaller constituents within a sentence (Grosjean & Collins, 1979). If the location of a breath is not at a typical boundary for a sentence or constituent, the prosodic pattern for that breath group may not be of the expected type. Unusual prosodic patterns would certainly contribute to alterations in speech naturalness. Future investigations should address the impact of respiratory patterning on the prosodic contour and speech naturalness.

Finally, the results of this study have certain clinical implications as well. Dysarthric speakers may benefit from intervention efforts directed toward increasing the variability of breath group lengths, as suggested by Bellaire et al. (1986), and also toward shifting breaths to appropriate syntactic boundaries.

REFERENCES

Annoni, J., Chevrolet, J., & Kesselring, J. (1993). Respiratory problems in chronic neurologic disease. *Critical Reviews in Physical and Rehabilitation Medicine, 5,* 155–192.

Bellaire, K., Yorkston, K.M., & Beukelman, D.R. (1986). Modification of breath patterning to increase the naturalness of a mildly dysarthric speaker. *Journal of Communication Disorders, 19,* 271–280.

Beukelman, D.R., Yorkston, K.M., Dowden, P.A., & Minifie, F.D. (1986). *Impact of speaking rate reduction of respiratory patterns of nonimpaired and dysarthric speakers.* Paper presented at the third Biennial Clinical Dysarthria Conference, Tucson, AZ.

Grosjean, F., & Collins, M. (1979). Breathing, pausing, and reading. *Phonetica, 36,* 98–114.

Hammen, V.L., Yorkston, K.M., & Minifie, F.D. (1994). The effect of temporal alterations on speech intelligibility in parkinsonian dysarthria. *Journal of Speech and Hearing Research, 37,* 244–253.

Hixon, T.J. (1982). Speech breathing kinematics and mechanism inferences therefrom. In S. Grillner, A. Persson, B. Lindblom, & J. Lubker (Eds.), *Speech motor control* (pp. 75–93). New York: Pergamon Press.

Hixon, T.J. (1987). *Respiratory function in speech and song.* San Diego: College-Hill Press.

Hixon, T.J., Goldman, M.D., & Mead, J. (1973). Kinematics of the chest wall during speech production: Volume displacements of the ribcage, abdomen, and lung. *Journal of Speech and Hearing Research, 16,* 78–115.

Hoit, J.D., & Hixon, T.J. (1986). Body type and speech breathing. *Journal of Speech and Hearing Research, 28,* 313–324.

Hoit, J.D., & Hixon, T.J. (1987). Age and speech breathing. *Journal of Speech and Hearing Research, 30,* 351–366.

Hoit, J.D., Hixon, T.J., Altman, M.E., & Morgan, W.J. (1989). Speech breathing in women. *Journal of Speech and Hearing Research, 32,* 353–365.

Hoit, J.D., Hixon, T.J., Watson, P.J., & Morgan, W.J. (1990). Speech breathing in children and adolescents. *Journal of Speech and Hearing Research, 33,* 51–69.

Huggins, A.W.E. (1978). Speech timing and intelligibility. In J. Requin (Ed.), *Attention and performance VII* (pp. 279–297). Hillside, NJ: Lawrence Erlbaum Associates.

Lieberman, P. (1967). *Intonation, perception, and language* (Research monograph No. 38). Cambridge, MA: MIT Press.

Murdoch, B.E., Chenery, H.J., Bowler, S., & Ingram, J.C.L. (1989). Respiratory function in Parkinson's subjects exhibiting a perceptible speech deficit: A kinematic and spirometric analysis. *Journal of Speech and Hearing Disorders, 54,* 610–626.

Putman, A.B. & Hixon, T.J. (1984). Respiratory kinematics in speakers with motor neuron disease. In M. McNeil, J. Rosenbek, & A. Aronson (Eds.), *The dysarthrias* (pp. 37–67). San Diego: College-Hill Press.

Solomon, N.P., & Hixon, T.J. (1993). Speech breathing in Parkinson's disease. *Journal of Speech and Hearing Research, 36,* 294–310.

Winkworth, A.L., Davis, P.J., Ellis, E., & Adams, R.G. (1994). Variability and consistency in speech breathing during reading: Lung volumes, speech intensity, and linguistic factors. *Journal of Speech and Hearing Research, 37,* 535–556.

Chapter 11

Progression of Respiratory Symptoms in Amyotrophic Lateral Sclerosis
Implications for Speech Function

Kathryn M. Yorkston,
Edythe A. Strand, and Robert M. Miller

AMYOTROPHIC LATERAL SCLEROSIS (ALS) is a progressive degenerative disease of unknown etiology involving the motor neurons of the cortex, brain stem, and spinal cord. Bulbar symptoms are the initial feature in approximately one third of individuals with ALS (Rosen, 1978), and dysarthria and dysphagia are among the most frequent near-terminal symptoms of the disease regardless of the pattern of initial symptoms (Gubbay, Kahana, Zilber, & Cooper, 1985). Because bulbar involvement occurs so frequently, speech-language pathologists regularly manage communication and swallowing needs of this population.

ALS has been described as a relentlessly progressive disease, with some individuals progressing more rapidly than others. For example, younger patients have a substantially better prognosis than those who are diagnosed after the age of 50 years, and those with initial spinal symptoms have a threefold better 5-year survival rate than those with initial bulbar symptoms (Rosen, 1978). Research that tracks disease progression with objective measures such as strength and movement rates reports a steady, linear deterioration by individuals with ALS (Prada et al., 1993). Clinical reports, however, suggest that functional performance on global measures such as speech intelligibility may reflect a stepwise decline rather than linear decline (Yorkston, Strand, Miller, Hillel, & Smith, 1993). Changes in speech intelligibility may be characterized by a threshold effect wherein intelligibility is maintained in the face of steadily declining oral movements rates. At some critical threshold point, speech intelligibility changes rapidly in the presence of only small changes in the level of underlying impairment, as measured with objective measures such as oral movement rates.

Typically, bulbar involvement of the tongue, lips, and soft palate is associated with early dysarthria in ALS (DePaul & Abbs, 1987). As dysarthria becomes more severe, oral articulatory problems are compounded by changes in respiratory status. Although respiratory decline is not the sole, or even the chief, feature of dysarthria associated with ALS, a number of deviant speech features implicate the respiratory system. For example, shortness of phrase, breathiness, and audible inspiration were among the most prominent perceptual features of dysarthria in ALS (Darley, Aronson, & Brown, 1975). These features suggest an important respiratory/phonatory component in dysarthric speakers with ALS. Clinical experience suggests that a speaker's perceived level of effort steadily increases as the disease progresses. Even before changes in speech intelligibility are noted, patients often complain of fatigue while speaking and will indicate that they change their messages (typically making them more telegraphic) because of the effort required to produce long utterances. One potential explanation for the increase in perceived effort is a gradually worsening level of respiratory support. Another explanation is an increased central drive, caused by weak muscles, which may increase the sense of effort as a result of central fatigue (Robin, Goel, Somodi, & Luschei, 1992; Somodi, Robin, & Leschei, in press).

Monitoring respiratory status in individuals with ALS is critical in staging of interventions. Although breathing problems are typically not one of the presenting symptoms of ALS, failure of the respiratory system is the most common cause of death in this disease (Tandan & Bradley, 1985). Weakening of the respiratory muscles causes a number of complications, including respiratory muscle fatigue, respiratory failure, ineffective cough, and failure to protect the lungs from aspiration (Braun, 1987; Tidwell, 1993). Objective measures of respiratory status are important, because patients' reports may not be sensitive to early respiratory problems at least in part because of their general reduction in level of physical activity. In a series of 36 individuals with ALS, 86% demonstrated respiratory muscle weakness while only 7% complained of respiratory symptoms (Schiffman & Belsh, 1993). Changing respiratory status in individuals with ALS has been documented with a variety of measures (Annoni, Chevrolet, & Kesselring, 1993). Both maximum inspiratory pressure and maximum expiratory pressure decrease. Lung volumes, such as vital capacity, decrease while residual volumes increase. The average rate of decline of respiratory muscle strength, as measured by vital capacity, was -3.5% per month in a series of 36 individuals followed by Schiffman and Belsh (1993).

The purpose of this study was to explore the respiratory status of individuals with ALS, especially as it relates to bulbar involvement and speech function. Specifically, we sought answers to the following questions:

- What is the relationship between level of bulbar function and respiratory status, as measured by vital capacity, and does this relationship change as a function of the patient's initial symptoms (i.e., bulbar versus spinal)?
- What is the rate of change in respiratory status, and does it vary as a function of the patient's initial symptoms (i.e., bulbar versus spinal) or gender?
- What is the relationship between rate of progression in respiratory status and change in speech function in women and men with ALS?

METHODS

Clinical Assessment

Data in this study were derived from a clinical database collected as part of an outpatient clinic focusing on management of adults with neurologic speech and swallowing disorders. During each visit, information regarding level of severity in the areas of speech, swallowing, and lower and upper extremity function was assessed using the ALS Severity Scale (Yorkston et al., 1993). One portion of this scale is the Speech Scale, a 10-point scale of function including the general categories of normal speech processes, detectable speech disturbance, behavioral modifications, use of augmentative communication, and loss of useful speech (Table 1). A scale score is assigned on the basis of an interview and brief clinical examination.

During each clinic visit, vital capacity was measured in the seated position using a hand-held Wright Respirometer. Patients were asked to take a deep breath and to exhale steadily as much air as possible. The measure reported represents the highest value produced during three trials. When considerable lip weakness was present, a second examiner manually assisted the patient to achieve a complete lip seal. An attempt was made to obtain a measure of vital capacity during each clinic visit. However, as respiratory status declines, a number of problems make these measurements difficult, including 1) adductor spasms of the larynx associated with audible exhalation during the measurement maneuver, and 2) inability to perform a deep inhalation/forced exhalation maneuver. Typically these prob-

Table 1. Speech Scale from the Amyotrophic Lateral Sclerosis Severity Scale

Normal Speech Processes

10—**Normal Speech**—Individual denies any difficulty speaking. Examination demonstrates no abnormality.

9—**Nominal Speech Abnormality**—Only the individual with ALS or spouse notices that speech has changed. Maintains normal rate and volume.

Detectable Speech Disturbance

8—**Perceived Speech Changes**—Speech changes are noted by others, especially during fatigue or stress. Rate of speech remains essentially normal.

7—**Obvious Speech Abnormalities**—Speech is consistently impaired. Affected are rate, articulation, and resonance. Remains easily understood.

Behavioral Modifications

6—**Repeats Messages on Occasion**—Rate is much slower. Repeats specific words in adverse listening situations. Does not limit complexity or length of message.

5—**Frequent Repeating Required**—Speech is slow and labored. Extensive repetition or a "translator" is commonly needed. Person probably limits the complexity or length of messages.

Use of Augmentative Communication

4—**Speech Plus Augmentative Communication**—Speech is used in response to questions. Intelligibility problems need to be resolved by writing or a spokesman.

3—**Limits Speech to One Word Response**—Vocalizes one word response beyond yes/no, otherwise writes or uses a spokesman. Initiates communication non-vocally.

Loss of Useful Speech

2—**Vocalizes for Emotional Expression**—Uses vocal inflection to express emotion, affirmation and negation.

1—**Non-Vocal**—Vocalization is effortful, limited in duration, and rarely attempted. May vocalize for crying or pain.

X—**Tracheostomy**

From Yorkston, K.M., Strand, E., Miller, R.M., Hillel, A.D., & Smith, K. (1993). Speech deterioration in amyotrophic lateral sclerosis: Implications for the timing of intervention. *Journal of Medical Speech-Language Pathology, 1*(1), 35–46; reprinted by permission.

lems occurred in patients with a vital capacity of 1 liter or less, but occasionally they occurred in patients with relatively high vital capacities. When these problems were judged to be serious, those data were not included in the results reported here.

Subjects

Records for 140 individuals with a confirmed diagnosis of ALS were reviewed. Table 2 contains the demographic information for the clinical population. Note that patients were grouped into three types according to their report of initial symptoms. Individuals in the bulbar group (28 women and 20 men) reported speech or swallowing problems or both as the initial symptom. Individuals in the spinal group (28 women and 38 men) reported changes in arm or leg function or both as the initial symp-

Table 2. Demographic information for clinical population at initial evaluation (N = 140)

	Initial symptoms					
	Bulbar		Spinal		Mixed	
	Women	Men	Women	Men	Women	Men
Number	28	20	28	38	10	16
(% of total)	(20)	(14)	(20)	(27)	(7)	(11)
Age in years						
Mean	65	59	63	55	69	57
SD	10	13	8.3	13	6.7	17
Months postdiagnosis						
Mean	4.6	7.2	8.4	18.4	8.6	13.6
SD	6.7	7.7	8.1	19.5	10.4	16.1
Vital capacity (L)						
Mean	1.74	3.3	1.72	2.73	1.76	3.35
SD	0.7	1.1	0.5	1.15	0.87	0.98
Percentage of predicted vital capacity	64	82	62	66	66	82

tom. Individuals in the mixed group (10 women and 16 men) reported both spinal and bulbar changes as initial symptoms. The mean age of onset ranged from 55 to 69 years. This is consistent with larger epidemiologic studies (Juergens, Kurland, Okazaki, & Mulder, 1980). Although there was a trend for women to be older than men at age of onset, simple t-tests indicated that the trend was not statistically significant. On the average, initial clinic visits occurred from 4.6 to 18.4 months after diagnosis. Women were seen for their initial visits earlier than men. Those with initial bulbar symptoms were seen in the clinic earlier than those with initial spinal symptoms. Earlier clinic visits for the bulbar group would be expected because the clinic focused on management of speech and swallowing disorders. Also included in Table 2 are data related to the vital capacity (in liters) and the percentage of predicted vital capacity. Note that the percentages of predicted vital capacity for women range from 62% to 66% and those for men range from 66% to 82%. Thus, at the time of the initial clinic visit, all groups were experiencing some reduction in vital capacity as compared to estimates of normal function.

Figure 1 illustrates the pattern of function in the areas of bulbar and spinal function for the three groups: initial bulbar, initial spinal, and initial mixed symptoms. The Bulbar Cumulative Scale score was computed by adding the Speech and the Swallowing Scale scores; the spinal cumulative score was computed by adding the Lower and the Upper Extremity Scale scores (Yorkston, Miller, & Strand, 1995). Note that, as expected, individuals with initial bulbar symptoms continued to experience greater bulbar

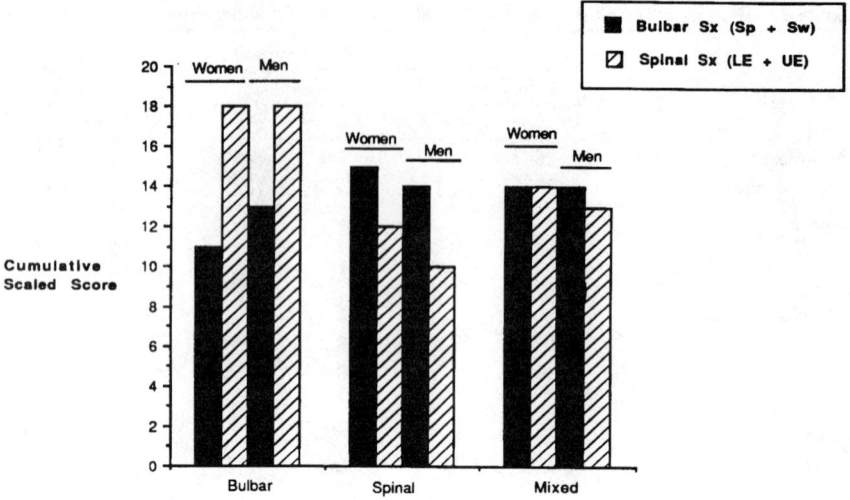

Figure 1. Cumulative scale scores for bulbar (black) and spinal (diagonals) symptoms for women and men with ALS. The subjects are grouped by pattern of initial symptoms: bulbar, spinal, or mixed. See text for description of cumulative scores. (Sp = speech; Sw = swallowing; LE = lower extremity; UE = upper extremity.)

than spinal involvement at the time of the first clinic visit. Likewise, those with initial spinal symptoms continued to experience greater spinal involvement at the time of the first clinic visit. The group with mixed initial symptoms exhibited roughly equivalent dysfunction across the bulbar and spinal scales.

RESULTS AND DISCUSSION

Recall that our first research question examined the relationship between the level of bulbar function and respiratory status (as measured by vital capacity). We were interested in two patient groups—those with initial bulbar symptoms versus those with initial spinal symptoms. Data from all patient visits for individuals with initial bulbar or spinal symptoms were examined (N = 114 subjects and 289 clinic visits). Figure 2 illustrates changes in Bulbar Scale scores (Speech plus Swallowing Scale scores) as a function of mean vital capacity. A review of the figure suggests that, for individuals with Bulbar Scale scores of 14 or less, there is a consistent decline in mean vital capacity. This decline in function occurs both for individuals with initial bulbar symptoms and for those with initial spinal symptoms. Furthermore, the slope of decline for those with initial spinal symptoms is similar to that for patients with initial bulbar symptoms. Thus, when bulbar function is severely compromised, one must also ex-

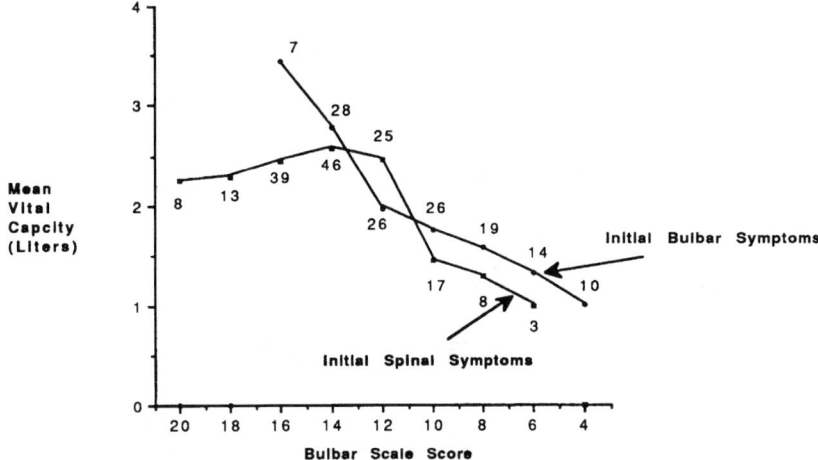

Figure 2. Mean vital capacity (in liters) as a function of Bulbar Scale scores for individuals with ALS with initial bulbar symptoms and with initial spinal symptoms. The data represent 114 patients and 289 clinic visits. The numbers adjacent to the lines indicate the number of patient visits represented by that point. (Sp = speech; Sw = swallowing.)

pect severe compromise in respiratory status, regardless of the pattern of initial symptoms.

The second question posed relates to longitudinal data: What is the rate of change in respiratory status over time, and does it vary as a function of the patient's initial symptoms or gender? In order to answer this question, data from the initial and most recent clinic visits were compared for individuals who were seen for at least three clinic visits. This population includes a total of 56 individuals, 19 with initial bulbar symptoms, 29 with initial spinal symptoms, and 8 with initial mixed symptoms. Table 3 presents the gender distribution of the groups.

Figure 3 illustrates mean initial and most current vital capacity for women and men in each initial symptom grouping (bulbar, spinal, and mixed). As points of comparison, the normal ranges of vital capacity for a 55-year-old woman and man are also illustrated. Examination of the figure suggests that, at the time of the initial clinic visit, both women and men with ALS tended to be at the low end of the normal range of respiratory function as measured by vital capacity. As progression occurs, the res-

Table 3. Gender distribution of subjects followed longitudinally

	Initial symptoms		
	Bulbar	Spinal	Mixed
Women	13	10	5
Men	6	19	3
Total	19	29	8

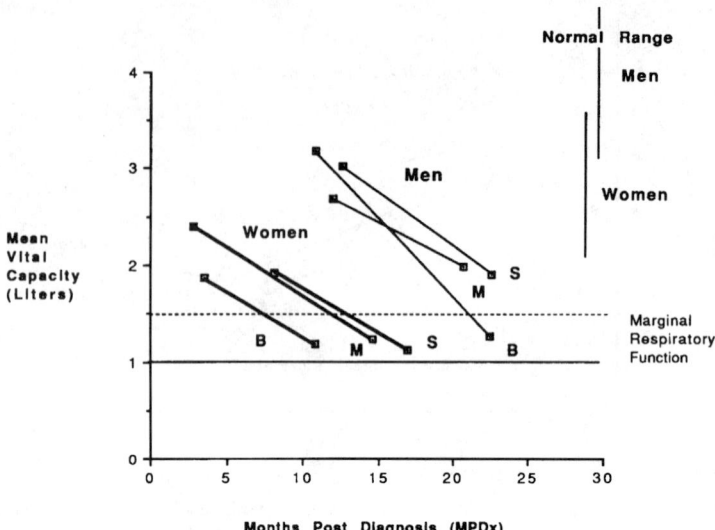

Figure 3. Mean vital capacity (in liters) as a function of months postdiagnosis for women and men. Subjects are grouped by type of initial symptoms: bulbar (B), spinal (S), and mixed (M). Group data are presented for the means of the initial (heavy lines) and most recent (light lines) clinic visits. Also included are the range of normal function for men and women and the range of respiratory function that is considered marginal.

piratory status of individuals with ALS may decline to the range of marginal adequacy (1.0–1.5 L). Note also that all groups decline, regardless of initial symptoms. For example, for women the slopes for the bulbar, mixed, and spinal groups are similar. Both women and men with initial bulbar symptoms tend to experience respiratory decline slightly earlier than those with initial spinal symptoms. Thus, clinically one must anticipate respiratory decline in *all* ALS patients regardless of initial symptoms.

Our final question relates to the relationship between rate of progression in respiratory status and change in speech function. In order to answer this question, median Speech Scale scores at initial and most current visits were plotted for the 56 individuals with ALS described above. Figure 4 illustrates the median Speech Scale scores for initial and most current visits for women and men in the bulbar, spinal, and mixed initial symptom groups. Also included is the point at which natural speech is no longer completely functional. In other words, a Speech Scale score of 4 indicates that natural speech is supplemented by writing or other means of resolving communication breakdowns. Of particular interest is the relatively rapid rate of functional speech decline in women. Note the more rapid rate of decline for women with initial bulbar symptoms as compared with the spinal or mixed groups. Recall that all three groups of women declined to the marginal range of respiratory function, yet only the bulbar group experienced a rapid loss of speech function. One is tempted to speculate

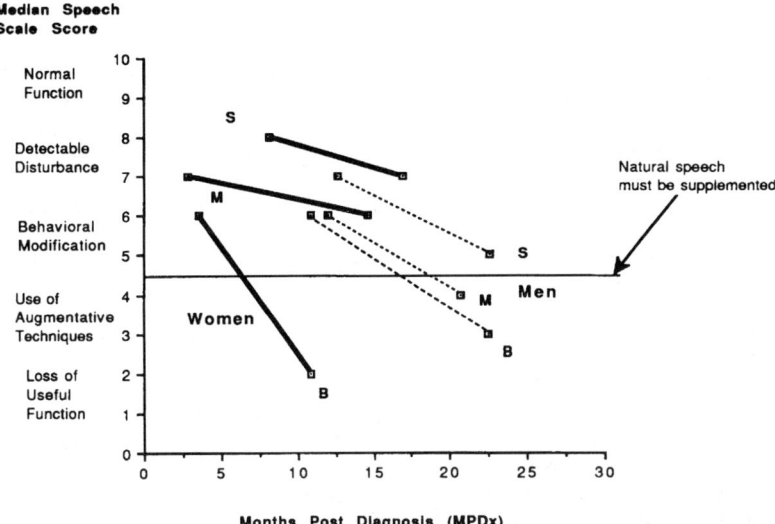

Figure 4. Median Speech Scale scores as a function of months postdiagnosis for women and men. Subjects are grouped by type of initial symptom: bulbar (B), spinal (S), and mixed (M). Group data are presented for the means of the initial (solid lines) and most recent (dashed lines) clinic visits. Also included is the point at which natural speech must be supplemented.

that the women with initial bulbar symptoms are challenged by both decline in respiratory support and rapid decline in oral movement. This dual impairment leads to a profound and rapid functional loss.

CONCLUSIONS

Our results suggest that decline in respiratory status must be anticipated in ALS regardless of the pattern of initial symptoms. Although individuals with initial bulbar symptoms experience this decline earlier than those with initial spinal symptoms, the respiratory status of individuals with initial spinal symptoms must also be carefully monitored. Knowledge of changes in respiratory status is necessary for the adequate timing of speech and swallowing intervention for a number of reasons. First, poor respiratory support exaggerates the oral movement problems of individuals with bulbar symptoms and contributes to vocal changes in individuals with spinal symptoms. Second, respiratory decline must be considered in management of swallowing disorders in ALS. Optimal timing of surgical tube or percutaneous endoscopic gastrostomy placement is dependent not only on swallowing status but also on respiratory status (Strand, Miller, Yorkston, & Hillel, in press). Finally, knowledge of a patient's respiratory status is critical for the timing of patient education regarding ventilatory support.

REFERENCES

Annoni, J., Chevrolet, J., & Kesselring, J. (1993). Resiratory problems in chronic neurological disorders. *Critical Reviews in Physical and Rehabilitation Medicine, 5*(2), 155–192.

Braun, S.R. (1987). Respiratory systems in amyotrophic lateral sclerosis. *Neurologic Clinics, 5*(1), 9–31.

Darley, F.L., Aronson, A.E., & Brown, J.R. (1975). *Motor speech disorders.* Philadelphia: W. B. Saunders.

DePaul, R., & Abbs, J.H. (1987). Manifestations of ALS in the cranial motor nerves. *Neurologic Clinics, 5*, 231–250.

Gubbay, S.S., Kahana, E., Zilber, N., & Cooper, G. (1985). Amyotrophic lateral sclerosis: A study of its presentation and prognosis. *Journal of Neurology, 232*, 295–300.

Juergens, S.M., Kurland, L.T., Okazaki, H., & Mulder, D.W. (1980). ALS in Rochester, Minnesota, 1925–1977. *Neurology, 30*, 463–470.

Pradas, J., Finison, L., Andres, P.L., Thornell, B., Hollander, D., & Munsat, T.L. (1993). The natural history of amyotrophic lateral sclerosis and the use of natural history control in therapeutic trials. *Neurology, 43*, 751–755.

Robin, D.A., Goel, A., Somodi, L.B., & Luschei, E.S. (1992). Tongue strength and endurance: Relation to highly skilled movements. *Journal of Speech & Hearing Research, 35*, 1239–1245.

Rosen, A. (1978). Amyotrophic lateral sclerosis: Clinical features and prognosis. *Archives of Neurology, 35*, 638–642.

Schiffman, P.L., & Belsh, J.M. (1993). Pulmonary function at diagnosis of amyotrophic lateral sclerosis: Rate of deterioration. *Chest, 103*, 508–513.

Somodi, L.B., Robin, D.A., & Luschei, E.S. (in press). A model of sense of effort of the tongue. *Brain and Language.*

Strand, E.A., Miller, R.M., Yorkston, K.M., & Hillel, A.D. (in press). Progression of dysphagia symptoms in ALS: Implications for timing of intervention. *Dysphagia.*

Tandan, R., & Bradley, W.G. (1985). Amyotrophic lateral sclerosis: Part 1. Clinical features, pathology, and ethical issues in management. *Annals of Neurology, 18*, 271–280.

Tidwell, J. (1993). Pulmonary management of the ALS patients. *Journal of Neuroscience Nursing, 25*, 337–342.

Yorkston, K.M., Miller, R.M., & Strand, E.A. (1995). *Management of speech and swallowing in degenerational diseases.* Tucson, AZ: Communication Skill Builders.

Yorkston, K.M., Strand, E., Miller, R.M., Hillel, A.D., & Smith, K. (1993). Speech deterioration in amyotrophic lateral sclerosis: Implications for the timing of intervention. *Journal of Medical Speech-Language Pathology, 1*(1), 35–46.

SECTION VI

MOTOR SPEECH INVOLVEMENT IN TRAUMATIC BRAIN INJURY

Chapter 12

Differential Patterns of Hyperfunctional Laryngeal Impairment in Dysarthric Speakers Following Severe Closed Head Injury

Deborah G. Theodoros and Bruce E. Murdoch

A SEVERE CLOSED head injury (CHI) has the potential to cause widespread disruption to the speech production mechanism, resulting in the motor speech disorder of dysarthria. The laryngeal subsystem is one of several components of the speech mechanism that may be compromised by the effects of a severe CHI, resulting in phonatory disturbance or dysphonia. Dysphonia has frequently been observed following severe head trauma and is generally seen as part of a specific dysarthric syndrome involving deviant respiratory, articulatory, and resonatory features (Aronson, 1980; Darley, Aronson, & Brown, 1975; Greene, 1972; Hartman, 1984; Vogel & von Cramon, 1982).

In that phonation requires highly integrated neurophysiologic coordination, it is likely that laryngeal dysfunction may result from impairment at many levels of the central nervous system (Hanson, 1991). The biomechanics of a CHI are such that damage can occur to diverse areas of the brain and as a result cause impairment of components of the central nervous system associated with laryngeal function. In the individual with CHI, a broad spectrum of laryngeal dysfunction involving hyperfunctional, hypofunctional, and incoordinated laryngeal activity can be ex-

---

Reprinted with minor revisions from *Brain Injury*, 8, 669–684, 1994, by permission of the authors and Taylor & Francis Ltd.

This research was supported by a grant from the National Health and Medical Research Council, Australia (Grant No. 930957).

pected to result from bilateral lesions of the upper motor neurons, damage to specific lower motor neurons that supply laryngeal musculature, lesions of the extrapyramidal system and its connections, lesions of the cerebellum and its connecting pathways, and lesions involving several locations within the central and/or peripheral nervous system. As a result of these lesions, the CHI subject may exhibit features of spastic, flaccid, hypokinetic, or ataxic dysphonia, or a combination of these, respectively (Aronson, 1980; Hartman, 1984).

Specific investigation of laryngeal dysfunction in dysarthric speakers following CHI has received minimal attention in the research literature. Previous studies have mainly focused on the etiology of aphonia following CHI (Sapir & Aronson, 1985; Scholefield, 1987), the acoustic measurement of the vocal quality in central dysphonia (Hartmann & von Cramon, 1984), and the documentation of the recovery of phonation following traumatic mutism (Vogel & von Cramon, 1982; von Cramon, 1981). Recently, a comprehensive study by Theodoros, Murdoch, and Chenery (1994) involving a perceptual analysis of the dysarthric speech of 20 severe CHI subjects found that 75% of the subjects were perceived to exhibit laryngeal dysfunction to some degree, based on five deviant laryngeal characteristics (harshness, strained–strangled quality, hoarseness, glottal fry, and intermittent breathiness). The finding of a high incidence of dysphonia in a group of CHI subjects is significant in that phonation is known to play an important role in the production and intelligibility of speech. The laryngeal subsystem not only provides the acoustic medium through which speech is delivered but also contributes to the suprasegmental and articulatory features of speech (Ramig, 1992).

Although perceptual analysis is commonly used as a primary clinical tool in the assessment of laryngeal function and voice, the validity of this method of evaluation is questionable, given the lack of definition of the concept of "normal" voice and its deviations, the low reliability and standardization difficulties associated with perceptual judgments, and the limitations of perceptual analysis in identifying specific deviant perceptual features (Blaustein & Bar, 1983; Fex, 1992; Hoodin & Gilbert, 1989; Kearns & Simmons, 1988; Kent & Rosenbek, 1982; Lethlean, Chenery, & Murdoch, 1990; Ludlow & Bassich, 1983; Zyski & Weisiger, 1987). Perceptual analysis essentially identifies and describes the characteristics of a speech or voice disorder but in effect does not define the nature of the physiologic impairment involved (Orlikoff, 1992). As a result, the reliance on perceptual assessment of laryngeal function alone may lead to inaccurate assumptions regarding the true nature of the phonatory disturbance (Theodoros et al., 1994).

The inadequacy of perceptual analysis and the complex neuromotor coordination involved in the phonatory process necessitate an objective physiologic evaluation of the laryngeal subsystem of speech in dysarthric CHI speakers. The aim of the current study, therefore, was to provide a detailed perceptual and physiologic evaluation of the laryngeal function of a group of severe CHI subjects with dysarthric speech to determine the frequency and severity of deviant laryngeal features, the nature of the vocal fold vibratory movements, and the laryngeal aerodynamics.

METHODS

Subjects

The subject group consisted of 19 individuals who had been clinically diagnosed by either a qualified neurologist or neurosurgeon as having suffered a severe CHI. All subjects were rated as having Glasgow Coma Scale (GCS) (Teasdale & Jennett; 1974) scores on admission of less than 8. A GCS score based on the medical history was assigned retrospectively to three subjects (3, 14, and 18) who had sustained head injuries prior to the introduction of the GCS rating scale. In addition to the neurologic diagnosis, each subject exhibited a perceptible speech deficit diagnosed as dysarthria by a qualified speech pathologist. Seventeen (89%) of the total sample of CHI subjects were male (mean age = 31.6 years; standard deviation [SD] = 7.82; range = 21–55 years) and two (10%) were female (mean age = 30.5 years; SD = 4.5; range = 26–35 years). The mean age of the total sample of CHI subjects was 31.5 years (SD = 7.54), with ages ranging from 21 to 55 years. All subjects were at least 3 months postonset of the CHI (see Table 1 for subjects' biographical details).

Subjects were excluded from the study if they had either a previous history of a speech disorder prior to the onset of the CHI, an existing neurologic disease or disorder other than that due to the CHI, or a speech disturbance due to another disorder coexisting post-CHI. Other criteria for exclusion of subjects included a positive history of either respiratory disease, drug and/or alcohol abuse, or dementia.

A further group of 19 nonneurologically impaired subjects matched for age (mean age = 31.2 years; SD = 7.70; range = 20–56 years) and sex served as controls. All control subjects had perceptually normal speech as judged by a qualified speech pathologist. Subjects were excluded from the control group if they had any previous or current history of respiratory disease, alcohol and/or drug abuse, traumatic brain injury, cerebrovascular accident, dementia, or other neurologic disorder.

Perceptual Assessment

Speech Sample Each subject was required to read a standard passage, the "Grandfather Passage" (Darley et al., 1975), to provide a sample of his

Table 1. Biographical and clinical details of closed head injury subjects (N = 19)

Subject	Age (years)	Sex	Year post-injury	Handedness	Nature of accident[a]	GCS score	Severity of CHI
1	21	M	2.5	Right	MVA	4	Severe
2	28	M	3.0	Left	STL	3	Severe
3	39	M	21.5	Right	MVA	3	Severe
4	32	M	8.0	Right	Fall	4	Severe
5	35	F	9.0	Right	MVA	4	Severe
6	25	M	7.0	Right	MVA	4	Severe
7	26	F	6.4	Right	MVA	4	Severe
8	26	M	7.0	Right	MVA	4	Severe
9	27	M	8.7	Right	MCA	6	Severe
10	55	M	2.0	Right	MVA	4	Severe
11	33	M	8.3	Right	RA	5	Severe
12	28	M	2.0	Left	MVA	5	Severe
13	25	M	0.6	Right	MVA	3	Severe
14	31	M	16.0	Right	FBI	3	Severe
15	25	M	8.7	Right	MCA	5	Severe
16	36	M	7.4	Right	MVA	6	Severe
17	32	M	0.4	Right	Fall	5	Severe
18	41	M	23.0	Right	Fall	3	Severe
19	34	M	5.2	Right	MVA	3	Severe

[a]FBI, football injury; MCA, motorcycle accident; MVA, motor vehicle accident; RA, railway accident; STL, struck by tree limb.

or her speech for perceptual analysis. An unlimited time period was allowed for each subject to familiarize himself or herself with the passage prior to reading. When the subject was fully prepared, he or she was instructed to speak in a natural manner, using a normal speaking rate, with a loudness level appropriate for speaking to one or two people in quiet surroundings. The speech sample was recorded onto audiotape using a JVC Radio Cassette Recorder (Model M60WH). The microphone was located 50 cm from the subject's mouth. One subject whose visual acuity was too poor to enable him to read the large print listened to a recording of the passage, and his repetition of each phrase was recorded on audiotape as described above.

Analysis of Speech Sample Each speech sample was rated by two judges (both qualified speech-language pathologists) on the series of dimensions used by Fitzgerald, Murdoch, and Chenery (1987). The series comprised 32 different dimensions of speech that pertained to five aspects of speech production (prosody, respiration, phonation, resonance, and articulation) and the overall intelligibility of speech. For the purposes of the current study, only the perceptual ratings for laryngeal function were extracted for further analysis.

Laryngeal function was assessed on five dimensions relating to hyperfunction (harshness and strained–strangled quality), hypofunction (hoarseness and glottal fry), and incoordination of the larynx (intermittent breathiness) (Darley et al., 1975). A descriptive 4-point equal-interval scale was used to rate the subjects' laryngeal function on each of the abnormal laryngeal perceptual features. A rating of 1 indicated an absence of the deviant laryngeal feature, 2 represented a just-noticeable presence of the dimension, 3 indicated the perception of a moderate degree of the deviant laryngeal feature, and a rating of 4 was indicative of the presence of the abnormal laryngeal feature to a severe degree.

Both judges listened independently to a recording of the speech sample. In all, two tapes of the speech samples were made, each with a randomized order of presentation of subjects. The judges had no knowledge regarding to which group each subject belonged. The judges were allowed unlimited time to listen to the tapes of the speech samples and rate each of the speech dimensions.

Following the judges' independent rating sessions, a further rating session was conducted during which both judges conferred to produce a single consensus rating for each of the laryngeal dimensions. The consensus ratings obtained from the two judges for each of the five deviant laryngeal dimensions were used in the analysis of the results.

Instrumental Assessment of Laryngeal Function

Instrumentation The laryngeal function of the 19 CHI and 19 control subjects was assessed instrumentally using electrolaryngographic and aerodynamic techniques. The assessments were performed on each subject on the same day.

While it is recognized that both of these techniques have inherent inadequacies, and caution should be exercised in the interpretation of results (Colton & Conture, 1990; Holmberg, Hillman, & Perkell, 1988), electrolaryngography and aerodynamic techniques are noninvasive and clinically available and provide useful information regarding laryngeal function. Electrolaryngography evaluates laryngeal microfunctions such as cycle-by-cycle periodicity and degree of vocal fold contact (Childers, Hicks, Moore, Eskenazi, & Lalwani, 1990; Childers & Krishnamurthy, 1985; Motta, Cesari, Iengo, & Motta, 1990), while aerodynamic techniques are designed to examine the macrofunctions of the larynx, which include laryngeal airway resistance, laryngeal airflow, and subglottal pressure (Holmberg, 1980; Holmberg et al., 1988; Netsell, Lotz, Du Chane, & Barlow, 1991).

Procedure for Electrolaryngographic Assessment Electrolaryngographic assessment of each subject was conducted using a Fourcin laryngograph interfaced with a Waveform Display System, Model 6091 (Kay Elemetrics

Corp.) running on a 486DX IBM-compatible computer. The system records the surface area of contact of the vocal folds and the subsequent vocal fold vibratory patterns during phonation. These features are displayed in the form of an Lx waveform (Baken, 1987). The Waveform Display System allows for acquisition and real-time viewing of the Lx waveform on the computer monitor as well as storage and analysis of segments of the waveform.

Laryngographic recordings were made with the subject seated in a straight-backed chair with his or her head positioned in the midline both horizontally and vertically. The subject was instructed not to flex or extend his/her neck and to remain in a steady position throughout the assessment. The duration of the procedure was approximately 15 minutes.

The surface electrodes, attached by Velcro to an elasticized neckband, were positioned over the laminae of the thyroid cartilage (Baken, 1987; Colton & Conture, 1990) and the neckband firmly fastened to ensure adequate electrode-to-skin contact. In that correct electrode placement is not always readily achieved (Colton & Conture, 1990), the subject was required to sustain the vowel /i/ while the gain level was adjusted to achieve the highest possible signal level. In cases in which the Lx signal remained very weak, the electrodes were moved up or down the neck in small increments or repositioned horizontally along the neckband. The researcher monitored the level of the Lx signal to determine which electrode position resulted in the highest possible signal level for each subject.

When the most suitable electrode position was determined, Lx waveforms were recorded as the subject repeated a series of vowels (/i/, /a/, /ɔ/, /u/, /ɜ/) and voiced continuant consonants (/m/, /n/, /r/, /z/, /v/). The subject was instructed to repeat each of the vowels and consonants for a duration similar to that demonstrated by the researcher (approximately 3 seconds). A waveform was recorded for each vowel and voiced consonant produced by the subject. One vowel, /i/, and a voiced consonant, /m/, were repeated three times each by the subject to determine intrasubject reliability. Mean values obtained for each of these sounds were used in the statistical analyses. In all, 14 Lx waveforms were recorded for analysis from each subject.

Lx Waveform Analysis The Lx waveforms recorded in the current study were displayed with the upward movement of the curve indicating increasing vocal fold contact (glottal closure) and the downward movement of the curve representing decreasing vocal fold contact (glottal opening). Although it is well recognized that the Lx waveform is difficult to quantify due to problems in determining the exact point on the waveform where vocal fold opening and closing commence and finish, Colton and Conture (1990) suggested that there are three basic measurements that can be made from the Lx waveform that may be useful in studying vocal fold vibration. These measures include fundamental frequency (F_0), duty cycle (DC), and closing time (CT). Analysis of the Lx waveforms recorded for each subject involved the calculation of these three parameters from each waveform. To obtain a reliable measure of each parameter, values were determined from each of three consecutive waveforms for each subject and the mean value for the parameter was used in further statistical analyses.

The F_0 for each waveform relates to the periodicity of the waveform and was determined by the calculation of the number of complete glottal cycles (the period/length of time necessary for the vocal folds to complete one vibratory cycle). The value for F_0 for each waveform was recorded in Hertz. The DC of the waveform is defined as the ratio of time that the vocal folds are open during the vocal period compared to the duration of the total vibratory cycle. A DC value was determined for each waveform by the statistical program of the Waveform Display System.

Closing time corresponded to the duration of the closing phase from totally open to totally closed. The CT was determined by positioning the cursors at the points on the waveform where the vocal folds could be reasonably assumed to be totally open and totally closed. The cursor positions were assigned to the lowest cursor counter number in the open phase and the highest cursor counter number in the closing phase. The duration of the total closing phase was recorded in milliseconds.

Procedure for Aerodynamic Assessment The aerodynamic assessment of each subject was performed using a voice function analyzer, the Aerophone II, Model 6800 (Kay Elemetrics Corp.). The Aerophone II consists of a hand-held transducer module together with a powerful data acquisition and processing software program for use in a 486DX IBM-compatible computer. The transducer module consists of miniaturized transducers that are capable of recording airflow, air pressure, and acoustic signals during speech. A disposable anesthetic face mask through which a thin flexible tube of silicon rubber was inserted to record intraoral pressure was attached to the hand-held transducer module. In the current study, a F300L flowhead was used for data collection.

The software program provided a real-time display of the subject's sound pressure level, air pressure, and airflow during speech. The subject's responses were instantly sampled 1,000 times per second and displayed in the form of color graphic traces on the monitor screen. The traces were subsequently analyzed to determine calibrated numerical values relating to sound pressure level, air pressure, and airflow.

The aerodynamic assessment was conducted with the subject seated comfortably in a straight-backed chair. Each subject was required to place the mask of the transducer module over his or her face with the thin tube positioned centrally over the top of the tongue. The subject was instructed to hold the mask firmly over his or her face to ensure an adequate seal around the face. Two tasks were selected to evaluate the aerodynamics of laryngeal function—a vocal efficiency task and a task involving rapid initiation and termination of voicing to determine the ad/abduction rate of the vocal folds.

The vocal efficiency task involved the subject's repetition of /ipipipi/ for several seconds until an adequate recording was obtained. The task enabled an estimation of subglottal air pressure (GP) (in centimeters of water) by measuring the intraoral air pressure during the pronunciation of /ipipipi/. The point of maximum oral pressure during the pronunciation of the /p/ was calculated automatically over six repetitions and used as an estimate of subglottal pressure. In addition to subglottal air pressure, three other parameters, average phonatory sound pressure level (SPL) (in decibels), laryngeal airway resistance (LR) (in centimeters of water per liter per second), and phonatory airflow (PF) (in liters per second) were determined from the vocal efficiency task and used in further statistical analyses.

In the second task, each subject was required to initiate and terminate voicing as quickly as possible by repeating /ʌʌʌ/, enabling an ad/abduction rate (AB) (in cycles per second) of the vocal folds to be determined. The task was demonstrated by the researcher, and the subject was instructed to ensure that voicing was initiated and then completely terminated before proceeding with the next vocalization. The duration of each task was approximately 5 minutes.

RESULTS

Perceptual Analysis

An analysis of the perceptual ratings for the CHI subjects for the deviant laryngeal features of harshness, strained–strangled vocal quality, hoarseness, glottal fry, and intermittent breathiness revealed that 16 (84%) CHI subjects were perceived by the judges as having some degree of laryngeal dysfunction, whereas the remaining 3 (16%) CHI subjects were not perceived to exhibit any abnormalities. Details of the severity and type of deviant laryngeal features exhibited by each of the CHI subjects are shown in Table 2. In the control group, all 19 (100%) of the subjects were rated as having perceptibly normal laryngeal function (i.e., no evidence of any of the above deviant laryngeal features).

Nine (47%) of the CHI subjects were perceived to exhibit harshness at varying degrees. A mild degree of harshness was evident in the vocal quality of 2 (22%) of the 9 CHI subjects, a moderate degree was present in 6 (66%) of the 9 subjects, and a severe degree of harshness was considered to be present in 1 (11%) of these CHI subjects. A strained–strangled vocal

Table 2. Type and severity of deviant laryngeal perceptual features for each CHI subject

Subject	Harshness	Strained–strangled	Hoarseness	Gottal fry	Intermittent breathiness
1	Absent	Absent	Just noticeable	Just noticeable	Just noticeable
2	Moderate	Moderate	Absent	Moderate	Just noticeable
3	Severe	Moderate	Just noticeable	Just noticeable	Absent
4	Absent	Absent	Moderate	Absent	Moderate
5	Just noticeable	Just noticeable	Just noticeable	Absent	Moderate
6	Absent	Absent	Absent	Absent	Absent
7	Absent	Absent	Absent	Absent	Absent
8	Absent	Absent	Absent	Absent	Absent
9	Absent	Absent	Just noticeable	Absent	Absent
10	Moderate	Moderate	Moderate	Moderate	Moderate
11	Just noticeable	Absent	Absent	Absent	Absent
12	Absent	Absent	Just noticeable	Absent	Just noticeable
13	Moderate	Moderate	Absent	Absent	Absent
14	Absent	Absent	Just noticeable	Absent	Absent
15	Absent	Absent	Moderate	Just noticeable	Just noticeable
16	Moderate	Absent	Absent	Absent	Absent
17	Moderate	Just noticeable	Absent	Absent	Absent
18	Moderate	Just noticeable	Absent	Absent	Absent
19	Absent	Absent	Severe	Absent	Moderate

quality was rated as being present in 7 (36%) of the 19 CHI subjects, with 3 (42%) of these 7 subjects exhibiting a mild degree of strained–strangled quality and 4 (57%) subjects displaying a moderate degree of this abnormal laryngeal feature.

Within the group of CHI subjects, 10 (52%) exhibited a hoarse vocal quality. Six (60%) of the 10 subjects were rated as having a mild hoarseness, 3 (30%) subjects were considered to be moderately hoarse, and 1 (10%) subject exhibited a severe hoarseness. The abnormal laryngeal characteristic of glottal fry was evident in 5 (26%) of the 19 CHI subjects, 3 (60%) of whom were considered to exhibit a mild degree of glottal fry while 2 (40%) were rated as displaying a moderate degree of glottal fry. Intermittent breathiness was perceived to be present in 8 (42%) of the CHI subjects, 4 (50%) of whom exhibited intermittent breathiness to a mild degree while the remaining 4 (50%) subjects were intermittently breathy to a moderate degree. The frequency of occurrence and severity of the deviant laryngeal features exhibited by the CHI subjects are presented in Table 3.

Instrumental Data Analysis

From each of the Lx traces recorded during the production of each of the five vowel and five consonant sounds, three separate waveforms were ana-

Table 3. Occurrence and severity of deviant laryngeal features in CHI subjects

Deviant laryngeal feature	Number of subjects	%	Mild		Moderate		Severe	
			n	%	n	%	n	%
Harshness	9	47	2	22	6	66	1	11
Strained–strangled	7	36	3	42	4	57	—	—
Hoarseness	10	52	6	60	3	30	1	10
Glottal fry	5	26	3	60	2	40	—	—
Intermittent breathiness	8	42	4	50	4	50	—	—

lyzed to obtain three sets of values, which were averaged to provide a measure of the F_0, DC, and CT for each sound. Statistical comparisons between each individual sound revealed that the F_0, DC, and CT values for all of the vowel and consonant sounds were not significantly different from each other and therefore could be collapsed to provide a mean value for F_0, DC, and CT for each subject. For statistical analysis, the parameters of GP, SPL, LR, PF, and AB from the aerodynamic assessment data were combined with the mean values for F_0, DC, and CT.

A preliminary examination of the instrumental data for the CHI subjects indicated a wide range of laryngeal performance within the subjects. As a result, it was considered inappropriate to directly compare the laryngeal performances of the CHI and control subjects on all of the instrumental measures as any difference between the two groups would be masked by the variability of laryngeal function in the CHI group. Of the eight variables, only four—F_0, CT, AB, and LR—demonstrated consistency across the CHI group. t-Tests for independent measures revealed that, as a group, the CHI subjects exhibited a significantly higher F_0 (t_{36} = −2.76, $p < .01$), faster CT (t_{36} = 5.74, $p < .01$), slower AB (t_{36} = 3.90, $p < .01$), and greater LR (t_{36} = −2.08, $p < .05$) than the control subjects (see Table 4).

In accordance with the suggestion by Holmberg et al. (1988) that analysis of laryngeal behavior in a subject group may need to involve the identification of subgroupings of subjects with similar vocal function to overcome intersubject variability, the instrumental data were subjected to an agglomerative hierarchical cluster analysis using complete linkage (SPSS/PC + Statistics 4.0; Norusis, 1990) to determine subgroups within the CHI group and to instrumentally define the laryngeal characteristics of each group. The cluster analysis, using all of the instrumental laryngeal variables (F_0, DC, CT, AB, GP, SPL, LR, and PF), identified the presence of five subgroups of CHI subjects, each with similar characteristics. The formation of the subgroups is displayed in the form of a dendrogram using complete linkage in Figure 1. From the dendrogram, it would appear that the clustering of the CHI subjects into five subgroups was the most appro-

Table 4. Comparison of means and standard deviations for CHI and control subjects for F_0, CT, AB, and LR

	Control subjects (n=19)		CHI subjects (n=19)		Difference between means	t	p
	Mean	SD	Mean	SD			
Fundamental frequency (F_0)	135.38	27.28	166.26	40.38	−30.88	−2.76	<.01
Closing time (CT)	2.97	0.62	1.96	0.45	1.01	5.74	<.01
Ad/abduction rate (AB)	3.75	1.29	2.39	0.80	1.36	3.90	<.01
Laryngeal airway resistance (LR)	24.52	15.77	40.03	28.26	−15.51	−2.08	<.05

priate distribution of subjects. The clusters were shown to be easily distinguishable and were formed within nine units from the origin (i.e., before the distances at which clusters were combined became too large).

An examination of the instrument measures obtained by each of the five subgroups identified hyperfunctional patterns of laryngeal activity in each subgroup. The subgroups differed, however, in the form in which the hyperfunctional laryngeal behavior was manifested. As there were limited numbers of subjects in each of the subgroups, the average performance of the members in each subgroup was compared to the mean and standard deviation of the control group for each variable. The means and standard deviations for the control group and the five CHI subgroups on the eight

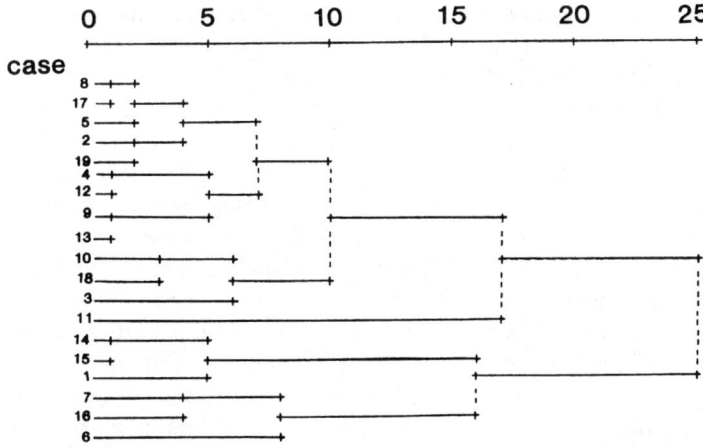

Figure 1. Dendrogram using complete linkage for the 19 CHI subjects.

variables (F_0, DC, CT, AB, GP, SPL, LR, and PF) are shown in Table 5. The characteristics of each subgroup are described in more detail below.

Subgroup 1 Subgroup 1 consisted of only one male subject (Subject 11), who remained isolated from the other CHI subjects following the cluster analysis (see Figure 1). Subject 11 exhibited F_0, DC, CT, and LR values that were within 1 *SD* of the controls. In addition, the subject exhibited a high GP (3.72 *SD* above the control mean), an elevated SPL (1.86 *SD* above the control mean), a very high PF (5.65 *SD* above the control mean), and a slow AB (1.34 *SD* below the control mean), which were largely consistent with a hyperfunctional pattern of laryngeal activity (see Table 5). The perceptual assessment of the laryngeal function of Subject 11 revealed the presence of a mild degree of harshness in the absence of any other deviant laryngeal features (see Table 2).

Subgroup 2 Three male subjects (Subjects 18, 10, and 3) were included in Subgroup 2. The instrumental measures obtained for the subjects in this subgroup indicated a presence of hyperfunctional laryngeal activity similar to that exhibited by the subject in Subgroup 1 but to a greater extent. For the subjects in Subgroup 2, only the mean values for DC and LR were within 1 *SD* of the control mean. The subjects differed from the controls on the basis of a high F_0 (1.96 *SD* above the control mean), fast CT (1.87 *SD* below the control mean), slow AB (1.18 *SD* below the control mean), very high GP (6.88 *SD* above the control mean), elevated SPL (2.99 *SD* above the control mean), and high PF (1.45 *SD* above the control mean) (see Table 5). Perceptually, the three subjects in Subgroup 2 exhibited a predominantly hyperfunctional pattern of laryngeal activity (see Table 2). Subject 18 was perceived to exhibit a moderate degree of harshness and a mild degree of strained–strangled vocal quality. The vocal quality of Subject 10 was considered to manifest hyperfunctional, hypofunctional, and incoordinated laryngeal characteristics, as indicated by the ratings of a moderate degree of harshness, strained–strangled vocal quality, hoarseness, glottal fry, and intermittent breathiness. The perceptual judges rated Subject 3 as predominantly displaying severe harshness and a moderate degree of strained–strangled vocal quality.

Subgroup 3 Subgroup 3 comprised nine subjects, eight male (Subjects 13, 9, 12, 4, 17, 8, 19, and 2) and one female (Subject 5). The instrumental measures recorded for the subjects in this subgroup generally reflected a mild hyperfunctional pattern of laryngeal activity that differed from the previous two subgroups in its presentation. The mean values for Subgroup 3 relating to GP, SPL, LR, and PF were found to be within 1 *SD* of the control mean. The subjects, however, differed from the controls in having a higher F_0 (1.48 *SD* above the control mean), shorter mean DC (1.20 *SD* below the control mean), faster CT (1.69 *SD* below the control mean), and slower AB (1.03 *SD* below the control mean) (see Table 5).

Table 5. Means and standard deviations for F_0, DC, CT, AB, GP, SPL, LR, and PF for control group and five CHI subgroups

Variable[a]	Control group (n=19)		Subgroup 1 (n=1)	Subgroup 2 (n=3)		Subgroup 3 (n=9)		Subgroup 4 (n=3)		Subgroup 5 (n=3)	
	Mean	SD	Mean	Mean	SD	Mean	SD	Mean	SD	Mean	SD
F_0	135.38	27.28	121.66	189.12	19.84	175.90	29.25	183.45	45.29	114.76	19.12
DC	0.55	0.05	0.54	0.52	0.07	0.49	0.04	0.49	0.01	0.58	0.008
CT	2.97	0.62	2.91	1.81	0.04	1.92	0.34	1.61	0.25	2.50	0.15
AB	3.75	1.29	2.01	2.22	0.72	2.41	0.56	1.75	0.68	3.40	0.65
GP	8.41	1.62	14.45	19.57	0.38	8.91	2.58	5.12	2.04	7.26	2.73
SPL	77.88	2.48	82.50	85.33	1.32	80.22	3.26	73.00	1.82	75.03	1.57
LR	24.52	15.77	9.13	28.26	8.08	31.84	12.34	73.03	39.11	53.66	28.28
PF	0.48	0.20	1.61	0.77	0.25	0.31	0.10	0.07	0.01	0.14	0.02

[a] F_0, fundamental frequency (Hz); DC, duty cycle; CT, closing time (ms); AB, adduction or abduction rate (cps); GP, glottal pressure (cm H_2O); SPL, sound pressure level (dB); LR, laryngeal airway resistance (cm H_2O/L/s); PF, phonatory flow rate (L/s).

The perceptual ratings for the subjects in Subgroup 3 revealed a wide range of laryngeal behaviors (see Table 2). Subject 13 was perceived to demonstrate a hyperfunctional pattern of laryngeal activity reflected in a rating of a moderate degree of harshness and strained–strangled vocal quality. The vocal quality of Subject 9 was perceived to be consistent with normal speakers except for the presence of a mild degree of hoarseness. Mildly hypofunctional and incoordinated laryngeal function was considered to be reflected in the vocal quality of Subject 12, whose ratings included mild hoarseness and intermittent breathiness. Similarly, Subject 4 was perceived to exhibit a moderate degree of hoarseness and intermittent breathiness. In contrast, Subject 17 was considered to display the hyperfunctional laryngeal features of harshness and strained–strangled vocal quality to a moderate and mild degree, respectively. Subject 8 was the only member of Subgroup 3 to be perceived by the perceptual judges as exhibiting normal laryngeal function. For Subject 5, the laryngeal perceptual assessment indicated the presence of predominantly incoordinated laryngeal function as identified by a rating of a moderate degree of intermittent breathiness. Subject 19 was perceived to exhibit a severe degree of hoarseness and a moderate degree of intermittent breathiness consistent with a hypofunctional and incoordinated larynx. Hyperfunctional and hypofunctional laryngeal function was considered to be present in Subject 2, who was rated as displaying a moderate degree of harshness, strained–strangled quality, and glottal fry.

Subgroup 4 The membership of Subgroup 4 included three subjects, two male (Subjects, 16 and 6) and one female (Subject 7). The subjects in this subgroup exhibited the most severe degree of hyperfunctional laryngeal activity for the five subgroups, dominated by the presence of a high mean LR (3.07 *SD* above the control mean) and a low mean PF (2.05 *SD* below the control mean). In addition, the subjects as a group exhibited a higher mean F_0 (1.76 *SD* above the control mean), shorter DC (1.20 *SD* below the control mean), faster CT (2.19 *SD* below the control mean), slower AB (1.55 *SD* below the control mean), lower GP (2.03 *SD* below the control mean), and lower SPL (1.96 *SD* below the control mean) (see Table 5). Of the three subjects in Subgroup 4, two (Subjects 7 and 6) were perceived by the perceptual judges to exhibit normal laryngeal function. The third (Subject 16) was considered to display a hyperfunctional pattern of laryngeal activity as indicated by a rating of moderate harshness (see Table 2).

Subgroup 5 Subgroup 5 comprised three male subjects (Subjects 15, 14, and 1), who were shown to have F_0, DC, CT, AB, and GP within 1 *SD* of the control mean. The high LR (1.84 *SD* above the control mean), the low PF (1.70 *SD* below the control mean), and the low SPL (1.16 *SD* below the control mean) determined for this subgroup were consistent with the hyperfunctional pattern of laryngeal activity exhibited by the subjects in Subgroup 4 but to a milder degree. The perceptual assessment of the three subjects in Subgroup 5 indicated that two (Subjects 15 and 1) exhibited laryngeal characteristics consistent with hypofunction and incoordination of the larynx, while the third (Subject 14) displayed hypofunctional laryngeal activity (see Table 2). Subject 15 was perceived to exhibit a moderate degree of hoarseness with a mild degree of both glottal fry and intermittent breathiness. Similarly, Subject 1 exhibited a mild degree of hoarseness, glottal fry, and intermittent breathiness. According to the perceptual judges, Subject 14 was considered to display a mild degree of hoarseness in the absence of any of the other deviant laryngeal features.

DISCUSSION

The perceptual and instrumental results of the present study identified the presence of a high incidence and wide range of laryngeal dysfunction in a group of severe CHI subjects with dysarthric speech. Perceptually deviant laryngeal characteristics were perceived to be present in 84% of the CHI subjects. The instrumental results, based on vocal fold vibration and aerodynamic measures, indicated the presence of a range of hyperfunctional laryngeal activity in the CHI subjects, with the emergence of different patterns of laryngeal hyperfunction. The identification of a predominately hyperfunctional pattern of laryngeal activity in the CHI subjects in the current study is consistent with the findings of von Cramon (1981) and Vogel and von Cramon (1982), who perceptually recorded hyperfunctional signs of spastic dysphonia in a group of CHI subjects during the latter stages of recovery from traumatic mutism following midbrain damage. Although the phonation of these subjects was not perceived to be strained and strangled, Vogel and von Cramon (1982) noted that the subjects utilized an effortful voice production.

In the neurologically impaired individual, laryngeal hyperfunction is presumed to indicate the presence of increased tone or spasticity in the laryngeal musculature that results in hyperadduction of the vocal folds, a reduction in the size of the laryngeal aperture, and an increase in resistance to airflow during phonation (Darley et al., 1975; Hartman, 1984). Spasticity or hypertonicity of the laryngeal muscles also results in a decrease in the range and rate of movements of the laryngeal muscles (Darley et al., 1975; Hanson 1991), in particular the intrinsic muscles of the larynx involved in the adduction and abduction of the vocal folds. At the level of vocal fold vibration, Hollien (cited in Holmberg, Hillman, & Perkell, 1989) found that the increased vocal fold tension that is usually associated with hyperfunctional laryngeal activity was related to an increase in fundamental frequency. In addition, laryngeal hyperfunction has been shown to be associated with decreases in the duty cycle and closing time of the vibratory cycle (Frokjaer-Jensen & Thyme-Frokjaer, 1989; Hanson, Gerratt, & Ward, 1983; Hillman, Holmberg, Perkell, Walsh, & Vaughan, 1989; Kitzing, Carlborg, & Lofqvist, 1982). Aerodynamically, laryngeal hyperfunction would be expected to result in an increase in laryngeal airway resistance and subglottal pressure and a decrease in the phonatory airflow and the ad/abduction rate of the vocal folds (Boone, 1977; Hanson, 1991; Hillman et al., 1989; Holmberg, 1980; Isshiki, 1965; Schutte, 1980, 1986; Smitheran & Hixon, 1981; von Leden, 1968).

In that a CHI has the propensity to cause both diffuse cortical and subcortical brain damage, there is a strong possibility that bilateral lesions of the upper motor neurons and corticobulbar fiber tracts, resulting in spasticity of the laryngeal musculature and hyperfunctional laryngeal activity, may occur following a severe CHI. Von Cramon (1981), in fact, suggested that the most probable site of the lesion resulting in spastic dysphonia and dysarthria in traumatically head-injured patients may prove to be at the most caudal level of the internal capsule. The hyperfunctional laryngeal features exhibited by the CHI subjects in the current study were consistent with the vocal fold vibratory patterns and laryngeal aerodynamics presumed to be associated with spasticity of the laryngeal musculature.

Each of these hyperfunctional characteristics was evident in the instrumental findings but never all together in any one subject. The cluster analysis, in fact, identified five subgroups of CHI subjects with varying degrees and combinations of hyperfunctional laryngeal features. Two subgroups (1 and 2) were identified on the basis of a high mean subglottal pressure, normal laryngeal airway resistance, high phonatory airflow and reduced ad/abduction rate, whereas Subgroups 4 and 5 were characterized by high laryngeal airway resistance and low phonatory airflow. Subgroup 4 also exhibited low subglottal pressures and reduced ad/abduction rates, whereas Subgroup 5 was characterized by normal subglottal pressures and ad/abduction rates. Subgroup 3 consisted of subjects for whom laryngeal hyperfunction was reflected in a high fundamental frequency, a short open phase, and a fast closing time in the vibratory cycle. Although the aerodynamic measures for this subgroup were within the normal range (except for adduction or abduction rate), the values indicated a trend toward an increase in laryngeal airway resistance and a reduction in phonatory airflow similar to the pattern exhibited by the subjects in Subgroups 4 and 5.

While the finding of hyperfunctional laryngeal activity in the CHI subjects as a group may be explained in terms of the presence of increased tone of laryngeal muscles due to upper motor neuron involvement, it is suggested that the different manifestations of hyperfunctional laryngeal activity reflect the various glottal and respiratory force adjustments deployed by the individual subjects in response to spasticity in the vocal folds. For example, the presence of spasticity in the vocal folds in the subjects in Subgroups 1 and 2 would seem to result in the subjects' generating very high subglottal pressures following hyperadduction of the vocal folds. The high pressures generated were sufficiently powerful to cause abduction of the vocal folds to such an extent that a high phonatory airflow was achieved and low to normal laryngeal airway resistance values were recorded for the two subgroups.

However, the subjects in Subgroup 4 appeared to exhibit different glottal and respiratory force settings during phonation in response to a possible increase in laryngeal tone. In contrast to Subgroups 1 and 2, subglottal pressures and phonatory airflow in Subgroup 4 remained very low while laryngeal airway resistance levels were high. In this instance, low subglottal pressure may be accounted for by inadequate adduction of the vocal folds due to reduced range and strength of movement of the hypertonic laryngeal muscles. The high laryngeal airway resistance and low phonatory airflow demonstrated by the subjects in Subgroup 4 would, in turn, tend to indicate a reduced abduction of the vocal folds during phonation due to reduced subglottal pressure and/or tension and stiffness of the vocal folds associated with spasticity. The suggestion of increased tone in the vocal folds was supported by the laryngographic findings for this subgroup, in which a high fundamental frequency, a short duty cycle, and a fast closing time were recorded.

While the subjects in Subgroup 5 demonstrated a response to the possible presence of laryngeal spasticity similar to that of the subjects in Subgroup 4, hypertonicity of the laryngeal musculature would appear to have been less in these subjects, as indicated by the lower mean laryngeal airway resistance value, the normal subglottal pressures, the higher phonatory airflow, and the normal vocal fold vibration values. The aerodynamic values for Subgroup 3 tended to indicate a trend in the subjects' responses to increased laryngeal tone similar to that of Subgroups 4 and 5, but it would appear that spasticity of the laryngeal muscles would be present to an even lesser extent in these subjects, apparently being manifested only at the level of vocal fold vibration.

For those CHI subjects in the present study who may demonstrate neurologic signs consistent with damage at levels of the central nervous system other than the upper motor neurons and corticobulbar tracts, the laryngeal hyperfunction in the subjects may not necessarily only indicate spasticity of the vocal folds per se, but may instead reflect compensatory behavior on the part of the speaker to overcome deficits in other subsystems of the speech production mechanism. For instance, the high subglottal pressures recorded for the subjects in Subgroups 1 and 2 may reflect a forceful and effortful voice production technique voluntarily employed by the speaker to compensate for reduced intelligibility of speech caused by impairments at other levels of the speech production apparatus (e.g., velopharyngeal and articulatory dysfunction).

A forceful, hyperfunctional approach to phonation involving the generation of a high subglottal pressure is commonly referred to as "hard glottal attack" (Boone, 1977; Kitzing et al., 1982; Prater & Swift, 1984). In the case of the subjects in Subgroups 1 and 2, the vocal folds did not appear to offer any increased resistance to the subglottal pressure and were readily abducted to produce a high phonatory airflow. The mean laryngeal airway resistance values recorded for both Subgroups 1 and 2, in fact, indicated that the laryngeal resistance for the subjects in these subgroups was within the normal range.

For the subjects in Subgroups 4 and 5, and to a lesser extent Subgroup 3, the high laryngeal airway resistance and low phonatory airflow recorded may similarly indicate the subjects' attempts to compensate for deficits in other subsystems of the speech production mechanism rather than reflect inherent spasticity of the vocal folds. In an attempt to compensate for wastage of expiratory airflow by other valving mechanisms, such as the velopharyngeal and articulatory valves, a subject may increase the tension of the laryngeal muscles and structures to conserve expiratory flow. Where the subject has reduced respiratory support for speech involving either reduced lung volume, inappropriate breathing patterns, or problems with respiratory control, laryngeal tension may be increased to compensate for respiratory deficits (LaBlance, Steckol, & Cooper, 1991). This situation may well be the case for the subjects in Subgroup 4, in whom the low subglottal pressures could be directly related to insufficient respiratory support rather than to the effects of spasticity of the vocal folds. In addition, it should be noted that the low mean subglottal pressure recorded for Subgroup 4 may be an underestimation of this parameter due to the instrumental method used to determine subglottal pressure. In that subglottal pressure is measured indirectly by the Aerophone II via an equivalent measurement of oral pressure during the production of a voiceless stop, /p/, it is possible that, in the dysarthric CHI subject, impairment of the velopharyngeal valve and/or the bilabial seal may cause a leakage of air from within the oral cavity, resulting in a recording of a reduced oral pressure and subglottal pressure (Smitheran & Hixon, 1981). In view of the fact that two out of the three subjects in Subgroup 4 had subglottal pressures greater than 1 SD below the control mean, it is recognized that the reduced subglottal pressures recorded for these subjects could be an outcome of velopharyngeal and/or articulatory dysfunction. Further investigation of the status of velopharyngeal and articulatory function in the subjects in this instance may be warranted to ascertain the contribution, if any, of velopharyngeal and/or articulatory dysfunction to the recording of low subglottal pressures for the subjects in Subgroup 4.

While the cluster analysis identified five subgroups of CHI subjects with similar vocal behavior based on the instrumental measures, the perceptual results for the individual subjects in the respective subgroups failed to concur with the instrumental findings in approximately half of the subjects. The inconsistencies between the instrumental and perceptual findings may possibly be explained in terms of the inherent inadequacies of perceptual evaluation of voice, the difference between the types of tasks used in the perceptual and instrumental assessments, the strategies utilized by the subjects to compensate for increased laryngeal tone, and the problems associated with the instrumental procedures.

The most likely explanation for the inconsistent results relates to the inadequacy of perceptual evaluation in identifying normal and abnormal voice as well as determining specific deviant laryngeal features at reduced levels of severity or against a background of other deviant speech features (Bassich & Ludlow, 1986; Blaustein & Bar, 1983; Fex, 1992). For example, in the subgroup with the most severe degree of hyperfunctional laryngeal activity (Subgroup 4), two of the three subjects were perceived to exhibit normal vocal quality while objectively exhibiting signs of laryngeal hyperfunction. It is suggested that, in the case of these subjects, the perceptual judges may have experienced difficulty in evaluating vocal quality due to the influence of other deviant perceptual features present in the dysarthric speech of these subjects (e.g., hypernasality, articulatory impairment, prosodic disturbances). Similarly, deviant laryngeal characteristics relating to hypofunction and incoordination of the larynx were perceived to be present in some of the subjects in Subgroups 2, 3, and 5, suggesting the possibility of inaccurate perceptual analysis.

The different types of tasks used in the perceptual and instrumental assessments may also have contributed to the inconsistencies between the perceptual and instrumental findings. The instrumental assessment involved a syllable-repetition task, while the perceptual evaluation was based on a reading passage. It is suggested that, in the case of the subjects in Subgroup 2, who instrumentally appeared to exhibit a forced and effortful pattern of voice production, the perceptual findings consistent with laryngeal hypofunction and incoordination in two of the subjects may reflect the inability of these subjects to consistently maintain the forced phonation throughout the duration of the passage of prose.

Alternatively, the irregularities between the instrumental and perceptual results within the subgroups may reflect voluntary attempts by some subjects to compensate for the hypertonicity of the vocal folds by producing a hypofunctional and breathy phonation requiring less muscular effort

(Aronson, Brown, Litin, & Pearson, 1968; Darley et al., 1975; von Cramon, 1981). This strategy may only become apparent in a longer speech sample (e.g., a reading task). The subjects in Subgroup 5 who demonstrated high laryngeal airway resistance and low airflow and were perceived to exhibit predominately hypofunctional and incoordinated laryngeal features may well have employed this strategy.

It is also possible that the discrepancies found to occur between the perceptual and instrumental findings may be, in part, due to the inherent inadequacies of the instrumental techniques used in the current study. Specifically, the difficulty in identifying the opening and closing phases on the Lx waveforms and the variability of aerodynamic measures may have contributed to the inconsistencies identified between the perceptual and instrumental results. Further research in this area, therefore, should include the use of direct measures of laryngeal function, such as videostroboscopy, to support the findings of indirect assessment techniques.

In conclusion, hyperfunctional laryngeal activity was identified as the predominant mode of laryngeal dysfunction in a group of CHI subjects, the manifestation of which differed across five subgroups. The various patterns of hyperfunctional laryngeal activity may be best explained in terms of the presence of spasticity in the laryngeal musculature, the glottal and respiratory force adjustments deployed by the subjects in response to increased laryngeal tone, and the strategies employed by the subjects to compensate for impairment in other subsystems of the speech production mechanism.

The findings of the current study have important implications for the rehabilitation of severe CHI persons with dysarthric speech. First, in that the laryngeal subsystem has considerable influence over the production and intelligibility of speech, the assessment and treatment of laryngeal dysfunction in CHI subjects with dysarthric speech should be actively addressed by speech pathologists. In addition to a perceptual assessment, it is essential that the assessment of laryngeal function in the CHI population involves an instrumental evaluation of laryngeal vocal fold and aerodynamic patterns to ascertain the nature of the underlying laryngeal pathophysiology and to determine the glottal and respiratory force settings that exist during phonation. Once the status of the laryngeal subsystem has been determined individually, therapy should be directed toward the aberrant laryngeal behaviors, with due consideration for the strategies employed by the subject to compensate for the laryngeal impairment, or for deficits in other subsystems of the speech mechanism. A comprehensive evaluation of other subsystems of the speech production mechanism may be necessary before therapy for laryngeal dysfunction in the CHI subject with dysarthric speech can be appropriately determined.

REFERENCES

Aronson, A.E. (1980). *Clinical voice disorders: An interdisciplinary approach.* New York: Thieme-Stratton.
Aronson, A.E., Brown, J.R., Litin, E.M., & Pearson, J.S. (1968). Spastic dysphonia I. Voice, neurologic, psychiatric aspects. *Journal of Speech and Hearing Disorders, 33,* 203–218.
Baken, R.J. (1987). Laryngeal function. In R.J. Baken (Ed.), *Clinical measurement of speech and voice* (pp. 197–240). London: Taylor and Francis.
Bassich, C.J., & Ludlow, C.L. (1986). The use of perceptual methods by new clinicians for assessing voice quality. *Journal of Speech and Hearing Disorders, 51,* 125–133.
Blaustein, S., & Bar, A. (1983). Reliability of perceptual voice assessment. *Journal of Communication Disorders, 16,* 157–161.
Boone, D.R. (1977). *The voice and voice therapy* (2nd ed.). Englewood Cliffs, NJ: Prentice Hall.
Childers, D.G., Hicks, D.M., Moore, G.P., Eskenazi, L., & Lalwani, A.I. (1990). Electroglottography and vocal fold physiology. *Journal of Speech and Hearing Research, 33,* 245–254.
Childers, D.G., & Krishnamurthy, A.K. (1985). A critical review of electroglottography. *CRC Critical Reviews in Biomedical Engineering, 12,* 131–161.
Colton, R.H., & Conture, E.G. (1990). Problems and pitfalls of electroglottography. *Journal of Voice, 4,* 10–24.
Darley, F.L., Aronson, A.E., & Brown, J.R. (1975). *Motor speech disorders.* Philadelphia: W. B. Saunders.
Fex, S. (1992). Perceptual evaluation. *Journal of Voice, 6,* 155–158.
Fitzgerald, F.J., Murdoch, B.E., & Chenery, H.J. (1987). Multiple sclerosis: Associated speech and language disorders. *Australian Journal of Human Communication Disorders, 15,* 15–33.
Frokjaer-Jensen, B., & Thyme-Frokjaer, K. (1989). *Changes in respiratory and phonatory efficiency during an intensive voice training course.* Paper presented at the Congress of the International Association of Logopedics and Phoniatrics, Prague, Czechoslovakia.
Greene, M.C.L. (1972). *The voice and its disorders.* London: Pitman Medical.
Hanson, D.G. (1991). Neuromuscular disorders of the larynx. *Otolaryngologic Clinics of North America, 24,* 1035–1051.
Hanson, D.G., Gerratt, B.R., & Ward, P.H. (1983). Glottographic measurement of vocal dysfunction: A preliminary report. *Annals of Otology, Rhinology and Laryngology, 92,* 413–420.
Hartman, D.E. (1984). Neurogenic dysphonia. *Annals of Otology, Rhinology and Laryngology, 93,* 57–64.
Hartmann, E., & von Cramon, D. (1984). Acoustic measurement of voice quality in central dysphonia. *Journal of Communication Disorders, 17,* 425–440.
Hillman, R.E., Holmberg, E.B., Perkell, J.S., Walsh, M., & Vaughan, C. (1989). Objective assessment of vocal hyperfunction: An experimental framework and initial results. *Journal of Speech and Hearing Research, 32,* 373–392.
Holmberg, E. (1980). Laryngeal airway resistance as a function of phonation type [Abstract No. ZZ4]. *Journal of the Acoustical Society of America, 68*(Suppl. 1), S101.

Holmberg, E.B., Hillman, R.E., & Perkell, J.S. (1988). Glottal airflow and transglottal air pressure measurements for male and female speakers in soft, normal and loud voice. *Journal of the Acoustical Society of America, 84*, 511–529.

Holmberg, E.B., Hillman, R.E., & Perkell, J.S. (1989). Glottal airflow and transglottal air pressure measurements for male and female speakers in low, normal and high pitch. *Journal of Voice, 3*, 294–305.

Hoodin, R.B., & Gilbert, H.R. (1989). Parkinsonian dysarthria: An aerodynamic and perceptual description of velopharyngeal closure for speech. *Folia Phoniatrica, 41*, 249–258.

Isshiki, N. (1965). Vocal intensity and air flow rate. *Folia Phoniatrica, 17*, 92–104.

Kearns, K.P., & Simmons, N.N. (1988). Intraobserver reliability and perceptual ratings: More than meets the ear. *Journal of Speech and Hearing Research, 31*, 131–136.

Kent, R.D., & Rosenbek, J.C. (1982). Prosodic disturbance and neurologic lesion. *Brain and Language, 15*, 259–291.

Kitzing, P., Carlborg, B., & Lofqvist, A. (1982). Aerodynamic and glottographic studies of the laryngeal vibratory cycle. *Folia Phoniatrica, 34*, 216–224.

LaBlance, G.R. Steckol, K.F., & Cooper, M.H. (1991). Non-invasive assessment of phonatory and respiratory dynamics. *Ear, Nose and Throat Journal, 70*, 691–696.

Lethlean, J.B., Chenery, H.J., & Murdoch, B.E. (1990). Disturbed respiratory and prosodic function in Parkinson's disease: A perceptual and instrumental analysis. *Australian Journal of Human Communication Disorders, 18*, 83–98.

Ludlow, C.L., & Bassich, C.J. (1983). The results of acoustic and perceptual assessment of two types of dysarthria. In W.R. Berry (Ed.), *Clinical dysarthria* (pp. 121–154). San Diego: College-Hill Press.

Motta, G., Cesari, U., Iengo, M., & Motta, G. (1990). Clinical application of electroglottography. *Folia Phoniatrica, 42*, 111–117.

Netsell, R., Lotz, W.K., Du Chane, A.S., & Barlow, S.M. (1991). Vocal tract aerodynamics during syllable productions: Normative data and theoretical implications. *Journal of Voice, 5*, 1–9.

Norusis, M.J. (1990). *SPSS/PC + Statistics 4.0.* Chicago: SPSS Inc.

Orlikoff, R.F. (1992). The use of instrumental measures in the assessment and treatment of motor speech disorders. *Seminars in Speech and Language, 13*, 25–37.

Prater, R.J., & Swift, R.W. (1984). *Manual of voice therapy.* Boston: Little, Brown.

Ramig, L.O. (1992). The role of phonation in speech intelligibility: A review and preliminary data from patients with Parkinson's disease. In R.D. Kent (Ed.), *Intelligibility in speech disorders: Theory, measurement and management* (pp. 119–155). Philadelphia: John Benjamins Company.

Sapir, S., & Aronson, A.E. (1985). Aphonia after closed head injury: Aetiological considerations. *British Journal of Disorders of Communication, 20*, 289–296.

Scholefield, J.A. (1987). Aetiologies of aphonia following closed head injury. *British Journal of Disorders of Communication, 22*, 167–172.

Schutte, H.K. (1980). *The efficiency of voice production.* Groningen: Kemper.

Schutte, H.K. (1986). Aerodynamics of phonation. *Acta Oto-Rhino-Laryngology Belgica, 40*, 344–357.

Smitheran, J.R., & Hixon, T.J. (1981). A clinical method for estimating laryngeal airway resistance during vowel production. *Journal of Speech and Hearing Disorders, 46*, 138–146.

Teasdale, G., & Jennett, B. (1974). Assessment of coma and impaired consciousness: A practical scale. *Lancet, 2*, 81–84.

Theodoros, D.G., Murdoch, B.E., & Chenery, H.J. (1994). Perceptual speech characteristics of dysarthric speakers following severe closed head injury. *Brain Injury, 8,* 101–124.

Vogel, M., & von Cramon, D. (1982). Dysphonia after traumatic midbrain damage: A follow-up study. *Folia Phoniatrica, 34,* 150–159.

von Cramon, D. (1981). Traumatic mutism and the subsequent reorganization of speech functions. *Neuropsychologia, 19,* 801–805.

Von Leden, H. (1968). Objective measures of laryngeal function and phonation. *Annals of the New York Academy of Sciences, 155,* 56–67.

Zyski, J.B., & Weisiger, B.E. (1987). Identification of dysarthria types based on perceptual analysis. *Journal of Communication Disorders, 204,* 367–378.

Chapter 13

Laryngeal Airway Resistance Following Traumatic Brain Injury

Monica A. McHenry

A HALLMARK OF traumatic brain injury (TBI) is diffuse damage that may affect various aspects of speech production. An individual's speech breathing, voice, resonance, and articulation may be differentially affected. Effective therapeutic intervention may be enhanced by objective knowledge of an individual's speech physiology. Several authors have suggested prioritizing therapeutic intervention strategies based on physiologic assessments (Coehlo, Gracco, Fourakis, Rosetti, & Oshima, 1994; McHenry & Wilson, 1994; Netsell & Daniel, 1979). Monitoring of physiologic change is also useful to document the effects of long-term treatment (Simpson, Till, & Goff, 1988; Workinger & Netsell, 1992). Furthermore, Barlow and Burton (1990) have speculated that physiologic assessment, such as orofacial force testing, may provide insight into an individual's underlying neuromotor control impairment.

There is a paucity of data regarding speech physiology following TBI, although data exist regarding the impact of TBI on orofacial force generation (Barlow & Burton, 1990; McHenry, Minton, Wilson, & Post, 1994), resonance (Theodoros, Murdoch, Stokes, & Chenery, 1993), and perceived dysarthria (Theodoros, Murdoch, & Chenery, 1994). Limited data are available regarding laryngeal function following TBI. Theodoros et al. (1994), in perceptual analyses of 20 dysarthric subjects with severe TBI, found that 75% of their dysarthric subjects evidenced some degree

---

This work was supported by Grant No. 91-15 from the Moody Foundation of Galveston, TX.

The technical support of John Minton and Yolanda Post is gratefully acknowledged.

of perceived dysphonia. Theodoros and Murdoch (see Chapter 12) obtained a variety of measures in 19 subjects with severe TBI. They used electroglottography to determine fundamental frequency, duty cycle, and closing time. Aerodynamic measures included estimated subglottal pressure and laryngeal airway resistance. Average sound pressure level and ad/abduction rates were also obtained. They determined that the majority of subjects evidenced some manifestation of laryngeal hyperfunction.

Earlier work (Vogel & von Cramon, 1982; von Cramon, 1981) suggested that individuals with TBI may manifest different vocal symptoms depending on the stage of recovery. The vocal symptoms typically begin with low intensity and breathiness and progress to effortful phonation more typical of spastic dysphonia. The voice symptoms finally resolve. This pattern of change in voice symptoms was apparent in a single subject followed from 14 to 24 months postinjury (McHenry, Wilson, & Minton, 1994). The results of other TBI investigations are less definitive. Although specific voice symptoms were not described, Groher (1977) reported that 9 of the 14 males he studied initially evidenced spastic dysarthria. After 4 months, all subjects demonstrated functional communication, with four patients evidencing mixed spastic–ataxic dysarthria. Other investigators (Najenson, Sazbon, Fiselzon, Becker, & Schechter, 1978) made a distinction between subjects whose dysarthria resolved and those for whom it persisted. Their study included 15 patients, 6 of whom remained in a persistent vegetative state and 9 of whom evidenced various degrees of recovery. Subjects were followed for differing lengths of time, some up to 2 years postinjury. The speech of the eight patients whose dysarthria persisted was characterized by harshness and hypernasality. Furthermore, they evidenced reduced vital capacities compared with normal controls. The authors suggested that the reduction was due to deficits of motor control that affected recruitment and coordination of respiratory muscles. They speculated that these deficits may "reflect similar or related difficulties in coordinating respiration, articulation and phonation" (p. 19).

It can be seen that accounts of voice disorders in persistent dysarthria following severe TBI vary along the continuum from breathiness to harshness, with time postinjury being a possible contributing variable. Because dysphonia may affect speech intelligibility (Ramig, 1992), a greater understanding of its occurrence is critical to the treatment of individuals with TBI.

This study was designed to determine the frequency and type of abnormal laryngeal airway resistance following TBI. Laryngeal function may be inferred from aerodynamic measures (Smitheran & Hixon, 1981). Laryngeal airway resistance has been investigated in relation to gender

(Langhans, 1981; Netsell, Lotz, Du Chane, & Barlow, 1991; Shaughnessy, Lotz, & Netsell, 1981), loudness (Hillman, Holmberg, Perkell, Walsh, & Vaughan, 1989; McHenry & Reich, 1985), phonation type (Holmberg, 1980; McHenry, Kuna, Vanoye, Roberts-Seibert, & Minton, in press) and voice disorders (Netsell, Lotz, & Shaughnessey, 1984; see also Chapter 12). Low laryngeal airway resistance has been associated with breathy or soft voices or both, whereas increased laryngeal airway resistance has been associated with strained or hyperfunctional voice production. The present data provide further insight into the nature of voice disorders following severe TBI.

METHODOLOGY

Subjects

The records of 68 individuals who completed a motor speech evaluation over a 3-year period were reviewed. Subjects were included only if they had an etiology of severe TBI. Severity was based on the diagnosis in the acute care medical records, when available, or on the results of neuropsychological testing. Sixteen records were deleted for various reasons, including subjects' inability to achieve bilabial closure and irretrievable data. Of the 52 remaining subjects, laryngeal airway resistance data are reported for 18 men and 8 women, with velopharyngeal resistance values of 100 cm $H_2O/L/s$. Because adequate velopharyngeal closure is required for valid laryngeal airway resistance estimation, this conservative criterion was applied.

Subject characteristics are shown in Table 1. The mean age for men and women was 26.8 (standard deviation [SD] = 7.64) and 25.5 (SD = 5.98) years, respectively. The mean coma duration for men and women was 7.33 (SD = 5.59) and 8 (SD = 7.97) weeks, respectively. The subjects completed a comprehensive battery of tests, including a visual examination of the structure and function of the lips, tongue, jaw, and soft palate; orofacial force testing, video- and audiotaping of conversational speech and phonatory tasks, including intelligibility testing; and estimation of velopharyngeal resistance and laryngeal airway resistance. Intelligibility and severity of perceived dysarthria also are provided in Table 1. These data are included to provide a rough estimate of the individual's functioning. Intelligibility is based on the subject's Computerized Assessment of Intelligibility of Dysarthric Speech (CAIDS) sentence test results (Yorkston, Beukelman, & Traynor, 1984). Tests were scored by various individual naive listeners. Reliability data are not available. Severity was determined by the examiner based on perceived dysarthria and is a subjective determination.

Table 1. Subject characteristics and sentence intelligibility based on CAIDS sentence test

Subject	Sex	Coma (weeks)	Sentence intelligibility (%)	Dysarthria severity	Initial head CT and medical results
BK	M	8	97	Mild	Multiple hemorrhagic contusions, specifically in the right frontal, left parietal, and left occipital horn areas. Significant edema in the right cerebral hemisphere.
CL	M	12	90	Mild	Small hemorrhagic contusions, the sequelae of deep white matter contusions. Primarily a brain stem injury with a right frontotemporal linear skull fracture.
GC	M	5	97	Mild	Bilateral parietofrontal lobe contusions (R>L); right temporal, parietal, and occipital lobe injuries.
DH	M	1	NA	Mild	Skull fracture, cerebral contusion, localized brain atrophy in the right parietal area, encephalomalacia, and mild hydrocephalus. Development of seizure disorder subsequent to injury.
DM	M	12	100	Mild	Subdural fluid collection in right frontal region. Focal atrophic changes. Bilateral and brain stem contusions.
EG	M	6	87	Mild	Multiple contusions and hemorrhages. Decerebrate posturing.
JB	M	2	NA	Mild	Extensive right frontal and temporal contusion. Hematoma evacuated from the right frontal and temporal lobes. Epidural and subdural hematomas.
JJ	M	18	95	Moderate	Diffuse brain damage with major lesions in both the left and right temporoparietal regions.
JK	M	18	99	Mild	Bilateral frontal lobe and left temporal lobe contusions with basal ganglia and brain stem hemorrhages. A pneumocephalus with air entering a large crack in the frontal sinus was also noted.
KL	M	1	98	Mild	Multiple petechial hemorrhages; atrophy and frontal hygromas.
LJ	M	None	NA	Mild	Evidence of brain hemorrhage and bilateral frontal cerebral dysfunction.
LW	M	7	73	Mild	Left frontal temporal contusion and right temporal contrecoup injury; compression of both ventricles.

MC	M	8	95	Mild	Diffuse edema with a midbrain contusion.
SM	M	8	99	WNL	Diffuse cerebral edema and small epidural collection in right hemisphere.
TR	M	2	92	Moderate	Interventricular hemorrhage in occipital horns and right frontal lobe with ventriculostomy in place for drainage.
TW	M	6.5	100	Mild	Bilateral frontal fractures with lateral fractures, subarachnoid hemorrhage and edema, and left lateral ventricle effacement.
WG	M	3.5	100	Mild	Hemorrhagic contusions in corpus callosum and bimedial temporal lobe; multiple scattered petechiae and some degree of edema without any shift.
CY	M	14	49	Moderate	Diffuse brain injury. Hemiparesis.
DAC	F	8	100	Mild	Bifrontal contusions at the level of the lateral ventricles and just above them. Evidence of swelling on the left. Right internal capsule and left parietal lobe and body of the left corpus callosum lesions.
DC	F	4	86	Mild	Basilar skull fracture; cerebral hemorrhage; possible subdural effusion. Small, dense enhancing lesion in the left frontal parasagittal area.
DE	F	3.5	100	WNL	Left epidural and subdural hematomas; intraparenchymal hematoma of left temporal lobe; right frontal contusions.
JR	F	4	95	Mild	Left frontal and ventricular intracerebral hematoma.
KS	F	4	100	Mild	Blows to the right frontal area, with possible contrecoup effects to the left.
MS	F	16	94	Moderate	Diffuse slowing and frequent recurring seizure activity localized in the right temporal region; subarachnoid hemorrhage, subdural hematoma, brain stem contusion; encephalomalacia in the right basal ganglia.
SD	F	0.5	NA	Mild	Left-side paresis and blindness in left eye.
TH	F	24	99	Mild	Several areas of cerebral contusion with bleeding in left temporal lobe, right lentiform nucleus, and posterior left thalamus.

Note: CT, computed tomography; NA, not available; WNL, within normal limits.

Instrumentation

To obtain the laryngeal airway resistance data, subjects wore a tight-fitting face mask (Bird) attached to a pneumotachograph (Hans Rudolph 4719) and differential pressure transducer (Honeywell 163PC01D36). Intraoral pressure was measured just inside the lips using a polyethylene catheter (2-mm inner diameter) attached to a pressure transducer (162PC016). The catheter was advanced through the face mask and positioned just inside the incisors so that its distal open tip was perpendicular to airflow and was not occluded by the tongue. Aerodynamic data were low-pass filtered at 20 Hz (Biocommunications) and digitized at 3,571 Hz. At a typical pitch and at self-perceived, nonrandomized comfortable, soft, and loud levels, subjects produced /pi/ syllable trains at approximately 1.5 syllables per second.

Three trials were obtained for each condition. The subjects were instructed before each trial to "take a big breath." The tasks were modeled, and the subjects were provided with practice trials. Trials that did not meet the criteria of increased prephonatory inspiration and smooth and connected syllable pulsing were rerun. Data were analyzed using automated software (RC Electronics; Barlow & Suing, 1991; Barlow, Suing, Grossman, Bodmer, & Colbert, 1989). Laryngeal airway resistance was calculated as intraoral pressure (used to estimate translaryngeal pressure) divided by translaryngeal flow. The three trials were averaged to determine each subject's laryngeal airway resistance.

Reliability was determined by recalculating laryngeal airway resistance data for three men and three women. The results for pressure, flow, and resistance were identical to the original data.

RESULTS

The data from this study are presented in Table 2 and are comparable to those of Netsell et al. (1991). Their normative study was based on 15 adult men and 15 adult women, with a mean age of 32 for the men and 27 for the women. Although these mean ages are not identical to those of the present subjects, Netsell et al.'s data may be considered representative of young adults and, as such, appropriate for comparative purposes. In their study, the mean normal laryngeal airway resistance was 31.71 cm H_2O/L/s (SD = 7.8) for men. One SD from the norm will be considered to be within normal limits.

Only 28% (5) of the 18 men in the present study fell within 1 SD of this norm, with 55% (10 of 18) evidencing laryngeal airway resistance less than 23.91 cm H_2O/L/s. The mean airflow for the subjects with reduced laryngeal airway resistance was 487 cc/s. This value is well beyond the normative flow mean of 193 cc/s (SD = 47). Figure 1 illustrates a male subject's translaryngeal airflow, intraoral pressure as an estimate of subglottal

Table 2. Translaryngeal flow, intraoral pressure (P_o), and laryngeal airway resistance (R_{LAW}) for each subject

Subject	Months post-injury	Flow (cc/s) Mean	SD	P_o (cm H_2O) Mean	SD	R_{LAW} (cm H_2O/L/s) Mean	SD
BK	23	60.65	10.24	6.60	0.20	116.80	21.33
CL	28	216.66	55.57	6.29	0.16	37.40	9.60
GC	31	397.35	31.69	2.95	0.47	9.10	1.70
DH	96	187.06	1.76	5.78	0.14	28.00	4.70
DM	34	248.87	55.19	4.83	0.96	21.70	1.80
EG	82	319.66	19.63	4.62	0.15	14.50	1.30
JB	9	264.77	30.31	8.48	0.15	32.30	4.40
JJ	64	140.46	32.47	9.33	0.18	87.10	14.00
JK	9	618.80	46.64	7.81	0.45	12.31	0.96
KL	13	732.31	146.94	8.67	1.74	11.90	0.20
LJ	82	293.61	23.89	9.09	0.59	25.50	1.30
LW	14	370.11	30.30	6.06	0.66	16.80	2.10
MC	7	135.30	39.49	6.18	0.59	49.05	12.05
SM	127	327.21	58.59	8.19	0.30	25.90	3.50
TR	41	337.60	33.50	6.36	0.09	19.90	2.90
TW	17	367.96	28.45	7.13	0.09	18.70	1.50
WG	7	790.76	44.51	6.82	0.46	10.23	0.53
CY	49	684.51	63.70	7.94	0.77	10.99	1.22
DAC	10	214.65	53.89	6.22	0.42	112.80	70.10
DC	6	212.96	15.18	6.13	0.18	28.50	2.80
DE	35	448.66	26.72	10.00	0.90	24.06	2.70
JR	69	225.80	18.69	6.85	0.06	30.80	2.00
KS	28	273.20	56.13	6.61	0.29	27.80	7.60
MS	42	409.42	75.78	9.17	0.55	21.80	6.90
SD	348	31.01	11.24	8.18	0.18	203.30	63.40
TH	45	483.88	145.67	10.36	0.25	24.60	6.50

pressure, and laryngeal airway resistance. The trace, typical of reduced laryngeal airway resistance, is characterized by very high translaryngeal airflow.

Three men (17%) evidenced laryngeal airway resistance values greater than 1 *SD* from the norm. Data from an illustrative subject who produced very low translaryngeal airflow are shown in Figure 2. It is of interest that the three subjects with high laryngeal airway resistance evidenced translaryngeal airflow values more than 1 *SD* lower than normal.

Normal mean laryngeal airway resistance for women was 42.6 cm H_2O/L/s (*SD* = 9.2) (Netsell et al. 1991). Of the eight female subjects, six evidenced laryngeal airway resistance less than 33.4 cm H_2O/L/s, or 1 *SD* from the norm. The two remaining female subjects' mean values were greater than 51.8 cm H_2O/L/s, again more than 1 *SD* from the norm,

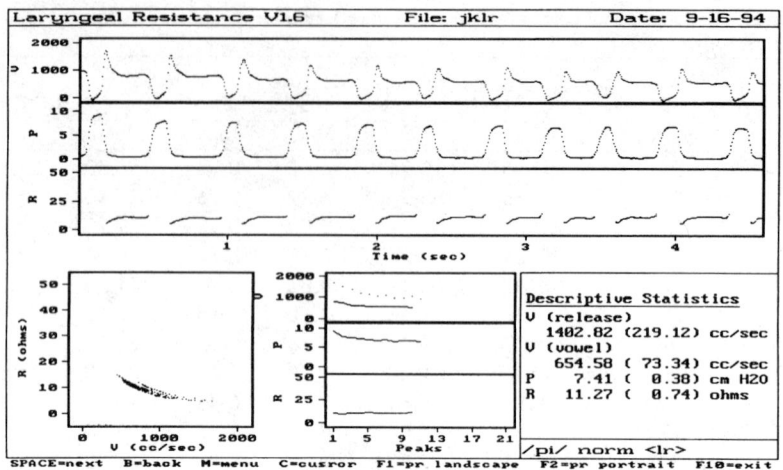

Figure 1. Subject evidencing reduced laryngeal airway resistance, characterized by very high translaryngeal airflow.

leaving no female subjects with normal velopharyngeal resistance having normal laryngeal airway resistance.

To determine the degree to which an individual can compensate for laryngeal deficits, data for the loud productions were reviewed. Of the 10 men with laryngeal airway resistance more than 1 *SD* lower than normal, data for increased loudness are available for eight. Of the eight, five were able to increase laryngeal airway resistance in the loud condition. A further issue, however, is whether the subjects were able to increase laryngeal airway resistance to the point of being within normal limits. Only one (TW) was able to do so.

Data on the increased loudness condition are available for four of the eight women whose velopharyngeal resistance was within normal limits. Although all four of the subjects increased laryngeal airway resistance in the loud condition, only one was within normal limits.

Given the investigations that suggest that dysphonia changes with time postinjury (Vogel & von Cramon, 1982; von Cramon, 1981), the data in Table 2 were examined to determine if this could be a factor in the present subjects. Of the three men (BK, JJ, and MC) with laryngeal airway resistance values greater than 1 *SD* from the norm, two (BK and MC) had been injured less than 2 years earlier. Ten of the 18 men had been injured more than 2 years ago, yet they evidenced lower than normal laryngeal airway resistance associated with breathiness. Among the women, the only woman *(SD)* whose laryngeal airway resistance exceeded the norm was indeed the one injured the longest ago; however, all but one woman had been injured more than 2 years earlier. These data are plotted in Figure 3.

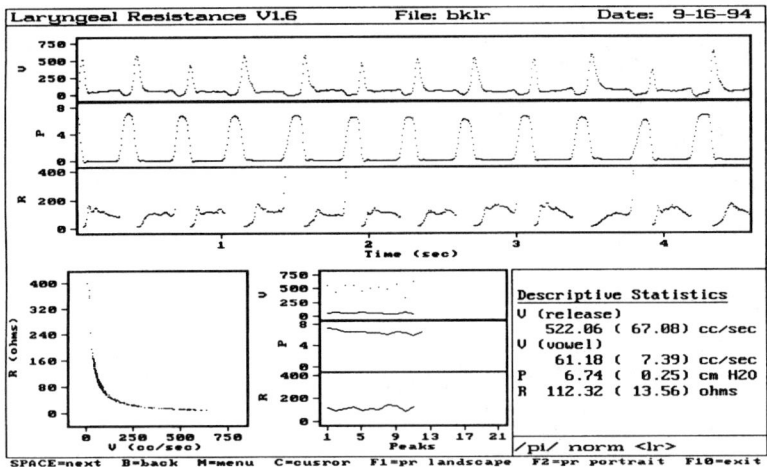

Figure 2. Subject evidencing high laryngeal airway resistance, characterized by very low translaryngeal airflow.

With the exception of a few outliers, it appears, then, that these subjects do not fit the suggested pattern of hypofunction gradually changing to hyperfunction.

DISCUSSION

It can be seen in the present investigation that hypolaryngeal valving, as evidenced by reduced laryngeal airway resistance, predominated following severe TBI. This results in unusually high translaryngeal airflows, yielding excessive air wastage, reduced loudness, breathiness, and loss of spectral energy.

In therapy, a subject with low laryngeal airway resistance is taught to reduce translaryngeal airflow by increasing vocal fold adduction. Clinically, this often may be accomplished by eliciting increased loudness (Countryman & Ramig, 1993; McHenry et al., 1994; Ramig, in press; Ramig, Horii, & Bonitati, 1991). The three subjects (DM, KL, and TR) whose laryngeal airway resistance decreased in the loud condition evidenced difficulty fine-tuning the increased vocal effort required and exacerbated the problem. For example, subject TR, in the normal condition, evidenced laryngeal airway resistance of around 20 cm H_2O/L/s, with translaryngeal airflow around 300 cc/s. In the loud condition, rather than being able to reduce airflow by increasing laryngeal adduction, he increased airflow to 1,000 cc/s, evidencing very inefficient laryngeal valving. Therapeutic intervention designed to increase both respiratory and laryngeal effort, as suggested by Ramig (in press) may be of benefit in these cases.

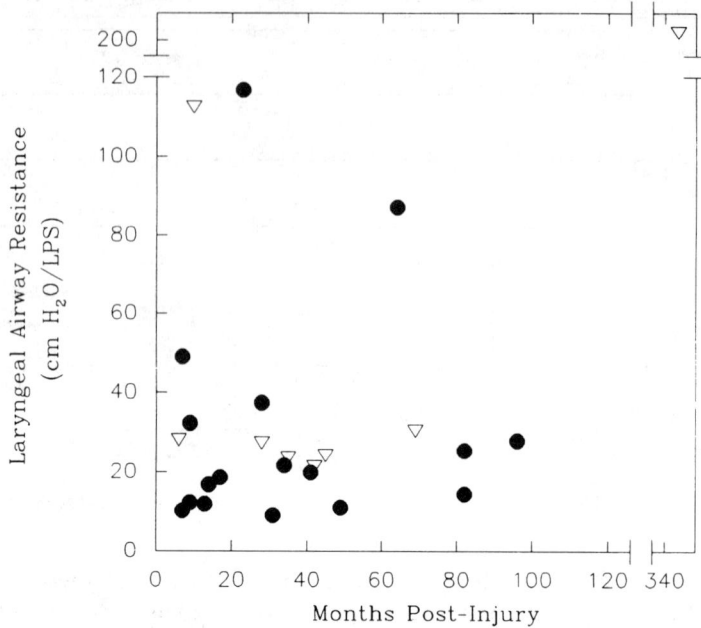

Figure 3. The relationship between months postinjury and laryngeal airway resistance. Men are represented by filled circles and women by open triangles.

It is of interest that the present study does not corroborate the preponderance of hyperfunctional voice production following severe TBI found by Theorodos and Murdoch (see Chapter 12). However, it is difficult to determine a given individual's place along the continuum of recovery, making it challenging to compare across studies. For example, measures of time postinjury imply an equivalence between two individuals at 30 months postinjury; however, one person may have spent 15 of the 30 months in a coma, whereas the second individual may have been in a coma for only 2 days. It is possible that the time after emergence from coma, or time after emergence from posttraumatic amnesia, may provide a more common starting point in tracking the course of physiologic and cognitive recovery. The other variable that cannot be discounted is the diffuse nature of the lesion. There may be subtleties in angle of injury, the degree to which structures are damaged, and the composite effect of the various forces at the time of injury that render it impossible to truly compare groups of individuals with severe TBI. Based on the present study and that of Theodoros and Murdoch (see Chapter 12), it can at least be stated that laryngeal function deficits are common following severe TBI and may persist long after the injury.

REFERENCES

Barlow, S.M., & Burton, M.K. (1990). Ramp-and-hold force control in the upper and lower lips: Developing new neuromotor assessment applications in traumatically brain injured adults. *Journal of Speech and Hearing Research, 33,* 660–675.

Barlow, S.M, & Suing, G. (1991). Aerospeech: Automated digital signal analysis of speech aerodynamics. *Journal for Computer Users in Speech and Hearing, 7,* 211–227.

Barlow, S.M., Suing, G., Grossman, A., Bodmer, P., & Colbert, R. (1989). A high-speed data acquisition and protocol control system for vocal tract physiology. *Journal of Voice, 3,* 283–293.

Coehlo, C.A., Gracco, V.L., Fourakis, M., Rosetti, M., & Oshima, K. (1994). Application of instrumental techniques in the assessment of dysarthria: A case study. In J.A. Till, K.M. Yorkston, & D.R. Beukelman (Eds.), *Motor speech disorders: Advances in assessment and treatment* (pp. 103–118). Baltimore: Paul H. Brookes Publishing Co.

Countryman, S., & Ramig, L.O. (1993). Effects of intensive voice therapy on voice deficits associated with bilateral thalamotomy in Parkinson disease: A case study. *Journal of Medical Speech-Language Pathology, 1,* 223–250.

Groher, M. (1977). Language and memory disorders following closed head trauma. *Journal of Speech and Hearing Research, 20,* 212–223.

Hillman, R.E., Holmberg, E.B., Perkell, J.S., Walsh, M., & Vaughan, C. (1989). Objective assessment of vocal hyperfunction: An experimental framework and initial results. *Journal of Speech and Hearing Research, 32,* 373–392.

Holmberg, E.B. (1980). Laryngeal airway resistance as a function of phonation type. *Journal of the Acoustical Society of America, 68* (Suppl.), S101.

Langhans, J. (1981). Laryngeal airway resistance during vowel production in adult females. *ASHA, 23,* 745.

McHenry, M.A., Kuna, S.T., Vanoye, C.R., Roberts-Seibert, N., Minton, J.T. (in press). Comparison of direct and indirect calculations of laryngeal airway resistance in various voicing conditions. *European Journal of Disorders of Communication.*

McHenry, M.A., Minton, J.T., Wilson, R.L., & Post, Y.V. (1994). Intelligibility and nonspeech orofacial strength and force control following traumatic brain injury. *Journal of Speech and Hearing Research, 37,* 1271–1283.

McHenry, M.A., & Reich, A.R. (1985). Effective airway resistance and vocal sound pressure level in cheerleaders with a history of dysphonic episodes. *Folia Phoniatrica, 37,* 223–231.

McHenry, M.A., & Wilson, R.L. (1994). The challenge of unintelligible speech following traumatic brain injury. *Brain Injury, 8,* 363-375.

McHenry, M.A., Wilson, R.L., & Minton, J.T. (1994). Management of multiple physiological deficits following traumatic brain injury. *Journal of Medical Speech-Language Pathology, 2,* 58–74.

Najenson, T., Sazbon, L., Fiselzon, J., Becker, E., & Schechter, I. (1978). Recovery of communicative functions after prolonged traumatic coma. *Scandinavian Journal of Rehabilitation Medicine, 10,* 15–21.

Netsell, R., & Daniel, B. (1979). Dysarthria in adults: Physiologic approach to rehabilitation. *Archives of Physical Medicine and Rehabilitation, 60,* 502–508.

Netsell R., Lotz, W.K., Du Chane, A.S., & Barlow, S.M. (1991). Vocal tract aerodynamics during syllable productions: Normative data and theoretical implications. *Journal of Voice, 5,* 1–9.

Netsell, R., Lotz, W.K., & Shaughnessey, A.L. (1984). Laryngeal aerodynamics associated with selected voice disorders. *American Journal of Otolaryngology, 5,* 397–403.

Ramig, L.O. (1992). The role of phonation in speech intelligibility: A review and preliminary data from patients with Parkinson's disease. In R.D. Kent (Ed.), *Intelligibility in speech disorders* (pp. 119–156). Amsterdam: John Benjamins.

Ramig, L.O. (in press). Speech therapy for patients with Parkinson's disease. In W. Koller & G. Paulson (Eds.), *Therapy of Parkinson's disease.* New York: Marcel Dekker.

Ramig, L.O., Horii, Y., & Bonitati, C.M. (1991). The efficacy of voice therapy for patients with Parkinson's disease. *NCVS Status and Progress Report, 1,* 61–86.

Shaughnessy A.L., Lotz W.K., & Netsell, R. (1981). Laryngeal resistance for syllable series and word productions. *ASHA, 23,* 745.

Simpson, M.B., Till, J.A., & Goff, A.M. (1988). Long-term treatment of severe dysarthria: A case study. *Journal of Speech and Hearing Disorders, 53,* 433–440.

Smitheran, J.R., & Hixon, T. (1981). A clinical method for estimating laryngeal airway resistance during vowel production. *Journal of Speech and Hearing Disorders, 46,* 138–146.

Theodoros, D.G., Murdoch, B.E., & Chenery, H.J. (1994). Perceptual speech characteristics of dysarthric speakers following severe closed head injury. *Brain Injury, 8,* 101–124.

Theodoros, D.G., Murdoch, B.E., Stokes, P.D., & Chenery, H.J. (1993). Hypernasality in dysarthric speakers following severe closed head injury: A perceptual and instrumental analysis. *Brain Injury, 7,* 59–69.

Vogel, M., & von Cramon, D. (1982). Dysphonia after traumatic midbrain damage: A follow-up study. *Folia Phoniatrica, 34,* 150–159.

von Cramon, D. (1981). Traumatic mutism and the subsequent reorganization of speech functions. *Neuropsychologia, 19,* 801–805.

Workinger, M.S., & Netsell, R. (1992). Restoration of intelligible speech 13 years post-head injury. *Brain Injury, 6,* 183–187.

Yorkston, K.M., Beukelman, D.R., & Traynor, C.D. (1984). *Computerized assessment of intelligibility of dysarthric speech.* Austin, TX: PRO-ED.

Chapter 14

Tongue Strength and Endurance
Relation to the Speaking Ability of Children and Adolescents Following Traumatic Brain Injury

Julie A.G. Stierwalt, Donald A. Robin, Nancy Pearl Solomon, Amy L. Weiss, and Jeffrey E. Max

RECENT STUDIES HAVE investigated the role of strength and endurance in motor speech disorders. In our laboratory, we have studied this topic in people with hypokinetic (Solomon, Lorrell, Robin, Rodnitzky, & Luschei, 1995; Solomon, Robin, & Luschei, 1994) and mixed (Robin, Somodi, & Luschei, 1991) dysarthrias. In addition, we have explored the relation between muscle strength and endurance in normal and supranormal (skilled debaters) speakers (Robin, Goel, Somodi, & Luschei, 1992). Results from these studies have suggested that strength and/or endurance of the tongue may be related to speech proficiency.

Whereas the communication deficits presented by adults who have sustained a traumatic brain injury (TBI) have been reported in the recent literature (Beukelman & Yorkston, 1991; Sarno, 1980, 1984; Sarno, Buonaguro, & Levita, 1986; Ylvisaker & Szekeres, 1994), relatively little information exists on dysarthria following TBI. In a series of investigations exploring the nature of verbal impairment following TBI in a total of 250

This research was supported by Grant No. P60 DC 00976 from the National Institute on Deafness and Other Communication Disorders.

We would like to acknowledge Elisa Mordue, Mary Morrisey, and Tara Temperly for their invaluable assistance in the data collection and analysis for this investigation.

adults (Sarno, 1980, 1984; Sarno et al., 1986), approximately one third presented with dysarthria.

Enderby and Crow (1990) described four adults who demonstrated severe dysarthria that affected multiple speech production systems following a severe TBI. In all subjects, tongue function, as assessed by the Frenchay Dysarthria Assessment (Enderby, 1980), was impaired. McHenry, Minton, Wilson, and Post (in press) examined maximal strength and sustained force control for the upper lip, lower lip, tongue, and jaw in 20 adult subjects with dysarthria following TBI. In addition to measuring maximal strength through maximum voluntary contraction for each of the articulatory structures, these authors also measured dynamic and sustained force levels at 0.25, 0.5, 1.0, and 2.0 N. Compared to control subjects, the group of subjects with TBI was different only in their ability to sustain a 2-N force level for 5 seconds with the tongue. This level of force represented approximately 30% of a maximum contraction in their study (range 10%–106%).

The exploration of communication impairment following TBI in the pediatric population has only been explored recently (Ewing-Cobbs, Levin, Eisenberg, & Fletcher, 1987; Jordan, Cannon, & Murdoch, 1992; Jordan & Murdoch, 1992). As with the investigations of adults, studies of children and adolescents who had sustained TBI revealed a variety of communication disorders. The emphasis of research, however, has been on language impairment. We found no published studies on the speaking ability of children following TBI. More specifically, there are no data in the literature regarding the strength or endurance of the muscles of the speech system for children and adolescents who have sustained a TBI. Thus, the current investigation was designed to examine tongue strength and endurance in relation to speech in a group of children and adolescents who had sustained a TBI. We were particularly interested in addressing the following questions:

- Is tongue strength reduced following TBI?
- Is tongue endurance reduced following TBI?
- Is there a relationship between tongue strength/endurance and speaking ability following TBI?

METHOD

Subjects

The children who served as subjects in this investigation were admitted to the University of Iowa Hospitals and Clinics in Iowa City with the primary diagnosis of TBI. The subjects were selected from a chart review that dated back to July 1987. The present study is a portion of a larger project investigating neuropsychological, psychiatric, and communication impairment following TBI in children and adolescents. Children with a preexisting diagnosis of mental retardation, a history of documented child abuse, or a previous clinical history of TBI were excluded from the study. Twenty-three children were included in the investigation.

The subjects had sustained a mild or a severe TBI. The severity of TBI was based on the lowest postresuscitation Glasgow Coma Scale (Teasdale, & Jennett, 1974) score (3–8, severe; 9–12, moderate; 13–15, mild) and results from the neuroimaging studies conducted emergently or soon after admission. Demographic information for individual TBI subjects is listed in Table 1. Data from age- and gender-matched control subjects were obtained from the normative sample of the Iowa Oral Performance Instrument (IOPI) data base located in the Laboratory of Speech and Language

Table 1. Demographic information for individual TBI subjects

Subject	Gender	Severity	Age	MPO[a]	Lesion data
1	M	Severe	11	32	No focal lesions
2	M	Severe	14	15	Superior parietal lobule
3	M	Severe	10	52	Right temporoparietal region
4	F	Severe	16	32	Right superior frontal gyrus, temporoparietal region
5	M	Severe	16	66	Basal temporo-occipital region
6	M	Mild	16	40	Normal
7	M	Mild	9	29	Normal
8	F	Severe	8	24	Bilateral frontal, right temporal region
9	M	Severe	9	34	Right frontal, temporal regions
10	M	Severe	15	42	Left frontotemporal region
11	M	Severe	9	40	Basal temporo-occipital region
12	M	Severe	16	12	Superior frontal gyrus, caudate nucleus
13	F	Severe	8	33	Basal temporo-occipital region
14	F	Severe	8	24	Shearing in left subcortex
15	F	Severe	7	30	Subarachnoid hemorrhage
16	M	Severe	17	14	Left cerebellar region, right frontoparietal, left medial temporal region
17	M	Severe	11	25	Left temporal region
18	F	Severe	7	14	Left superior frontal gyrus
19	F	Mild	6	16	Normal
20	M	Mild	8	32	Normal
21	F	Mild	9	45	Normal
22	M	Mild	16	41	Normal
23	F	Severe	6	16	Two right epidural hematomas

[a]Months post-onset.

Neuroscience, University of Iowa. The ages of the children/adolescents were matched to within 1 year for all subject–control pairs.

Strength and Endurance

Strength and endurance were assessed for the tongue and the hand[1] using the IOPI (available through Breakthrough, Inc., 131 Technology Innovation Center, Oakdale, IA 52319). The IOPI is a device that measures the amount of pressure exerted on an air-filled bulb with either the tongue or the hand (for details of the method, see Robin et al., 1991, 1992). The IOPI displays the peak pressure in kilopascals (kPa) obtained with a digital readout or continuous pressure via a light display.

Maximum strength was determined by having the subject perform a maximum voluntary contraction (MVC) with the tongue. The highest pressure obtained from three trials was recorded as the individual's maximum strength. The three trials were conducted one after another, with a short pause between each in order to record the number obtained. Endurance was determined by the length of time an individual was able to maintain 50% of his or her maximum strength. The light display on the IOPI was utilized as visual feedback to monitor the percentage of the maximum pressure. Endurance trials were timed with a stopwatch. When an individual was unable to maintain 50% of his or her maximum pressure, the trial was terminated and the time, to the nearest tenth of a second, was recorded.

Speech Samples

Following the strength and endurance tasks, speech samples were gathered from 22 of the subjects who had sustained a TBI (a speech sample was not collected from Subject 2). The samples consisted of repetition of the final 10 sentences from the Carrow Elicited Language Inventory (Carrow, 1974) and a 20-second segment of spontaneous speech, for a total of 11 separate samples per subject. The spontaneous speech sample was obtained using a cartoon description task (Weiss, Temperly, Stierwalt, Robin, & Max, 1993) that consisted of a description of one of five syndicated comic strips ranging in length from four to six panels. The selected cartoons involved minimal text, so the narrative was not based on the individual's reading ability. The 5 cartoons were selected from a group of 10 based on descriptions obtained by several normally developing 5- and 6-year-old children. To elicit the sample, the children were asked to look at the whole cartoon and then tell the examiner the "story" that was taking place in the cartoon.

---

[1]We routinely measure hand strength and endurance as a comparison to the tongue to provide an indication of generalized muscle dysfunction. It is also used to help orient subjects to the tasks because it is not as unusual to squeeze a hand bulb as it is to squeeze a tongue bulb.

The speech samples were recorded on high-quality audiotape with a Marantz (model PMD420) tape recorder and an external electric condenser microphone (Realistic 33-1063) clipped to the subject's shirt. In spite of these standard procedures for recording, the quality of the recordings varied across subjects. Although the speech signal was always audible, the judges noted that approximately 10% of the samples, mostly deriving from Subject 21, contained substantial background noise or interference. Fortunately, the interjudge reliability for these subjects' speech samples was comparable to that for the samples without background interference.

The original recordings were digitized at 22 kHz and low-pass filtered at 11 kHz using the C-Speech software program (Milenkovic & Read, 1992). Once the samples were digitized, the 220 sentences (10 from each subject) and 22 spontaneous speech segments (1 from each subject) were randomized for order and rerecorded on high-quality audiotape. This tape, consisting of a total of 242 speech samples, was used for obtaining perceptual judgments.

Perceptual Judgments

Five certified speech-language pathologists, each of whom had at least 5 years of clinical experience with children, served as judges for this investigation. Each judge performed this task independently and listened to the tape by headphones (Yamaha YH-2). The judges were asked to rate each sample for articulatory imprecision and overall speech defectiveness on a 7-point scale on which a rating of 1 indicated normal and 7 indicated a severe deviation from normal. Articulatory imprecision was selected as a parameter to provide an indication of tongue function. Overall speech defectiveness was selected in order to provide a general overview of speaking ability. The judges were provided with instructions regarding the interpretation of these two speech parameters and the use of the 7-point scale (see Table 2 for specific instructions). In addition, prior to listening to the

Table 2. Instructions for speech sample judgments

You will listen to speech samples of people repeating sentences and describing cartoons. Some of the speakers have a speech disorder and others do not.

You will judge the speech samples based on two parameters (which are not mutually exclusive): articulatory imprecision and overall speech defectiveness. For articulatory imprecision, listen to the accuracy and preciseness of the speech articulation. For overall speech defectiveness, listen to all aspects of the signal, including articulation, resonance, voice, prosody, and any other characteristics that affect the speech.

You will judge the speech based on a 7-point rating scale, where 1 = normal and 7 = severe deviation from normal. The points in between are at equal intervals between these extremes. Circle a single number for each sample and each parameter. Do not circle in between numbers or more than one number. Try to use the whole scale. Also, please do not refer to previous ratings as you continue the task. Use this sheet of paper to cover your previous responses. Do not go back and change answers.

experimental tape, the judges listened to a sample tape containing a range of the severity of speech samples. This procedure has been suggested as an alternative to anchoring the extremes and the midpoint of a perceptual judgment scale (Schiavetti, 1992).

Reliability measures across all five judges were obtained utilizing Pearson product-moment correlations. Average correlation coefficients were .83 (range .73–.92) for overall speech deficiency and .86 (range .76–.89) for articulatory imprecision. This was considered acceptable for the current study.

Statistical Analyses

Strength and endurance data were analyzed with a repeated-measures multivariate analysis of variance (MANOVA). The two dependent variables included in the analysis were maximal strength and endurance. For the MANOVA, the within-subjects variables were subject group (TBI and control) and structure (tongue and hand). This analysis preserved the pairing of matched subjects and of the structures for each subject. An alpha level of .05 was assigned for all statistical analyses.

Additional analyses were conducted to examine the relationship between perceptual judgments of the speech samples and tongue strength and endurance measures. Pearson product-moment correlations were obtained for articulatory imprecision and overall speech defectiveness, in relation to tongue strength and endurance.

RESULTS

Strength and endurance measures for the tongue and hand for all subjects can be found in Table 3. Analysis of the main effects revealed a significant group (TBI, control) main effect when all variables were considered ($F_{2,21} = 10.49$; $p = .0007$). Endurance contributed more to the group difference ($F_{2,21} = 13.22$; $p = .0002$) than did strength ($F_{2,21} = 3.27$; $p = .0578$). A significant main effect for structure (hand, tongue) was also found ($F_{2,21} = 33.59$; $p = .0001$). The difference between structures was due to both increased strength ($F_{1,22} = 38.10$; $p = .0001$) and increased endurance ($F_{1,22} = 33.10$; $p = .0001$) for the hand as compared to the tongue. The Group × Structure interaction did not reach statistical significance ($F_{2,21} = 0.86$; $p = .4374$).

Graphic representations of the differences between matched pairs of subjects for tongue strength and for endurance are provided in Figures 1 and 2, respectively. These graphs display the differences when measures of strength and endurance obtained from subjects with TBI were subtracted from those obtained from the matched control subjects. For each graph, the subject pairs were ordered to reflect the magnitude and direction (positive or negative) of the differences. Visual inspection of Figure 1 indicates

Table 3. Strength and endurance measures obtained from subjects with TBI and matched controls

	TBI group				Control group			
	Strength (kPa)		Endurance (s)		Strength (kPa)		Endurance (s)	
Subject	Tongue	Hand	Tongue	Hand	Tongue	Hand	Tongue	Hand
1	55	121	3	88	68	90	32	90
2	90	142	15	24	86	133	70	40
3	50	95	8	24	77	125	29	60
4	42	91	0	3	52	123	34	58
5	27	112	1	8	89	199	40	70
6	88	239	26	52	80	132	52	50
7	56	93	2	15	55	92	23	50
8	25	70	0	8	51	112	6	13
9	86	88	5	12	52	110	40	50
10	89	286	29	55	89	199	40	70
11	60	89	6	56	81	72	30	56
12	74	161	40	47	64	182	18	23
13	33	83	6	11	70	110	32	48
14	45	70	2	6	51	112	6	13
15	44	74	10	16	53	58	19	82
16	47	18	0	0	80	126	47	83
17	57	83	32	66	64	134	14	40
18	50	63	19	43	70	32	70	48
19	20	70	0	9	53	58	19	82
20	65	98	2	5	77	125	29	60
21	64	80	11	25	39	73	11	31
22	61	220	34	131	75	132	70	60
23	50	77	31	13	53	58	19	82
Mean	55.6	109.7	12.4	31.1	66.5	112.5	32.8	57.3
SD	19.7	62.5	13.1	32.2	14.2	43.5	19.4	24.5

that tongue strength was greater for the control subjects (reflected by positive-going bars) in the majority of subject pairs. However, this difference in tongue strength between groups approached but did not reach statistical significance ($p = .0578$). No difference between groups for hand strength was evident by examination of the data (Table 3) or statistical analysis. Figure 2 reveals greater tongue endurance (positive-going bars) for the control member of all but two subject pairs. Results for hand endurance were similarly striking.

The results of the perceptual study for each subject with TBI are provided in Table 4. Figures 3 and 4 plot tongue strength against articulatory imprecision and overall speech defectiveness, respectively. Figures 5 and 6 plot tongue endurance against these perceptual measures. Significant negative correlations were obtained for measures of tongue strength and ar-

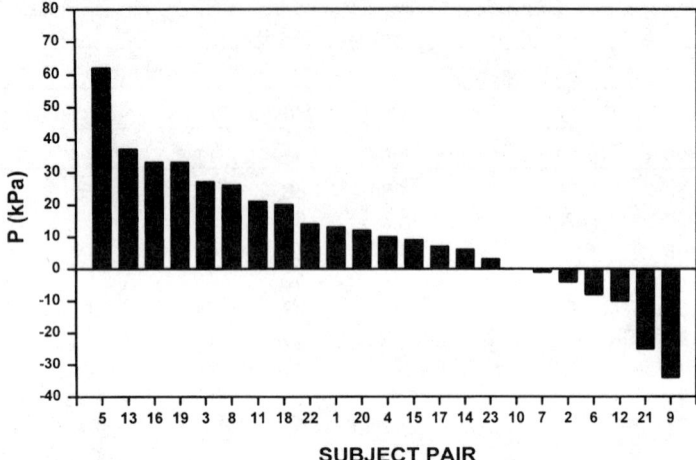

Figure 1. Differences in tongue strength (in kPa) for matched pairs of subjects (control minus TBI). Positive differences indicate that control subjects obtained greater pressures than did subjects with TBI.

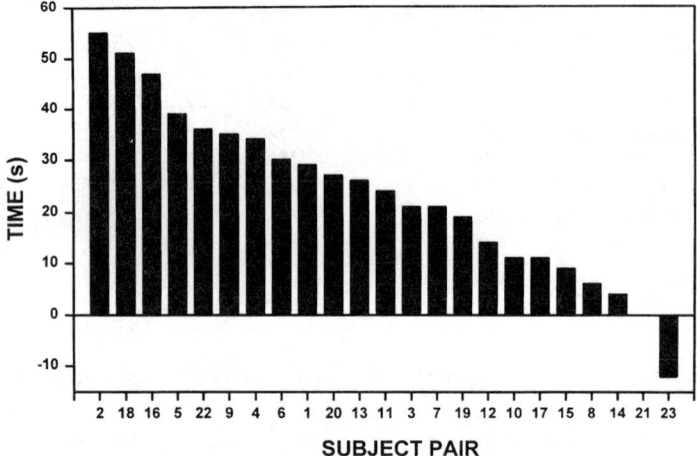

Figure 2. Differences in tongue endurance (in seconds) for matched pairs of subjects. Positive differences indicate that control subjects exerted pressure longer than did subjects with TBI.

ticulatory imprecision ($r = -.455, p < .001$) and overall speech defectiveness ($r = -.378, p = .003$). Similarly, significant negative correlations were found between tongue endurance and articulatory imprecision ($r = -.50; p < .001$) (Figure 3) and overall speech defectiveness ($r = -.317; p = .036$) (Figure 4). These correlations, although not strong, suggest that subjects with closer-to-normal speech generally had greater tongue strength and endurance. Conversely, subjects with more disordered

Table 4. Average ratings of articulatory imprecision and overall speech defectiveness for TBI speech samples

Subject	Articulatory imprecision	Overall speech defectiveness
1	2.39	1.00
3	3.00	2.75
4	4.42	2.67
5	4.05	2.67
6	2.04	1.04
7	1.97	1.47
8	5.15	2.27
9	2.32	1.0
10	1.13	1.0
11	4.75	4.25
12	1.20	1.00
13	3.75	1.75
14	3.17	2.32
15	2.97	2.55
16	1.42	1.15
17	1.57	1.37
18	2.10	1.45
19	1.40	1.15
20	2.07	1.85
21	3.37	1.06
22	2.42	1.72
23	2.00	2.0

speech tended to have lower tongue strength and endurance. This effect was particularly pronounced for the perceptual judgment of articulatory imprecision.

DISCUSSION

Tongue Strength and Endurance Following TBI

This investigation was designed to examine tongue strength and endurance following TBI in children and adolescents. Results from this study indicated that, as a group, the subjects with TBI did not differ from matched normal control subjects in terms of maximal strength of the tongue. This result is similar to that found by McHenry and colleagues (1994) for adults with TBI. Data from our study and the study by McHenry et al. indicate that, in this group of subjects, TBI does not affect the ability to perform a rapid MVC with the tongue (or with the lips and jaw). In addition, as a group, our subjects were no different than control subjects in terms of maximal hand strength, suggesting that generalized weakness may not be secondary to TBI.

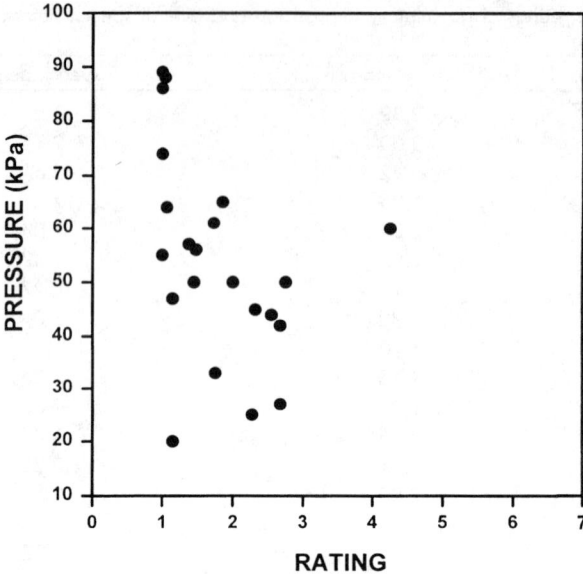

Figure 3. Scatter plot of perceptual ratings of articulatory imprecision and measures of tongue strength ($r = -.50$; $p < .001$).

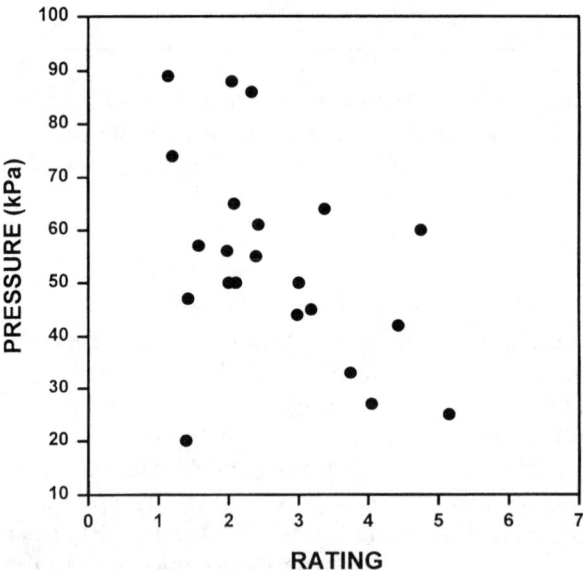

Figure 4. Scatter plot of perceptual ratings of overall speech defectiveness and measures of tongue strength ($r = -.317$; $p = .036$).

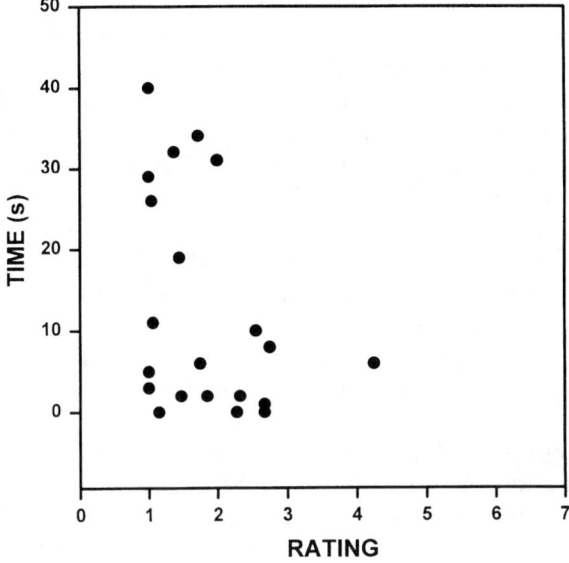

Figure 5. Scatter plot of perceptual ratings of articulatory imprecision and tongue endurance times ($r = -.455; p < .001$).

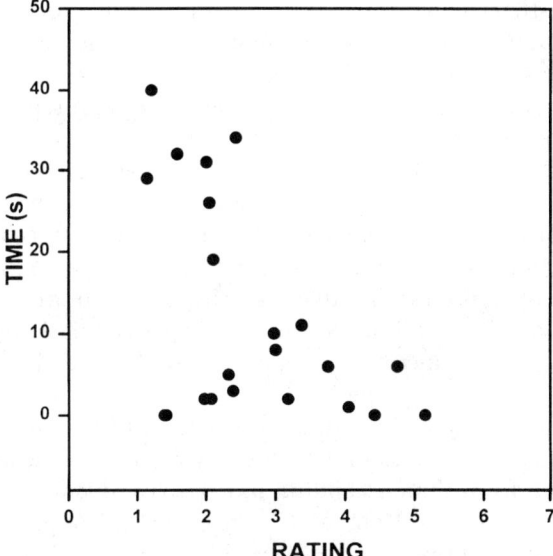

Figure 6. Scatter plot of perceptual ratings of overall speech and tongue endurance times ($r = -.378; p = .003$).

As mentioned previously, although the group difference in strength did not reach our a priori level of statistical significance, it did approach this level ($p=.0578$). Because the TBI population is heterogeneous by nature as a result of the wide range of lesions and severity of injuries, findings of large differences between individuals are not surprising. Inspection of the differences in tongue strength for matched pairs of subjects (Figure 1) reveals that a majority of subjects with TBI had weaker tongues than their matched control subjects. In fact, eight of the subjects with TBI demonstrated tongue strength that was more than 1 standard deviation below the mean of the control group. Likewise, inspection of the data provided by McHenry et al. (1994) reveals that a few of their subjects had substantially reduced tongue strength. Thus, one should examine each patient with TBI and not assume, based on group data, that strength will be normal.

A major finding of the current study was the markedly reduced tongue endurance for subjects with TBI. Inspection of the individual subject differences in the current study (Figure 2) reveals that, for the tongue, all but two of the TBI subjects fatigued more quickly (had lower endurance times) than their matched control subjects. This finding is not unlike that reported by McHenry et al. (1994), who found that their adult TBI subjects demonstrated difficulty sustaining a 2-N force with the tongue for 5 seconds.

Note that the subjects who demonstrated the greatest tongue strength were not those who had the longest tongue endurance times. It is possible that those individuals who demonstrated the greatest strength had lower endurance because of the high level of strength represented by 50% of their maximal pressure.

Finally, it is of interest to note that those individuals with mild injuries (Subjects 6, 7, 19, 20, 21, and 22) were not the ones who demonstrated the least amount of impairment in terms of strength and endurance. Mild injuries were classified as having a Glasgow Coma Scale score of 13–15 and neuroimaging that was within normal limits. This indicates that the severity of TBI as measured by typical clinical predictors is not predictive of performance on the tongue strength and endurance measures obtained in this investigation.

Explanations for increased fatigue following TBI may be related to central or peripheral factors. Central factors involved in fatigue may be related to feedback from the descending motor drive during a voluntary contraction (e.g., Gandevia, 1982; McCloskey, 1981). The perceptual result of this feedback is termed *sense of effort*. The reduction in the ability of the TBI subjects in this investigation to maintain a pressure output corresponding to 50% of their maximal strength compared to matched controls may be related to an increased sense of effort. The notion of an increased sense of effort was reinforced by comments from subjects (TBI and control) in the investigation. When the endurance trial was terminated, subjects often remarked that the task had become too difficult for them to continue. Another factor may be that central drive is adequate for producing a normal MVC (normal strength), but fatigue may occur sooner than normal as a result of more rapid adaptation of the motor neuron pool (Kernell & Monster, 1982).

Peripheral factors may also contribute to the increased fatigue exhibited by the subjects with TBI. Recall that, as a group, the subjects with TBI were not different from normal for maximal strength. Moreover, subjects with TBI who had the weakest tongues did not have the lowest endurance times. A possible explanation for these apparently paradoxical results involves the transformation of slow to fast motor unit types with changes in muscle innervation (Roy, Baldwin, & Edgerton, 1991). If such a transformation occurred in the subjects with TBI in the present investigation, strength would be expected to be greater or unchanged from prelesion levels, but endurance would be impaired because fast units are known to fatigue more quickly and slow units are fatigue resistant.

Relation Between Strength/Endurance and Speaking Ability in TBI

Significant correlations between the nonspeech measures of tongue performance and the perceptual judgments of overall speech defectiveness and articulatory imprecision in TBI subjects were found. This result was obtained for both tongue strength and endurance even though strength did not differentiate the TBI and control subjects as groups. This finding is in contrast to that reported by McHenry et al. (1994), who found no differences in their measures when their group of TBI subjects was divided into those with high intelligibility and those with low intelligibility. Two differences in the methodology between our study and the study by McHenry et al. should be mentioned. First, we did not use an intelligibility measure to index speaking ability, but rather used ratings of articulatory imprecision and overall speech defectiveness. It may be that intelligibility measures are not subtle enough to capture differences related to tongue performance on some tasks. Second, we did not divide our speakers into categories, but rather performed correlational analyses on the variables. Separation of the TBI subjects into two discrete groups may obscure potential relations among variables.

It is interesting to note that prevalence of dysarthria in children and adolescents for the subjects included in this study was 7 of 23, or 30%, similar to the reports of prevalance of dysarthria in adults following TBI (Sarno, 1980, 1984; Sarno et al., 1986). To identify dysarthric speech, we adopted a criterion of an average perceptual rating greater than 2 for overall speech deficiency. On our 7-point scale, a rating of 2 indicates a mild deviation from normal. Therefore, a rating greater than 2 would indicate an impairment that is easily apparent to speech-language pathologists.

The subjects included in this investigation were individuals with normal speech or with mild to moderate dysarthria. This fact was evidenced by the number of subjects who obtained a rating less than the midrange (19 of 23 subjects for the articulatory imprecision measure and 22 of 23 subjects for the overall speech defectiveness measure). If the subject group had contained more severely dysarthric individuals, it is possible that the correlations would have been even stronger. The perceptual ratings that were obtained in this investigation from the five independent judges matched the clinical impressions of two speech-language pathologists who interacted with the children in this study.

The findings of the current investigation suggest that measures of tongue strength and endurance may be related to speaking ability in people with dysarthria secondary to TBI. Given the number of diverse groups in which we have found that tongue endurance is associated with speaking ability, including the mixed dysarthria of TBI, adults with Parkinson's disease (Solomon et al., 1994), debaters (Robin et al., 1992), and children with developmental apraxia (Robin et al., 1991), further consideration of the clinical significance of fatigue in the speech system is warranted.

SUMMARY

We studied tongue and hand strength and endurance in 23 children and adolescents who had sustained TBI and 23 age- and gender-matched control subjects. Tongue strength and endurance were correlated with perceptual judgments of overall speech defectiveness and articulatory imprecision. Results showed that, as a group, the subjects with TBI were not significantly different from the control subjects for strength. By contrast, the subjects with TBI had significantly shorter endurance times compared to the control subjects. Significant negative correlations were found between measures of tongue strength and endurance and perceptual judgments of speech.

REFERENCES

Beukelman, D.R., & Yorkston, K.M. (1991). *Communication disorders following traumatic brain injury: Management of cognitive, language, and motor impairments.* Austin, TX: PRO-ED.

Carrow, E. (1974). *Carrow Elicited Language Inventory.* Austin, TX: Learning Concepts.

Enderby, P. (1980). Frenchay Dysarthria Assessment. *British Journal of Disorders of Communication, 15,* 165–173.

Enderby, P., & Crow, E. (1990). Long-term recovery patterns of severe dysarthria following head injury. *British Journal of Disorders of Communication, 25*, 341–354.
Ewing-Cobbs, L., Levin, H.S., Eisenberg, H.M., & Fletcher, J.M. (1987). Language functions following closed-head injury in children and adolescents. *Journal of Clinical and Experimental Neuropsychology, 9*, 575–592.
Gandevia, S.C. (1982). The perception of motor commands or effort during muscular paralysis. *Brain, 105*, 151–159.
Jordan, F.M., Cannon, A., & Murdoch, B.E. (1992). Language abilities of mildly closed head injured (CHI) children 10 years post-injury. *Brain Injury, 6*, 39–44.
Jordan, F.M., & Murdoch, B.E. (1992). Linguistic status following closed head injury in children: A follow-up study. *Brain and Language, 4*, 147–154.
Kernell, D., & Monster, A.W. (1982). Time course and properties of late adaptation in spinal motoneurons of the cat. *Experimental Brain Research, 46*, 191–196.
McCloskey, D.I. (1981). Corollary discharges: Motor commands and perception. In V.B. Brooks, (Ed.), *Handbook of physiology, Section 1; The nervous system, Vol. II: Motor control, Part 2* (pp. 1415–1447). Bethesda, MD: American Physiological Society.
McHenry, M.A., Minton, J.T., Wilson, R.L., & Post, Y.V. (1994). Intelligibility and nonspeech orofacial strength and force control following traumatic brain injury. *Journal of Speech and Hearing Research, 37*, 1271–1283.
Milenkovic, P.H., & Read, C. (1992). *C-Speech Version 4: User's Manual*. Madison: University of Wisconsin–Madison.
Robin, D.A., Goel, A., Somodi, L.B., & Luschei, E.S. (1992). Tongue strength and endurance: Relation to highly skilled movements. *Journal of Speech and Hearing Research, 35*, 1239–1245.
Robin, D.A., Somodi, L.B., & Luschei, E.S. (1991). Measurement of tongue strength and endurance in normal and articulation disordered subjects. In C. Moore, K. Yorkston, & D. Beukelman (Eds.), *Dysarthria and apraxia of speech: Perspectives on management* (pp. 173–184). Baltimore: Paul H. Brookes Publishing Co.
Roy, R.R., Baldwin, K.M., & Edgerton, V.R. (1991). The plasticity of skeletal muscle: Effects of neuromuscular activity. *Exercise and Sport Sciences Reviews, 19*, 269–312.
Sarno, M.T. (1980). The nature of verbal impairment after closed head injury. *Journal of Nervous and Mental Disease, 168*, 685–692.
Sarno, M.T. (1984). Verbal impairment after closed head injury, a report of a replication study. *Journal of Nervous and Mental Disease, 172*, 475–478.
Sarno, M.T., Buonaguro, A., & Levita, E. (1986). Characteristics of verbal impairment in closed head injured patients. *Archives of Physical and Medical Rehabilitation, 67*, 400–405.
Schiavetti, N. (1992). Scaling procedures for the measurement of speech intelligibility. In R.D. Kent (Ed.), *Intelligibility in speech disorders* (pp. 11–34). Philadelphia: John Benjamins Publishing Co.
Solomon, N.P., Lorell, D.M., Robin, D.A., Rodnitzky, R.L., & Luschei, E.S. (1995). Tongue strength and endurance in mild to moderate Parkinson's disease. *Journal of Medical Speech-Language Pathology, 3*, 15–26.
Solomon, N.P., Robin, D.A., & Luschei, E.S. (1994, March). *Strength, endurance and sense of effort: Studies of the tongue and hand in people with Parkinson's disease and accompanying dysarthria*. Paper presented at the Conference on Motor Speech, Sedona, AZ.

Teasdale, G., & Jennett, B. (1974). Assessment of coma and impaired consciousness: A practical scale. *Lancet, 2,* 81–84.

Weiss, A.L., Temperly, T.D., Stierwalt, J.A.G., Robin, D.A., & Max, J.E. (1993, June). *Use of cartoons to elicit narrative language samples from children and adolescents with severe TBI.* Paper presented at the Symposium for Research in Child Language Disorders, Madison WI.

Ylvisaker, M.S., & Szekeres, S.F. (1994). Communication disorders associated with closed head injury. In R. Chapey (Ed.), *Language intervention strategies in adult aphasia* (3rd ed.) (pp. 546–570). Baltimore: Williams & Wilkins.

SECTION VII

PARKINSON'S DISEASE

Chapter 15

Tongue Strength and Endurance in Mild to Moderate Parkinson's Disease

Nancy Pearl Solomon, Daryl M. Lorell, Donald A. Robin, Robert L. Rodnitzky, and Erich S. Luschei

WEAKNESS AND FATIGUE have been recognized as common symptoms of Parkinson's disease as early as its original description by James Parkinson in 1817. However, the few objective studies of muscle strength and endurance in Parkinson's disease have produced equivocal results. Wilson (1925) provided examples of reduced strength in various muscles of a few people with parkinsonism, but indicated that the more pervasive problem is slowness of muscle contraction and relaxation, and the inability to maintain contractions. Schwab, England, and Peterson (1959) argued that weakness is not a problem in Parkinson's disease, because with adequate motivation, normal amplitudes and directions of finger movements involving the first dorsal interosseous muscle were achieved voluntarily, and normal movement was elicited from electrical stimulation of the same muscle. They also noted that endurance was a primary problem.

Reprinted from the *Journal of Medical Speech-Language Pathology*, 3(1), 15–26, 1995, by permission of the authors and Singular Publishing Group, Inc.
  This research was supported by Grant No. R03 DC01182 and Grant No. P60 DC00976 from the National Institute on Deafness and Other Communication Disorders.
  We gratefully acknowledge Lori B. Somodi, Samuel K. Seddoh, Daniel L. Keyser, and Judith K. Dobson for their assistance with this project. We would like to thank two anonymous reviewers for their helpful comments on an earlier version of this chapter.

Additional studies have demonstrated normal maximal isometric strength of various muscle systems (hand, arm, foot, leg, respiratory) in subjects with Parkinson's disease (Koller & Kase, 1986; Saltin & Landin, 1975; Tzelepis, McCool, Friedman, & Hoppin, 1988), but weakness was apparent on repetitive tasks (Koller & Kase, 1986; Tzelepis et al., 1988). In contrast to these findings of normal isometric strength, Yanagawa, Shindo, and Yanagisawa (1990) reported decreased maximal strength for voluntary ankle dorsiflexion in 15 subjects with mild to moderate Parkinson's disease. However, as in the study by Schwab et al. (1959), electrical stimulation to the corresponding nerve (common peroneal) yielded normal results.

We are aware of only one study that systematically examined endurance in Parkinson's disease. Koller and Kase (1986) defined endurance as the number of repetitions of maximum extension/flexion movements of the wrist, arm, and knee to fatigue or until only 50% of the maximum strength could be generated. They found that endurance was greater for subjects with Parkinson's disease than for control subjects. This measure of endurance is difficult to interpret because the level of force (strength) and the rate of repetitions (movement velocity) can differ between subjects. Case study reports have clearly indicated a progressive decline in muscle strength over time that is quite different than that seen in healthy subjects (Schwab et al., 1959; Wilson, 1925).

Our research is directed toward understanding the nature of speech disorders of people with neurologic diseases. Common characteristics of the speech disorder of Parkinson's disease, hypokinetic dysarthria, are imprecision of articulation (Canter, 1965; Chenery, Murdoch, & Ingram, 1988; Darley, Aronson, & Brown, 1969; Ewanowksi, 1964; Laszewski, 1956; Logemann, Fisher, Boshes, & Blonsky, 1978; Morrison, Rigrodsky, & Mysak, 1970; Solomon & Hixon, 1993; Tanner, 1976) and abnormal speech rate (Canter, 1963; Darley et al., 1969; Hammen, Yorkston, & Beukelman, 1989; Hanson & Metter, 1983; Ludlow & Bassich, 1983; Peacher, 1950). The physiologic mechanisms responsible for these speech problems are not known. However, strength and endurance abnormalities in the orofacial musculature may contribute to articulatory and temporal abnormalities in the speech disorder of Parkinson's disease.

Examination of strength in the orofacial system of people with Parkinson's disease has been reported in a few studies. Dworkin and Aronson (1986) reported lower than normal maximum tongue "strength," measured by calculating the area under a force curve, in one subject with Parkinson's disease. Lip weakness has also been reported in Parkinson's disease (Netsell, Daniel, & Celesia, 1975; Wood, Hughes, Hayes, & Wolfe, 1992). Netsell et al. (1975) studied muscle activity of the upper lip in 22 people with Parkinson's disease (some of whom had been treated with thalamic surgery) and reported evidence of weakness (reduced amplitude and duration of electromyographic activity) in at least one representative subject. Wood et al. (1992) used a labial force transducer to assess maximum force generation and found weakness of the lower lip, but not the upper lip, in 10 subjects with Parkinson's disease, 8 of whom had dysarthria. Barlow and Abbs (1983) and Abbs, Hartman, and Vishwanat (1987) described subjects with Parkinson's disease who did not demonstrate orofacial weakness (although no quantitative data for this conclusion were provided) but exhibited instability in maintaining steady elevation forces for 4–5 seconds with the lower lip, the jaw, and especially the tongue. We are not aware of any studies that have examined endurance, per se, in the orofacial system in people with Parkinson's disease.

Although the mechanisms for movement difficulties in the orofacial system of people with Parkinson's disease are unknown, the tongue appears to be affected for speech (Logemann, Boshes, & Fisher, 1972). Acoustic data indicate that the center frequencies of vowel formants may be abnormal (Tanner, 1976) or the extent and speed of formant transitions are reduced for speakers with Parkinson's disease (Connor, Ludlow, & Schulz, 1989; Forrest, Weismer, & Turner, 1989).

In the present investigation, we tested strength and endurance of the tongue and hand in 19 people with mild to moderate idiopathic Parkinson's disease and 19 control subjects matched for physical characteristics. Assessing hand function was deemed informative as an indicator of general muscle functioning and because individuals with Parkinson's disease may demonstrate differential impairment of the extremities and midline structures. An additional purpose of this research was to address possible relations between tongue function and speech production.

METHODS

Subjects

Subjects were 19 adults diagnosed with idiopathic Parkinson's disease recruited from the Movement Disorders Clinic at the University of Iowa Hospitals and Clinics.[1,2] Individual data pertaining to physical characteristics and disease severity for the subjects with Parkinson's disease are provided in Table 1. The subjects were in mild to moderate stages of Parkinson's disease as judged on a modified Hoehn and Yahr scale (1967; Fahn et al., 1987) by a neurologist on the same day as data collection. Mild disease (Stages 1 or 2) was present in 12 subjects, mild to moderate (Stage 2.5) in

---

[1]In our original presentation of these data (Lorell et al., 1992), 23 subjects were included. For this final analysis, 2 subjects were eliminated because English was not their first language, 1 for having a history of drug abuse, and 1 for being in a severe stage of the disease (Hoehn & Yahr, 1967; Stage 4).

[2]Two of these subjects were described previously in a preliminary report (Subjects P-L ["Mrs. S."] and P-Q ["Mrs. H."]; Solomon, Robin, Lorell, Rodnitzky, & Luschei, 1993).

Table 1. Demographic information for subjects with Parkinson's disease, including stage of disease (Hoehn & Yahr, 1967), sex, age, weight, and height, and for the matched control subjects, including age, weight, and height (subjects were matched for sex)

	Parkinson's disease subjects					Control subjects		
Subject	Stage	Sex	Age (yr)	Weight (kg)	Height (cm)	Age (yr)	Weight (kg)	Height (cm)
A	1	F	54	75	175	55	76	163
B	1	F	72	70	163	72	75	158
C	1	M	64	106	185	62	105	185
D	2	F	49	90	172	49	95	163
E	2	M	58	99	185	61	100	183
F	2	F	61	79	160	58	74	168
G	2	M	73	87	179	71	86	183
H	2	F	76	59	160	73	60	158
I	2	M	64	72	172	64	68	173
J	2	M	66	97	185	67	97	178
K	2	M	73	76	181	70	78	183
L	2	F	65	79	161	64	78	168
M	2.5	F	46	78	173	49	80	163
N	2.5	F	64	87	165	65	85	163
O	2.5	M	73	108	170	72	96	178
P	2.5	M	66	76	178	65	76	183
Q	2.5	F	71	65	166	72	55	175
R	3	M	65	78	185	62	80	168
S	3	M	73	97	178	74	95	174

5, and moderate (Stage 3) in 2. The subjects had no neurologic or speech disorders other than those associated with Parkinson's disease. Sixteen subjects with Parkinson's disease were taking antiparkinsonism medications, although none experienced clinical fluctuations in their motor signs. Unfortunately, we were not able to coordinate data collection with the drug cycle because of scheduling constraints.

Nineteen neurologically normal adults were recruited from the community to match, one-to-one, subjects with Parkinson's disease for sex and age (within 3 years). In addition, subjects were matched as closely as possible for weight (all were within 5 kg with the exception of subject pair O) and height (within 10 cm except for subject pairs A and R). These variables have been found to correlate with strength in various skeletal muscles (Burke, Tuttle, Thompson, Janey, & Weber, 1953; Collumbine, Bibile, Wikramanayake, & Watson, 1950; Larsson & Karlsson, 1978; Petrofsky & Lind, 1975; Robin, Somodi, & Luschei, 1991). Control subjects had negative histories for neurologic, speech, or language disorders and were not taking medications that would affect motor performance. All subjects spoke General American English as their native language.

Procedures

The Iowa Oral Performance Instrument (IOPI) was used to assess strength and endurance. The IOPI has been described previously (Robin, Goel, Somodi, & Luschei, 1992; Robin et al., 1991). In brief, the IOPI measures pressure exerted on a small, air-filled bulb, and displays the result digitally (in kPa) or by a multilight LED display. For the tongue, a small bare plastic bulb[3] was placed against the hard palate immediately posterior to the alveolar ridge, and the subject, with lips together and teeth lightly resting on the bulb holder, pushed against the bulb in a rostral direction with the anterior portion of the tongue dorsum. External to the lips, the bulb was held gently in place by the experimenter's or the subject's hand. For the hand measurements, the subject gripped a hand bulb that was placed in the center of the palm of the dominant hand, and the fingers were wrapped around it. Care was taken to ensure that fingernails and fingertips did not press into the bulb as this would create artificial increases in pressure.

To measure maximum strength, subjects squeezed the bulb as hard as possible. Subjects were instructed to squeeze quickly to their maximum level and then to release the bulb. These instructions yielded the best results and minimized ensuing fatigue. The best of two trials was taken as the maximum. Hand strength was determined first, then tongue strength. Following the maximum strength maneuvers, endurance of the hand and then the tongue (one trial each) was measured. Subjects were instructed to maintain 50% of the maximum pressure as long as possible. Subjects monitored their own performance, using the LED display on the IOPI for visual feedback, and the experimenter provided loud verbal encouragement based on the visual display. Trials were timed with a stopwatch, and were terminated when the subject abruptly dropped the pressure or when 50% of the maximum pressure could not be maintained.

A speech sample was collected from all 38 subjects in a quiet patient examination room or speech research laboratory. A lapel-type electret microphone (Realistic 33-1063) was clipped to the subject's shirt, and speech was recorded onto high-quality cassette tape with a Marantz PMD420 tape recorder. Subjects described the Cookie Theft picture from the *Boston Diagnostic Aphasia Examination* (Goodglass & Kaplan, 1983). Later, approximately 20-s segments from each speech sample were recorded, from one Marantz tape recorder to another, onto a blank cassette tape in random order.

---

[3]Different tongue bulbs have been developed for use with the IOPI. In this study, the first-generation clear Silastic tongue bulb was used.

Four speech-language pathologists with 5 or more years of clinical experience (not the investigators involved in data collection) listened over Yamaha YH-2 headphones to the speech samples and rated them for articulatory imprecision and overall speech defectiveness on a 6-point scale (0 = normal, 1 = mild, 2 = mild to moderate, 3 = moderate, 4 = moderate to severe, 5 = severe). For articulatory imprecision, judges were instructed to attend to the articulation of the speech and to rate it for preciseness or lack thereof. For overall speech defectiveness, judges were told to take all characteristics of speech into account, including rate, phrasing, voice, resonance, and articulation. Judges rated the two variables for each speech sample before moving on to the next sample. Judges had no knowledge of the diagnostic category for each speaker when rating the samples. All four judges agreed within 1 scale point for 84% of the speech samples for articulatory imprecision and 87% of the samples for overall speech defectiveness. Judgments by the four listeners were averaged to provide a single numeric result for each speech sample.

Speech rate was determined for each of the speech samples by measuring the acoustic waveform with the C-Speech software program for personal computers (Milenkovic & Read, 1992). The duration of speech, with the exclusion of pauses greater than 250 ms, was determined. The number of syllables was divided by the duration of speech. This procedure resulted in a measure of "interpause speech rate."[4]

Statistical Analysis

A repeated-measures multivariate analysis of variance with one within-subjects factor was used to analyze the strength and endurance data. Two variables were included in the analysis: structure (tongue and hand) and function (strength and endurance). The within-subjects factor was Subject Group (Parkinson and control). This analysis allowed for paired comparisons of matched subjects. The Wilcoxon signed-rank test was used to test for differences between paired perceptual judgments of speech (equal judgments for a pair were considered missing data; a correction was conducted for tied ranks). Speech rate between pairs of subjects was compared with a one-sample t-test for paired data (two-tailed probability). Associations between disease and speech severity and strength and endurance measures were assessed with Spearman rank correlations. For all analyses, a probability level of .05 was assigned.

---

[4]Measures of speech rate that exclude pauses may provide more meaningful information for the speed of speech articulation than if pauses are included (Alp, 1988; Hammen, 1990; Metter & Hanson, 1986; Till & Goff, 1986). Recent studies in Parkinson's disease have excluded pauses from measures of speech rate (Hammen, 1990; Solomon & Hixon, 1993).

RESULTS

Measures of tongue and hand strength and endurance for each subject are provided in Table 2. A statistically significant difference between the subject groups was realized when all variables were considered ($F_{2,17} = 4.393$; $p = .029$). The difference was due to strength ($F_{2,17} = 4.645$; $p = .025$), not endurance ($F_{2,17} = 0.359$; $p = .704$). A significant difference between the structures (hand and tongue) was found for both strength and endurance ($F_{2,17} = 121.9$; $p = .0001$); both were greater for the hand. However, the interaction between subject group and structure was not significant ($F_{2,17} = 0.524$; $p = .601$), indicating that the structures were not affected differentially for the subject groups.

Differences between matched pairs of subjects for tongue strength are illustrated in Figure 1, and for tongue endurance in Figure 2. In the graphic displays, the result for the subject with Parkinson's disease was subtracted from that for the matched control subject. The data were ordered in terms of the magnitude and direction of the differences. There-

Table 2. Results for strength and endurance of the hand and the tongue for the subjects with Parkinson's disease and the matched control subjects

	Parkinson's disease subjects				Control subjects			
	Strength (kPa)		Endurance (s)		Strength (kPa)		Endurance (s)	
Subject	Tongue	Hand	Tongue	Hand	Tongue	Hand	Tongue	Hand
A	71	117	12	42	65	119	26	75
B	65	158	37	84	76	120	24	34
C	88	168	15	28	70	196	18	18
D	70	106	30	52	63	128	53	40
E	84	186	32	56	86	224	33	50
F	64	115	30	50	73	126	37	54
G	60	118	24	127	71	151	30	53
H	53	83	11	39	78	121	17	62
I	63	191	30	12	64	115	17	70
J	72	151	24	31	80	156	15	21
K	38	139	49	23	64	157	16	35
L	70	112	45	83	53	169	43	60
M	66	158	10	30	69	189	25	94
N	30	104	4	49	62	150	42	55
O	75	182	18	35	79	201	38	45
P	57	120	39	144	57	193	25	90
Q	29	149	55	52	50	126	32	30
R	26	143	23	38	90	195	51	60
S	46	110	13	21	66	137	23	37
M	59.3	137.4	26.4	52.4	69.3	156.5	29.7	51.7
SD	18.1	31.1	14.2	34.8	10.6	34.1	11.7	21.0

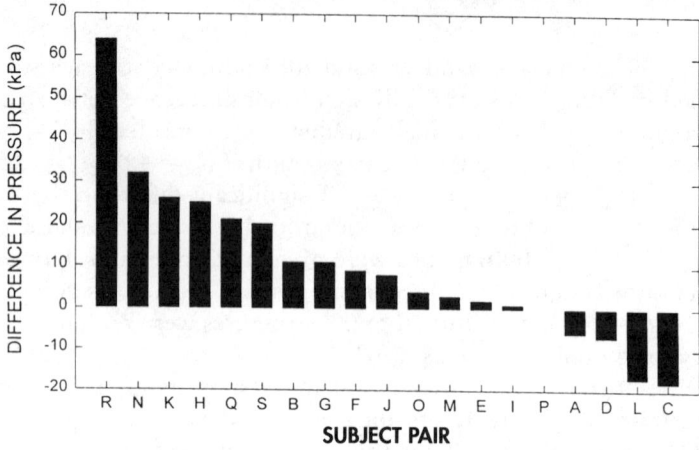

Figure 1. Differences in tongue strength (pressure, in kPa) plotted for matched pairs of subjects (control–Parkinson). Positive differences indicate that the control subjects exhibited greater pressures than did subjects with Parkinson's disease.

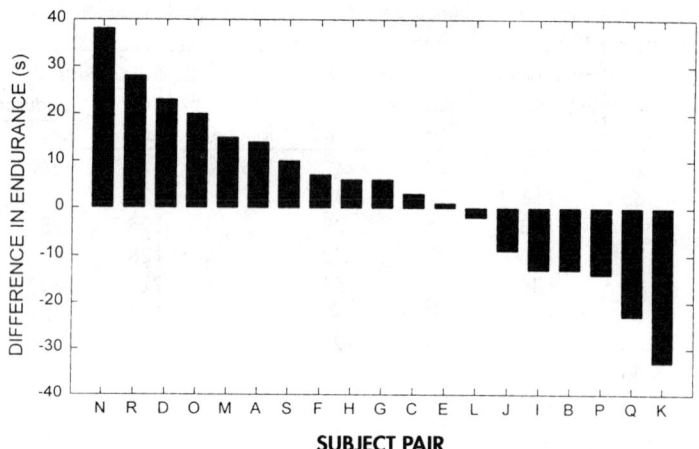

Figure 2. Differences in tongue endurance (duration, in seconds) plotted for matched pairs of subjects (control–Parkinson). Positive differences indicate that the control subjects exhibited greater endurances than did subjects with Parkinson's disease.

fore, the subject order is different for the two graphs. For tongue strength (Figure 1), it is clear that most of the data are positive (i.e., the control subject had greater tongue strength than the matched subject with Parkinson's disease). For tongue endurance (Figure 2), the data are more evenly split between positive and negative differences.

The results for the analyses of speech are provided in Table 3. Group analyses revealed slightly but significantly greater articulatory imprecision

Table 3. Results for the perceptual analyses of speech for articulatory imprecision and overall speech defectiveness

	Parkinson's disease subjects			Control subjects		
Subject	Articulation	Overall speech	Interpause speech rate (syl/s)	Articulation	Overall speech	Interpause speech rate (syl/s)
A	0	0	3.96	0.50	0.25	4.81
B	1.25	1.50	4.49	0	0.75	4.70
C	1.00	1.50	5.15	0.25	0.75	5.11
D	0	0	4.19	0	0.25	3.91
E	0	0	4.43	0.25	0	3.83
F	0	0	5.04	1.00	0.75	5.12
G	0.75	0.50	4.25	0.25	0.75	5.31
H	0.50	0.75	4.19	0.25	1.00	3.23
I	0.75	0.25	3.79	0.75	1.00	4.60
J	0.75	0	4.30	0.75	0.25	4.53
K	1.25	1.00	4.17	0.25	0.25	3.78
L	1.00	1.50	5.62	0	0	4.79
M	0	0	4.90	0	0	3.67
N	0	0	4.97	0.25	0.50	4.18
O	0.50	0.25	4.66	0.75	0.50	4.96
P	0.50	0.50	5.16	1.25	1.25	4.19
Q	0.75	0.50	4.98	0.50	0	5.27
R	2.25	2.00	5.43	0	0	3.80
S	2.25	2.50	5.44	0	0.25	5.07
M	0.694	0.671	4.691	0.368	0.447	4.465
SD	0.710	0.777	0.543	0.376	0.396	0.626

Average judgments (on a scale from 0 = normal to 5 = severe) and measures of interpause speech rate (syllables per second) for the subjects with Parkinson's disease and the matched control subjects.

for the subjects with Parkinson's disease as compared to the control subjects ($V = 35$, $n = 15$; $Z = -1.65$, $p = .049$, after correction for tied ranks). No difference was detected for overall speech defectiveness ($V = 63$, $n = 17$; $Z = -0.88$, $p = .188$, after correction). Inspection of the individual subject data indicated that all of the subjects were judged as having normal or mildly defective articulation and speech with the exception of Parkinson subjects R and S.

Correlations between disease and speech severity and strength and endurance measures were examined for the subjects with Parkinson's disease; the correlation coefficients and probability values are listed in Table 4. Only tongue strength resulted in a statistically significant correlation with stage of disease. Despite the fact that speech was perceived as normal or mildly affected for most subjects, tongue strength tended to be negatively correlated with overall speech defectiveness and articulatory imprecision.

Table 4. Spearman rank correlation coefficients and significance values for disease severity (Hoehn & Yahr scale) and speech (articulatory imprecision and overall speech defectiveness) correlated with hand and tongue strength and endurance for the subjects with Parkinson's disease

Correlations			r_S	p
Disease severity	×	Tongue strength	−0.56	.0001
		Hand strength	−0.12	.7940
		Tongue endurance	−0.15	.7090
		Hand endurance	−0.14	.7520
Articulatory imprecision	×	Tongue strength	−0.32	.0710
		Tongue endurance	0.29	.1480
Overall speech defectiveness	×	Tongue strength	−0.36	.0220
		Tongue endurance	0.19	.5160
Interpause speech rate	×	Tongue strength	−0.17	.6420
		Tongue endurance	0.05	.9720

Scatter plots illustrating these relations are provided in Figure 3. Speech did not correlate with tongue endurance for this group of subjects.

Interpause speech rate (Table 3) did not differ between subject groups ($t_{18} = 1.3179$; $p = .204$) and did not correlate with tongue strength or endurance (see Table 4).

DISCUSSION

Subjects with mild to moderate Parkinson's disease were found on average to have less strength in the tongue and hand than 19 matched control subjects. Strength was determined by the maximum pressure exerted on an air-filled bulb. Despite the contribution of subject pair R to the large difference in tongue strength between subject groups (Parkinson subject R had the lowest and control subject R had the greatest tongue strength of all subjects), the difference for strength remains when this subject pair is removed from statistical analysis ($F_{2,16} = 4.411$; $p = .0298$). Previous research generally has indicated that limb isometric strength (i.e., maximal force, torque, or pressure generated during a single maximal voluntary contraction) is not reduced in Parkinson's disease (Koller & Kase, 1986; Saltin & Landin, 1975; Tzelepis et al., 1988; for an exception, see Yanagawa et al., 1990). However, weakness has been reported in the tongue (Dworkin & Aronson, 1986) and lips (Netsell et al., 1975; Wood et al., 1992).

Endurance, defined in this investigation as the maximum duration for which 50% of the maximum pressure could be maintained, did not differ systematically between the subject groups. This finding was unexpected because people with Parkinson's disease often complain of fatigue (Friedman & Friedman, 1993). This perception of fatigue may relate to the

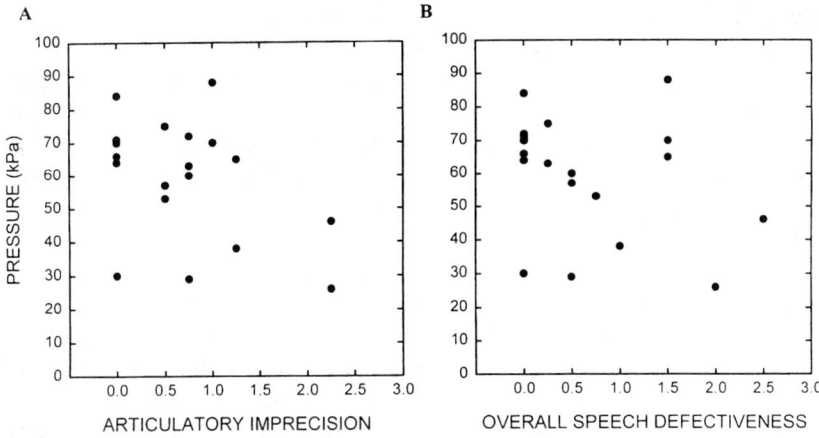

Figure 3. Tongue strength (maximal pressure) for subjects with Parkinson's disease plotted against average perceptual judgments of (A) articulatory imprecision ($r_s = -.32$; $p = .0710$) and (B) overall speech defectiveness ($r_s = -.36$; $p = .0220$); 0 = normal, 1 = mild, 2 = mild to moderate, 3 = moderate.

muscle weakness demonstrated for these subjects; muscle weakness corresponds with an increased sense of effort (Gandevia, 1982; McCloskey, 1981), a critical component of fatigue (Edwards, 1981; Enoka & Stuart, 1985). In addition, weakness may provide a possible explanation for the finding of normal endurance. That is, the target pressure during the endurance task would be lower in the subjects with Parkinson's disease than in the control subjects. Because of the lower target pressure, the task may require less effort and recruitment of more fatigue-resistant motor units than when strength is normal. Koller and Kase's (1986) finding of greater than normal endurance values in subjects with Parkinson's disease is consistent with this hypothesis.

It also may be important to consider a potential relation between endurance and instability. Previous reports of instability during tongue elevation have required subjects with Parkinson's disease to sustain a given level of force for 4–5 s (Abbs et al., 1987; Barlow & Abbs, 1983). Instability could cause our endurance task, for which tongue elevation is required at a target level for as long as possible, to be difficult for subjects with Parkinson's disease. Our subjective impression was that most of the subjects with Parkinson's disease in this study did not differ appreciably from the normal control subjects in their ability to control the tongue bulb during the endurance task. It is possible that the lingual contact arm of the force transducer described by Barlow and Abbs (1983) was more bothersome and difficult to control than the IOPI tongue bulb. In addition, the subjects in the previous studies may have had more severe Parkinson's disease and dysarthria than the present subjects. Although some of our subjects with Parkinson's disease did have trouble controlling the tongue bulb, it seems unlikely that this affected the overall result. That is, if trials were terminated prematurely due to motor instability, one would expect our endurance measure to show a deficit for the subjects with Parkinson's disease. On the contrary, tongue endurance did not differ significantly between the two subject groups. However, control may become an important methodological issue for subjects who have more severe impairments of the tongue.

We should not assume, however, that instability is simply an obstacle to understanding fatigue. Instability may, in fact, result from fatigue or contribute to it. Abbs et al. (1987) developed an instability index that is the standard deviation of forces generated during 10-ms intervals of the middle 3 s of the sustained-force trial. This index does not account for changes in instability over time. Visual inspection of the data for the tongue of the subject with Parkinson's disease in Figure 1 in the paper by Abbs et al. indicates a possible decrease in instability but no apparent fatigue during this 4-s trial. In trials that continue until fatigue ensues, changes in instability may provide a clue regarding the mechanisms affecting motor performance in Parkinson's disease. In our current research efforts with this population, we have been digitizing the entire endurance trial to examine the pressure data for instability.

A potential association between tongue strength and speech was suggested by the present data. That is, correlations were found such that the weaker the tongue, the greater the speech disorder in the subjects with Parkinson's disease. For example, the two subjects who were the most severe in terms of speech, as well as disease (Parkinson subjects R and S), had abnormally weak tongues. In fact, these subjects also had less tongue endurance than their matched control subjects. It is possible that these deficiencies in tongue function contributed to their speech disorder, but it must also be considered that these subjects were more severely involved in many measures and that the correlations have no causal implications. Exceptions to the tongue-function/speech link can be found as well. Parkinson subject N, for example, was rated by all judges to have perceptually normal speech, and yet her tongue strength and endurance were among the most impaired of all the subjects.

Because most of the subjects in the present investigation had speech that was perceived as normal or mildly disordered, it is difficult to assess the true relationship between nonspeech tongue function and speech proficiency. However, the correlations obtained are interesting and deserve attention in future investigations with more subjects who have a wider range of dysarthria severity. In support for this line of research, a small number of studies have found reduced tongue strength or endurance to be related to speech disorders in populations other than Parkinson's disease.

Children and adults with a variety of articulation and fluency disorders (Palmer & Osborn, 1940) and adults with amyotrophic lateral sclerosis (Dworkin, Aronson, & Mulder, 1980) have demonstrated lower than normal tongue strength. Children with developmental apraxia of speech were found to have normal tongue strength but reduced tongue endurance (Robin et al., 1991).

Speech rate did not correlate with tongue strength or endurance for the present subjects. Although people with Parkinson's disease can have abnormally slow or abnormally fast speech, the subjects in this study did not differ from normal for speech rate. In fact, no individual subject's speech rate was remarkably different than the speech rates for the control subjects. In studies with subjects who have markedly abnormal speech rates, perhaps this variable would relate to tongue function.

In a previous report, we had speculated that increased speech rate may correspond with better tongue endurance in people with Parkinson's disease (Solomon et al., 1993). We based this hypothesis on the finding that "supranormal" speakers (debaters) with fast speech rates ($M = 414$ words/min, or approximately 8.90 syllables/s) had supernormal tongue endurance (approximately 95 s at 50% of maximal pressure; Robin et al., 1992). It should be clarified that the debaters and control subjects in that study were asked to speak as fast as possible while maintaining intelligibility. In contrast, the present subjects' speech rate was determined from a task of habitual speech rate. We also acknowledge that the fast speech rate of supranormal speakers is unlikely to be comparable to the imprecise articulation, "fused" syllables, and relatively flat intensity profile that has been described for people with Parkinson's disease (e.g., Canter, 1965). It is important to note, however, that the subjects in the present investigation did not have speech characterized by rapid, indistinct syllables.

It it noteworthy that a significant positive correlation was found between tongue strength and disease severity. Conversely, it is as noteworthy that correlations were *not* found between disease severity and hand strength and endurance. Clinically, these subjects were not more impaired for midline structures than for peripheral structures. In addition, speech (presumably involving tongue function) is one of the few signs of Parkinson's disease that does not necessarily progress along with the disease (Metter & Hanson, 1986; Morrison et al., 1970). Replication of these findings, particularly with subjects with a greater range of disease severity, is necessary before conclusions can be drawn.

In summary, reduced strength of the tongue and hand was found in 19 subjects with mild to moderate Parkinson's disease in comparison to matched control subjects. Group comparisons failed to detect differences for endurance. Speech generally was mildly affected for the subjects with Parkinson's disease. Nevertheless, a negative correlation between tongue strength and speech defectiveness was suggested. Whether these findings will be replicated for subjects with more severe Parkinson's disease and dysarthria is a topic of our current research.

REFERENCES

Abbs, J.H., Hartman, D.E., & Vishwanat, B. (1987). Orofacial motor control impairment in Parkinson's disease. *Neurology, 37*, 394–398.

Alp, L.A. (1988). *The effects of imposed speech rate reductions on linguistic parameters and speech characteristics.* Unpublished master's thesis, University of California, Santa Barbara.

Barlow, S.M., & Abbs, J.H. (1983). Force transducers for the evaluation of labial, lingual and mandibular function in dysarthria. *Journal of Speech and Hearing Research, 26,* 616–621.

Burke, W.E., Tuttle, W.W., Thompson, C.W., Janey, C.D., & Weber, R.J. (1953). The reduction of grip strength and grip-strength endurance to age. *Journal of Applied Physiology, 5,* 628–630.

Canter, G.J. (1963). Speech characteristics of patients with Parkinson's disease: I. Intensity, pitch, and duration. *Journal of Speech and Hearing Disorders, 28,* 221–229.

Canter, G.J. (1965). Speech characteristics of patients with Parkinson's disease: III. Articulation, diadochokinesis, and over-all speech adequacy. *Journal of Speech and Hearing Disorders, 30,* 217–224.

Chenery, H.J., Murdoch, B.E., & Ingram, J.C.L. (1988). Studies in Parkinson's disease: I. Language and perceptual speech analyses. *Australian Journal of Human Communication Disorders, 16,* 17–29.

Collumbine, H., Bibile, S.W., Wikramanayake, T.W., & Watson, R.S. (1950). Influence of age, sex, physique and muscular development on physical fitness. *Journal of Applied Physiology, 2,* 488–511.

Connor, N.P., Ludlow, C.L., & Schulz, G.M. (1989). Stop consonant production in insolated and repeated syllables in Parkinson's disease. *Neuropsychologia, 27,* 829–838.

Darley, F.L., Aronson, A.E., & Brown, J.R. (1969). Differential diagnostic patterns of dysarthria. *Journal of Speech and Hearing Research, 12,* 246–269.

Dworkin, J.P., & Aronson, A.E. (1986). Tongue strength and alternate motion rates in normal and dysarthric subjects. *Journal of Communication Disorders, 19,* 115–132.

Dworkin, J.P., Aronson, A.E., & Mulder, D.W. (1980). Tongue strength in normal subjects and dysarthric patients with amyotrophic lateral sclerosis. *Journal of Speech and Hearing Research, 23,* 828–837.

Edwards, R.H.T. (1981). Human muscle function and fatigue. In R. Porter & J. Whelan (Eds.), *Human muscle fatigue: Physiological mechanisms* (pp. 1–18). London: Pitman Medical.

Enoka, R.M., & Stuart, D.G. (1985). The contribution of neuroscience to exercise studies. *Federation Proceedings, 44,* 2279–2285.

Ewanowski, S.J. (1964). Selected motor-speech behavior of patients with parkinsonism. *Dissertation Abstracts International, 24/11,* 4860. (University Microfilms No. AAC6407081)

Fahn, S., Elton, R.L., & Members of the UPDRS Development Committee. (1987). Unified Parkinson Disease Rating Scale. In S. Fahn, C.D. Marsden,

D.B. Calne, & M. Goldsteing (Eds.), *Recent developments in Parkinson's disease* (Vol. 2, pp. 153–163). New York: Macmillan.

Forrest, K., Weismer, G., & Turner, G.S. (1989). Kinematic, acoustic, and perceptual analyses of connected speech produced by parkinsonian and normal geriatric adults. *Journal of the Acoustical Society of America, 85*, 2608–2622.

Friedman, J., & Friedman, H. (1993). Fatigue in Parkinson's disease. *Neurology, 43*, 2016–2018.

Gandevia, S.C. (1982). The perception of motor commands or effort during muscular paralysis. *Brain, 105*, 151–159.

Goodglass, H., & Kaplan, E. (1983). *The assessment of aphasia and related disorders* (2nd ed.). Philadelphia: Lea & Febiger.

Hammen, V.L. (1990). The effects of speaking rate reduction in parkinsonian dysarthria. *Dissertation Abstracts International, 51/09B*, 4304. (University Microfilms No. AAC9104243)

Hammen, V.L., Yorkston, K.M., & Beukelman, D.R. (1989). Pausal and speech duration characteristics as a function of speaking rate in normal and parkinsonian dysarthric individuals. In K.M. Yorkston & D.R. Beukelman (Eds.), *Recent advances in clinical dysarthria* (pp. 213–224). Boston: College-Hill Press.

Hanson, W.R., & Metter, E.J. (1983). DAF speech rate modification in Parkinson's disease: A report of two cases. In W.R. Berry (Ed.), *Clinical dysarthria* (pp. 231–251). San Diego, CA: College-Hill Press.

Hoehn, M.M., & Yahr, M.D. (1967). Parkinsonism: Onset, progression, and mortality. *Neurology, 17*, 427–442.

Koller, W., & Kase, S. (1986). Muscle strength testing in Parkinson's disease. *European Neurology, 25*, 130–133.

Larsson, L., & Karlsson, J. (1978). Isometric and dynamic endurance as a function of age and skeletal muscle characteristics. *Acta Physiologica Scandinavia, 104*, 129–136.

Laszewski, Z. (1956). Role of the department of rehabilitation in preoperative evaluation of parkinsonian patients. *Journal of the American Geriatrics Society, 4*, 1280–1284.

Logemann, J., Boshes, B., & Fisher, H. (1972). The steps in the degeneration of speech and voice control in Parkinson's disease. In J. Siegfried (Ed.), *Parkinson's disease: Rigidity, akinesia, behavior. Vol 2: Selected communications on topic* (pp. 101–111). Bern Stuttgart Vienna: Hans Huber.

Logemann, J.A., Fisher, H.B., Boshes, B., & Blonsky, E.R. (1978). Frequency and co-occurrence of vocal tract dysfunctions in the speech of a large sample of Parkinson patients. *Journal of Speech and Hearing Disorders, 43*, 47–57.

Lorell, D.M., Solomon, N.P., Robin, D.A., Somodi, L.B., Rodnitzky, R., & Luschei, E.S. (1992, April). *Tongue strength and endurance in individuals with Parkinson disease*. Paper presented at the Conference on Motor Speech, Boulder, CO.

Ludlow, C.L., & Bassich, C.J. (1983). The results of acoustic and perceptual assessment of two types of dysarthria. In W.B. Berry (Ed.), *Clinical dysarthria* (pp. 121–153). San Diego, CA: College-Hill Press.

McCloskey, D.I. (1981). Corollary discharges: Motor commands and perception. In V.B. Brooks (Ed.), *Handbook of physiology: Section 1, Vol. II. The nervous system: Motor control, Part 2* (pp. 1415–1447). Bethesda, MD: American Physiological Society.

Metter, E.J., & Hanson, W.R. (1986). Clinical and acoustical variability in hypokinetic dysarthria. *Journal of Communication Disorders, 19*, 347–366.

Milenkovic, P.H., & Read, C. (1992). *CSpeech Version 4: User's manual.* Madison: University of Wisconsin–Madison.

Morrison, E.B., Rigrodsky, S., & Mysak, E.D. (1970). Parkinson's diseases: Speech disorder and released infantile oroneuromotor activity. *Journal of Speech and Hearing Research, 13,* 655–666.

Netsell, R., Daniel, B., & Celesia, G.G. (1975). Acceleration and weakness in parkinsonian dysarthria. *Journal of Speech and Hearing Disorders, 40,* 170–178.

Palmer, M.F., & Osborn, C.D. (1940). A study of tongue pressures of speech defective and normal speaking individuals. *Journal of Speech Disorders, 52,* 133–140.

Parkinson, J. (1817). An essay on shaking palsy. London: Serwood, Nelly & Jones. Reprinted in *Archives of Neurology and Psychiatry, 7,* 681–710, with a bibliographic note by A.J. Ostheimer (1922).

Peacher, W.G. (1950). The etiology and differential diagnosis of dysarthria. *Journal of Speech and Hearing Disorders, 15,* 252–265.

Petrofsky, J.S., & Lind, A.R. (1975). Isometric strength, endurance, and the blood pressure and heart rate responses during isometric exercise in healthy men and women with special reference to age and body fat content. *Pflügers Archiv: European Journal of Physiology, 360,* 49–61.

Robin, D.A., Goel, A., Somodi, L.B., & Luschei, E.S. (1992). Tongue strength and endurance: Relation to highly skilled movements. *Journal of Speech and Hearing Research, 35,* 1239–1245.

Robin, D.A., Somodi, L.B., & Luschei, E.S. (1991). Measurement of strength and endurance in normal and articulation disordered subjects. In C.A. Moore, K.M. Yorkston, & D.R. Beukelman (Eds.), *Dysarthria and apraxia of speech: Perspectives on management* (pp. 173–184). Baltimore: Paul H. Brookes Publishing Co.

Saltin, B., & Landin, S. (1975). Work capacity, muscle strength and SDH activity in both legs of hemiparetic patients and patients with Parkinson's disease. *Scandinavian Journal of Clinical and Laboratory Investigation, 35,* 531–538.

Schwab, R.S., England, A.C., & Peterson, E. (1959). Akinesia in Parkinson's disease. *Neurology, 9,* 65–72.

Solomon, N.P., & Hixon, T.J. (1993). Speech breathing in Parkinson's disease. *Journal of Speech and Hearing Research, 36,* 294–310.

Solomon, N.P., Robin, D.A., Lorell, D.M., Rodnitzky, R.L., & Luschei, E.S. (1993). Tongue function testing in Parkinson's disease: Indications of fatigue. In J. Till, K. Yorkston, & D. Beukelman (Eds.), *Motor speech disorders: Advances in assessment and treatment* (pp. 147–160). Baltimore: Paul H. Brookes Publishing Co.

Tanner, D.C. (1976). Spectrographic, pausimetric, and intelligibility measures in Parkinson's disease. *Dissertation Abstracts International, 37/09,* 4415. (University Microfilms No. AAC7705901)

Till, J.A., & Goff, A.M. (1986, November). Task variables affecting temporal structure and respiratory patterns in speech [Abstract]. *Asha, 28,* 102.

Tzelepis, G.E., McCool, F.D., Friedman, J.H., & Hoppin, F.G., Jr. (1988). Respiratory muscle dysfunction in Parkinson's disease. *American Review of Respiratory Disease, 138,* 266–271.

Wilson, S.A. (1925). The Croonian lectures on some disorders of motility and of muscle tone, with special reference to the corpus striatum. *Lancet, 2*(209), 1–10, 53–62.

Wood, L.M., Hughes, J., Hayes, K.C., & Wolfe, D.L. (1992). Reliability of labial closure force measurement in normal subjects and patients with CNS disorders. *Journal of Speech and Hearing Research, 35,* 252–258.

Yanagawa, S., Shindo, M., & Yanagisawa, N. (1990). Muscular weakness in Parkinson's disease. *Advances in Neurology, 53,* 259–269.

Chapter 16

Communication Disability of Parkinson's Disease
Perceptions of Dysarthric Speakers and Their Primary Communication Partners

Kim Antonius, David R. Beukelman, and Robert Reid

THE MOTOR SPEECH disorder known as dysarthria is commonly experienced by persons with Parkinson's disease. Solomon and Hixon (1993) report that "approximately 60% to 80% of individuals with Parkinson's disease have disordered speech" (p. 294). Mlcoch (1987) reported that approximately half of all persons with Parkinson's disease exhibit a speech disorder and, toward the later stages, the prevalence of the speech disorder increases. Depending on the severity of the dysarthria and the speaker's social situation, the disability resulting from the dysarthria of Parkinson's disease can be extensive. This study investigated the perception of disability by speakers with Parkinson's disease and their primary communication partners.

Dysarthria is a neurologically based motor speech disorder that is usually associated with diseases and conditions that are chronic or long term, such as Parkinson's disease. Yorkston, Beukelman, and Bell (1988) suggested models of chronic disability that are helpful in developing a

---

Portions of this chapter are based on the master's thesis of the first author at the University of Nebraska–Lincoln under the direction of the second and third authors. This research was supported in part by the Barkley Trust and Grant MCJ 319152 from the Maternal and Child Bureau, Health Resources Administration.

The authors wish to thank Marsha Sullivan and Kathryn Yorkston for their assistance with this project. Special appreciation is extended to the participants for their involvement in the study.

clinical perspective for the management of individuals with dysarthria. They found the framework adapted by the World Health Organization to be a useful framework from which to assess the disorder of dysarthria at four distinct levels. In 1991, Nagi revised the chronic disability framework slightly. The revised framework is reviewed here.

The *pathology* level involves the dysfunction of the neuronal mechanisms at a cellular or tissue level. For example, the pathology of Parkinson's disease is a "loss of dopaminergic neurons in the basal ganglia" (Yorkston et al., 1988).

The *impairment* level is the "loss and or abnormality of mental, emotional, physiological or anatomical structure or function" (Nagi, 1991, p. 314). An impairment is reflected at the subsystem level. The neurobiologic view of dysarthria proposed by Netsell (1986) focuses on the assessment of subsystem performance (respiration, phonation, articulation, and velopharyngeal function). Most descriptions of parkinsonian speech include monopitch, reduced stress, monoloudness, imprecise consonants, inappropriate silences, short inappropriate silences, short rushes, harsh voice quality, breathy voice (continuous), pitch level, and variable rate. Often, all of the subsystems of speech are affected (Darley, Aronson, & Brown, 1975).

The *functional limitation* level of a disorder is defined as the restriction of performance or inability to perform an activity in the manner or within the range considered normal as a result of the impairment. Functional limitations are reflected at the level of the organism (individual), and for dysarthric speakers are usually reported as the level of intelligibility, speaking rate, and/or naturalness of speech.

The *disability* level of a disorder refers to the inability to perform or limitation in performing socially defined activities and roles expected of individuals within a social or physical environment. At this level the reference changes from the individual (organism) to the society in which he or she is functioning and involves the perceptions and reactions of both the person with a disorder and the society around him or her. Nagi (1991) described three contributing factors to the differing patterns of disability in individuals with similar impairments: 1) the individual's definition (perception) of the situation and reactions; 2) the definition (perception) of the situation by others, and their reactions and expectations; and 3) the characteristics of the environment and the degree to which it is free from or encumbered with physical and sociocultural barriers.

Mlcoch (1987) suggested that individuals with Parkinson's disease have difficulty monitoring their own speech and applying the necessary corrections or compensations learned in the clinic to everyday speaking situations. Yorkston, Bombardier, and Hammen (1994) studied the perceptions of dysarthric speakers by examining dysarthria from the viewpoint of mildly, moderately, and severely dysarthric speakers with various etiologies. They found that the subjects did differ in their perceived reactions of others to their speech. Yorkston et al. (1994, p. 2) stated that this finding possibly "suggests that asking questions about perceived reactions of others may be a reasonable means of assessing the [disability] associated with dysarthria." Results of the study also indicated differences in the number of situations endorsed as difficult by parkinsonian speakers, with the most severely dysarthric speakers endorsing fewer speaking situations as difficult than the mild group. Yorkston et al. (1994, p. 30) suggested that "an explanation of these responses may be that some parkinsonian speakers do not have a proper appreciation of the extent of their disability." The differences between the mildly and severely dysarthric speakers, and the explanations given for the differences, indicate that further research should focus on the perception of dysarthria by mildly or severely dysarthric parkinsonian speakers. Yorkston et al. (1994) also suggested that future research be directed toward examining the perception of the dysarthric speakers' communication partners.

The purpose of the present study was to compare the perceptions of disability by speakers with Parkinson's disease and their primary communication partners. The specific research question was, "Do adults with hypokinetic dysarthria secondary to Parkinson's disease perceive the communicative disability caused by their dysarthria differently than do their primary communication partners?"

METHODOLOGY

Participants

Fifteen individuals who had been diagnosed as having Parkinson's disease at least 15 months ago, and their primary communication partners, participated in this study. The group included 16 men and 14 women who ranged in age from 49 to 79 years. The relationships of the individual with dysarthria to the primary communication partner included wife, husband, brother, and sister. All subjects spoke American English as a first language and had at least an eighth-grade education. Any subjects with concomitant language deficits, severe hearing loss, and/or psychological disorders were excluded from this study. All the above criteria were determined using an inclusionary screening form that was administered to the subjects prior to participation in this study. Subjects were recruited from three sources: the Meyer Rehabilitation Institute, the Omaha Parkinson's Support Group, and the Lincoln Parkinson's Support Group.

Speech intelligibility was measured using the Computerized Assessment of the Intelligibility of Dysarthric Speech (CAIDS) (Yorkston, Beukelman, & Traynor, 1984). The CAIDS samples were audio recorded and transcribed by three graduate students in speech-language pathology. The perceptions of the subjects and their primary communication partners were measured using the Communication Profile for Speakers with Motor Speech Disorders (Yorkston & Bombardier, 1992a) and the Communication Profile for Spouses of Speakers with Motor Speech Disorders (Yorkston & Bombardier, 1992b).

Procedures

The first author and a research assistant, both of whom were speech-language pathology graduate students with academic training pertaining to Parkinson's disease and its concomitant speech disorders, were trained to administer the questionnaires. They were also instructed in the administration of the CAIDS according to the guidelines provided in the manual. The speech samples were audiorecorded by a member of the research team and transcribed by three judges. The distribution of sentence intelligibility scores is reported in Table 1. Scores ranged from 74% to 99%, with a mean sentence intelligibility score across all speakers of 85.9%.

The participants with dysarthria completed the Communicaton Profile for Speakers with Motor Speech Disorders (Yorkston & Bombardier, 1992a). Their primary communication partners completed the Communication Profile for Spouses of Speakers with Motor Speech Disorders (Yorkston & Bombardier, 1992b), with assistance from the research staff if required. If participants had visual deficits, questions were read orally and the researchers recorded the participants' verbal responses. If participants

Table 1. Distribution of CAIDS scores for participants with Parkinson's disease

CAIDS scores	Frequency
74.0[a]	1
85.0	1
86.0	1
87.0	1
92.0	2
93.0	1
94.0	4
96.0	1
97.0	2
98.0	1
99.0	1

[a]Mean score for three judges.

had writing deficits, the researchers recorded the participants' verbal responses.

Dependent Variables

The dependent variables for this study consisted of the 15 different domains within the two communication profiles: one profile for the dysarthric speakers and one for their primary communication partners. These domains were divided into four areas: 1) situational difficulty, 2) compensatory strategies, 3) perceived reactions of others, and 4) dysarthric characteristics.

Situational Difficulty This area includes six domains that examine a range of situations encountered by a dysarthric individual, from difficult to easy:

- *Partner familiarity:* The speaker finds communication in situations in which he or she is unfamiliar with the communication partner more difficult.
- *Size of audience:* The speaker finds communication more difficult in large groups.
- *Demand for intelligibility:* The speaker has more difficulty when the demand for intelligibility increases (e.g., talking on the telephone).
- *Demand for speed:* The speaker has more difficulty when the listener requires the message to be quick.
- *Emotional load:* The speaker has more difficulty in situations that are emotionally involved.
- *Environmental adversity:* The speaker has more difficulty in an environment that does not facilitate communication (e.g., a large room).

Compensatory Strategies This area includes five domains that target the ability to use techniques or strategies to resolve communication breakdowns:

- *Improved precision:* The speaker will repeat the same message and modify speech output in a way that would improve precision and hence intelligibility.
- *Environmental manipulation:* The speaker will eliminate environmental aspects that contribute to communication breakdowns.
- *Avoidance:* The speaker simply avoids communication situations that may be difficult.
- *Message modification:* The speaker will change the mode of communication or the wording of the message.
- *Partner instruction:* The speaker will instruct communication partners to better facilitate their communication success.

Perceived Reactions of Others This area contains three domains that focus on the reactions of listeners:

- *Helpful:* The speaker receives a constructive or beneficial response from the communication partner.
- *Solicitous:* The speaker finds that the communication partner has excessive concern for his or her well-being.
- *Punishing:* The speaker finds that he or she is being penalized for the speech difficulties.

Dysarthric Characteristics This area contains only a single domain that focuses on a number of dysarthric speech characteristics, including intelligibility, rate, loudness, naturalness, voice quality, and nasality.

Scoring

Total scores were compiled for informants in each group, across each of the domains. Answers for all 100 items on the questionnaire were compiled into the 15 different domains, resulting in a summary sheet that reported the number of items endorsed by each subject in each domain.

Analysis

Data were analyzed using a two-stage process. First, a multivariate analysis of covariance (MANCOVA) was used to compare group differences for the speaker and primary communication partners in the areas of situational difficulty, compensatory strategies, and perceived reaction of others. Significant multivariate effects were then followed up with univariate analyses of covariance (ANCOVAs) to determine differences across individual domains within the areas. This analysis allowed group differences to be detected while comparing the dependent variables simultaneously. An ANCOVA design, with intelligibility scores as a covariate, was used to control statistically for any differences in the speaker group that might have been due to differing levels of intelligibility. Alpha was set at the .05 level for all tests.

RESULTS

Descriptive Statistics

Means and standard deviations for speakers and their communication partners for each domain are shown in Table 2.

Multivariate and Univariate Tests

In initial comparisons of the two subject groups (parkinsonian speakers and primary communication partners) using MANCOVAs, a significant

Table 2. Means and standard deviations (SD) for participants with Parkinson's disease and their primary communication partners

Variable	Group 1 (speaker)		Group 2 (partner)	
	Mean	SD	Mean	SD
Partner familiarity	58.06	29.57	52.31	27.41
Size of audience	54.88	27.77	43.87	28.67
Demand for intelligibility	57.56	27.79	48.81	24.89
Demand for speed	54.94	27.85	45.88	25.58
Emotional load	53.81	28.29	46.69	24.34
Environmental adversity	53.00	29.48	39.13	28.25
Improved precision	78.75	23.63	52.50	34.93
Environmental manipulation	43.75	32.02	27.50	17.70
Avoidance	53.75	36.31	47.50	35.68
Message modification	31.25	30.08	17.50	19.15
Partner instruction	30.44	26.62	12.50	15.71
Others helpful	54.94	19.82	46.56	24.61
Others punishing	0	0	0	0
Others solicitous	30.81	24.11	29.00	22.57
Dysarthric characteristics	52.88	18.68	33.94	14.31

difference was found for the area of compensatory strategies ($df = 15,15$, $p = .026$) (Figure 1). A review of Figure 1 reveals that the speakers with dysarthria endorsed more items in each situation as difficult than did their communication partners. The extent of the perceived differences was quite similar across the various situations. MANCOVAs revealed no significant differences between the perceptions of the two participant groups for the areas of situational difficulty (Figure 2) and perceived reactions of others (Figure 3). The mean domain scores for the area of compensatory strategies were then compared using an ANCOVA. The results indicated significant differences between groups on improved precision ($F_{1,29} = 6.02$, $p = .02$) and partner instruction ($F_{1,29} = 5.41$, $p = .027$), with the dysarthric speakers endorsing more items in all three of the domains than the primary communication partners. The difference in dysarthric characteristics was also significant ($F_{1,29} = 10.04$, $p = .004$), with the dysarthric speakers endorsing more items than their partners (Table 2).

DISCUSSION

As previously noted, the two groups differed in their perceptions of the impact of dysarthria on communication. However, there were significant differences for only 3 of the 15 domains: dysarthric characteristics, improved precision, and partner instruction. For all significant differences, the speakers endorsed more items than the primary communication part-

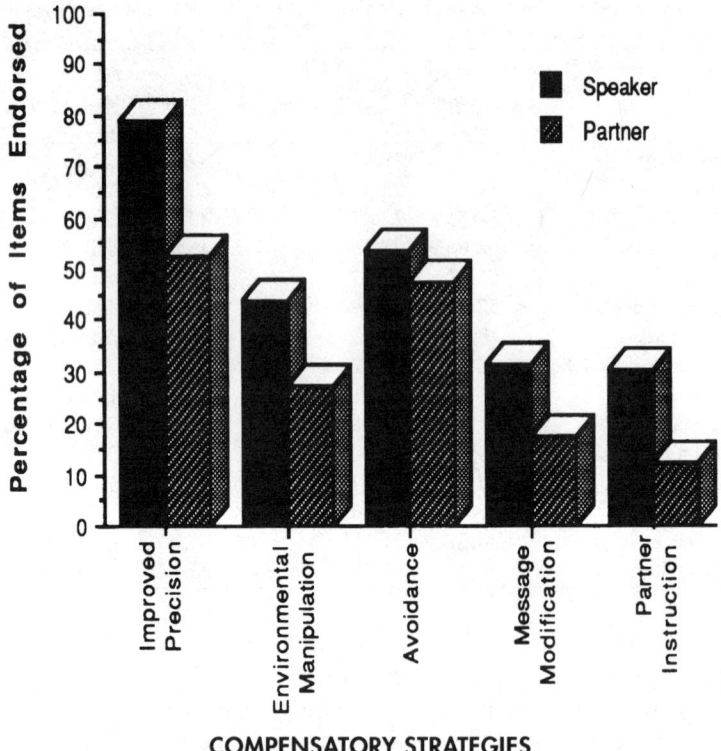

Figure 1. Percentage of items endorsed for the area of compensatory strategies by the parkinsonian speakers and their primary communication partners.

ners. The following sections discuss the possible reasons behind the differences in perceptions of the two groups and the differences in the number of items endorsed for each domain in the main areas.

Compensatory Strategies

Our findings are in general agreement with those of Yorkston et al. (1994), who also found that improved precision of speech was a frequently endorsed strategy for mildly, moderately, and severely dysarthric speakers. They suggested two possible reasons for this trend. First, it is possible that improved speech production actually was an effective strategy for the dysarthric speakers. Therefore, they endorsed a strategy that was effective for them. A second possibility is that speakers with dysarthria had never learned strategies other than improved precision of speech. Perhaps this strategy was sufficient to resolve communication breakdowns when they were normal speakers and, as their speech deteriorated, the strategy be-

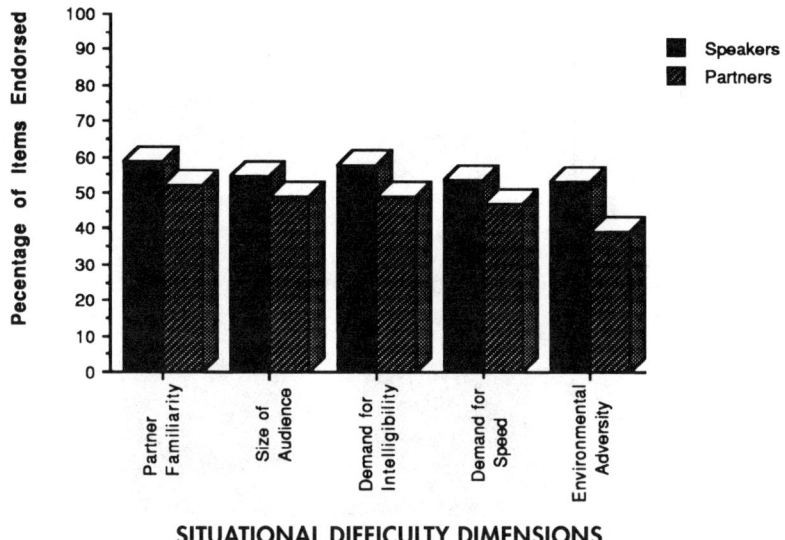

Figure 2. Percentage of items endorsed for the area of situational difficulty by the parkinsonian speakers and their primary communication partners.

came less effective but continued to be used because they had not been taught other strategies.

These explanations can be further examined when considering the results of the current study, almost exclusively obtained from mildly dysarthric speakers. For these speakers, improved precision of speech may be the best strategy. Based on the extent of the pathology and impairment, it may be easier for a speaker with a mild disablity to use the strategy of improved precision than it would be for someone with a more severe disability. Another explanation may be that a person with a mild disability may not see a need to use other compensatory strategies, such as partner instruction or message modification, because improved precision is effective to compensate for their current level of disability, whereas someone with a moderate or severe disability may no longer find improved precision a useful strategy and, therefore, would utilize a different strategy. Finally, the speaker with mild dysarthria may require training to use compensatory techniques such as partner instruction, which may not be as natural and automatic to use as trying to improve the intelligibility of natural speech.

Situational Difficulty

No differences were found across all domains within the situational difficulty area (Figure 2). Even though the speakers endorsed a slightly higher

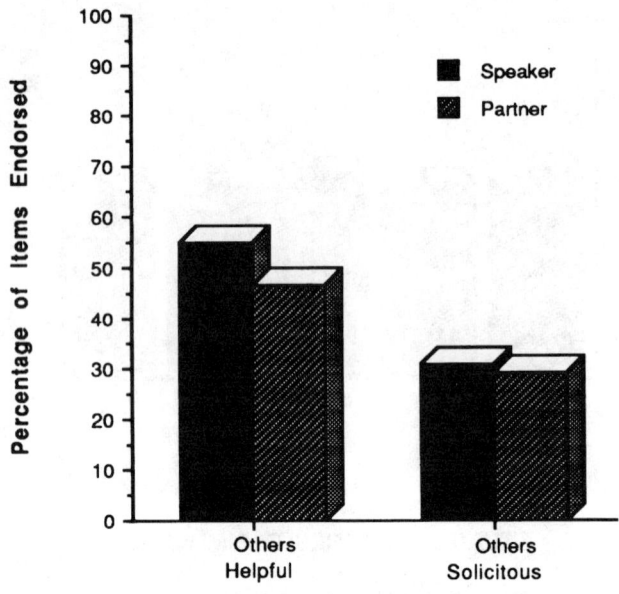

Figure 3. Percentage of items endorsed for the area of perceived reactions of others by the parkinsonian speakers and their primary communication partners.

percentage of items than the primary communication partners for all domains, these differences were not statistically significant. This supports the conclusion that persons with mild or moderate dysarthria do not perceive differential effects of situational difficulty. The consistency of ratings across domains may indicate that the speakers and primary communication partners view all speaking situations as similarly difficult. Variables other than the speaking situation may affect communication effectiveness. For example, the fluctuating course of increasing/decreasing performance observed in parkinsonian patients as a result of medication changes or physiologic/biologic changes may more extensively influence functional communication than the speaking situation itself.

Perceived Reactions of Others

In the area of perceived reaction of others, the speakers endorsed a slightly higher percentage of items than the primary communication partners in two domains (Figure 3). However, these differences were not found to be statistically significant. These results are in agreement with those of a similar study done by Yorkston et al. (1994) in which endorsements of mildly, moderately, and severely dysarthric speakers were compared across all domains. They also found that the domain "others helpful" was the most frequently endorsed by all speakers.

Dysarthric Characteristics

Past clinical observations have described parkinsonian speakers as having a lack of awareness regarding their speech deficits. However, our results suggest that they perceived themselves as having significantly more dysarthric characteristics than did their primary communication partners. This can be explained in two ways. First, perhaps these mildly-to-moderately dysarthric speakers are correct in perceiving themselves as having more dysarthric characteristics than do their primary communication partners. The dysarthric speakers may be more aware of their speech deficits because these deficits are internalized and not so easily observed by the communication partners. For example, the speakers may have to expend a great deal of effort in order to participate in a conversation, yet, when the primary communication partners view their conversational interactions, the partners do not perceive indications of this expended effort (i.e., fatigue, unintelligibility). Second, the speakers may have inaccurate perceptions of the extent of their speech disorder. Considering the fact that the majority of the subjects were only mildly dysarthric, a high endorsement of speech characteristics may not be expected. It is possible that the speakers, being in an early stage of their communicative disorder, view their mild impairments as substantial, whereas their primary communication partners do not perceive as extensive an impairment.

SUGGESTIONS FOR FUTURE RESEARCH

The current study evaluated the perceptions of speakers with dysarthria and their primary communication partners regarding the nature and extent of the communication disability associated with hypokinetic dysarthric speech. However, there are still questions that must be considered. First, it is uncertain whether or not significant differences would be evident across more domains of the questionnaire if the number of participants were increased. As mentioned above, a replication of this study with an increased number of subjects may increase the power enough to show significant results across more of the variables. Second, future researchers should examine whether or not individuals with differing levels of unintelligibility (e.g., mild, moderate, severe) and their primary communication partners have differing perceptions of how much dysarthria contributes to the overall communicative disability. It would be interesting to know if results of this study involving mildly dysarthric subjects would be similar to those of a study involving mildly, moderately, and severely dysarthric subjects and their primary communication partners. A third possibility for future research would be to examine whether or not individuals with dysarthria associated with an etiology other than Parkinson's disease perceive the impact of dysarthria on communication similarly.

The last suggestion for future research would be to document the impact of treatment on the perceptions of the impact of dysarthria on communication. As mentioned above, speakers may require treatment in order to make use of some of the strategies suggested in the Communication Profile for Speakers with Motor Speech Disorders. It would be interesting to give subjects similar to the ones in this study treatment, which would include teaching of compensatory strategies, improving physiologic support for speech, and improving the attitudes of people in the speakers' environment, and compare the results of a study after treatment with those of this study to see if the subjects endorse more items across all the domains.

REFERENCES

Darley, F., Aronson, A., & Brown, J. (1975). *Motor speech disorders.* Philadelphia: W.B. Saunders.

Mlcoch, A.G. (1987). Diagnosis and treatment of parkinsonian dysarthria. In W.C. Koller (Ed.), *Handbook of Parkinson's disease* (pp. 181–207). New York: Raven Press.

Nagi, S.Z. (1991). Disability concepts revisited: Implications for prevention. In A.M. Pope & A.R. Tarlov (Eds.), *Disability in America: Toward a national agenda for prevention* (pp. 309–327). Washington, DC: National Academy Press.

Netsell, R. (1986). *A neurobiological view of speech production and the dysarthrias.* Austin, TX: PRO-ED.

Solomon, N., & Hixon, T.J. (1993). Speech breathing in Parkinson's disease. *Journal of Speech and Hearing Research, 36,* 294–310.

Yorkston, K.M., Beukelman, D.R., & Bell, K.R. (1988). *Clinical management of dysarthric speakers.* Austin, TX: PRO-ED.

Yorkston, K.M., Beukelman, D.R., & Traynor, C. (1984). *Computerized assessment of intelligibility of dysarthric speech* [Computer program]. Tigard, OR: C.C. Publications.

Yorkston, K.M., & Bombardier, C. (1992a). *The Communication Profile for Speakers with Motor Speech Disorders.* Unpublished questionnaire, University of Washington, Seattle.

Yorkston, K.M., & Bombardier, C. (1992b). *The Communication Profile for Spouses of Speakers with Motor Speech Disorders.* Unpublished questionnaire, University of Washington, Seattle.

Yorkston, K.M., Bombardier, C., & Hammen, V. (1994). Dysarthria from the viewpoint of individuals with dysarthria. In J.A. Till, K.M. Yorkston, & D.R. Beukelman (Eds.), *Motor speech disorders: Advances in assessment and treatment* (pp. 19–36). Baltimore: Paul H. Brookes Publishing Co.

Chapter 17

Maintenance of Speech Changes Following Group Treatment for Hypokinetic Dysarthria of Parkinson's Disease

*Marsha D. Sullivan,
Patrick J. Brune, and David R. Beukelman*

THE INCIDENCE OF Parkinson's disease (PD) increases with age until approximately 1% of the population over the age of 50 years exhibits the disorder (Hull, 1970). Speech disorders are experienced by 60%–80% of persons with PD at some point during the course of their progressive disease (Solomon & Hixon, 1993). Phonatory impairment is often an initial symptom (Logemann, Fisher, Boshes, & Blonsky, 1978), with monopitch, reduced stress, monoloudness, harsh or breathy voice, lower than normal fundamental frequency, and variable speaking rate as commonly reported speech characteristics (Darley, Aronson, & Brown, 1975).

Early reports of behavioral interventions for hypokinetic dysarthria of PD were not too promising. For example, Sarno (1968) concluded that none of the persons with PD seen in her speech clinic over a 15-year period benefited from speech therapy. Sarno reported improvement in the treatment environment that did not transfer to other contexts. A close review of this retrospective study reveals that there was no control for the consistency or type of treatment.

Several research groups have subsequently reported immediate improvement in the speaking patterns of persons with PD as a result of behavioral interventions. Downie, Low, and Lindsay (1981), Hanson and

Metter (1983), Hanson, Metter, and Riege (1984), and Yorkston, Beukelman, and Traynor (1984) reported the positive impact of delayed auditory feedback (DAF) on selected persons with hypokinetic dysarthria. In most cases, the improvements reflected in increased speech intelligibility scores and reduced speaking rate were obtained only when these individuals utilized the DAF equipment and did not generalize to speaking tasks without the equipment. In subsequent work, Yorkston, Hammen, Beukelman, and Traynor (1990) reported the positive impact on speech intelligibility of speaking rate reduction using a computer pacing program. This study did not investigate generalization beyond the experimental situation.

Several prospective studies of behavioral intervention have reported immediate improvement and some maintenance of these gains (Johnson & Pring, 1990; LeDorze, Dionne, Ryalls, Julien, & Ouellet, 1992; Ramig, Horri, & Bonitati, 1991; Robertson & Thomson, 1984; Scott & Caird, 1983). Ramig and her colleagues reported long-term success, if the goal of intervention is the maintenance of phonatory function through a very intensive, although short-term, intervention program. Johnson and Pring reported improvement in PD speakers who received group speech treatment and deterioration of speech in a control group of PD speakers who received no treatment.

At the encouragement of a local PD support group, the current authors initiated a group intervention program for persons with PD. The purposes of this project were to develop a group intervention program for persons with hypokinetic dysarthria caused by PD and to investigate the impact of the group intervention program on the speaking performance of the participants by addressing the following questions:

- What changes in speech performance occurred as a result of group speech treatment?
- What evidence is there to support maintenance of speech changes following group treatment as evaluated by speech-language pathologists and speaker and spouse reports?

METHODOLOGY

Participants

Six participants (five men and one woman) with PD were included in the study. The age of the participants ranged from 55 to 77 years, and the time since onset of the disease ranged from 4 to 16 years. All individuals in the group displayed some type of motor speech deficit, including reduced speech volume, excessive speech rate, and reduced intelligibility.

All of the participants were evaluated as to the extent of their disability at the time of treatment using the Hoehn and Yahr scale (Hoehn & Yahr, 1967) (Table 1), with which each participant was rated on an arbitrary scale (Stages 1–5) based on the level of clinical disability.

At the initiation of treatment, each participant and his or her spouse completed a pure-tone screening to determine hearing acuity. This information was helpful in planning treatment strategies, particularly when the participant tended to blame his or her spouse's hearing ability as the cause of the participant's communication breakdown.

Measures of Communication Ability

Several measures were administered to the participants prior to and following intervention. All of the participants were taking prescribed medications for the symptoms of PD. The types and dosages of medications taken by each participant were not documented. There were no changes in the medication regimen for any of the participants between the pre- and postintervention measures. Medication status was not confirmed at the 5- or 10-month intervals. Reports of the benefits of the medications on communication ability varied according to the participant. In an attempt to keep medication effects stable during treatment measures, the neurologist who supervised all of the participants instructed each participant to take his or her medication 30 minutes prior to data collection, so that the benefits from the medication would be maximal at the time of data collection. Because each participant had a different medication schedule and length of medication benefit, no control of medication effects was attempted during the group treatment sessions.

Speech Intelligibility The sentence portion of the Computerized Assessment of Intelligibility of Dysarthric Speech (CAIDS) (Yorkston et al., 1984) was administered to assess speech intelligibility and speaking rate.

Table 1. Hoehn and Yahr scale of clinical disability in PD

Stage 1	Unilateral involvement only, usually with minimal or no functional impairment.
Stage 2	Bilateral or midline involvement, without impairment of balance.
Stage 3	First sign of impaired righting reflexes. This is evident by unsteadiness as the patient turns or is demonstrated when he is pushed from standing equilibrium with the feet together and eyes closed. Functionally the patient is somewhat restricted in his activities but may have some work potential depending upon the type of employment. Patients are physically capable of leading independent lives, and their disability is mild to moderate.
Stage 4	Fully developed, severely disabling disease; the patient is still able to walk and stand unassisted but is markedly incapacitated.
Stage 5	Confinement to bed or wheelchair unless aided.

From Hoehn, M.M., & Yahr, M.D. (1967). Parkinsonism: Onset, progression and mortality. *Neurology, 17,* 427–442; reprinted by permission.

Participant speech performance was audiorecorded, with the microphone worn by each participant on a headset 15 cm anterior to the lips. The CAIDS audiotapes were judged by three graduate students in speech-language pathology who were unfamiliar with the participants and were unaware of the interval during the study at which speech samples had been recorded. The interjudge correlation for 50% of the CAIDS samples was .83.

Perceptual Perceptual judgments were completed by three experienced speech-language pathologists who listened to recorded samples of the "Rainbow Passage." These passages were audiorecorded with the microphone mounted on a headset placed at a fixed distance (15 cm) from the participants' lips and with the tape-recording setting the same for all participants. The listeners rated each participant on a 5-point scale, with 1 as normal for vocal tone, appropriateness of pitch, and loudness. The listeners were required to listen to the passages at a fixed loudness level. The order of tape presentation was randomized across participants and recording intervals. Interjudge reliability studies for the three judges were completed for all of the rating tasks in the study. For vocal tone, 60% of the judgments were the same and 100% of the judgments were within ±1 scale point. For loudness, 80% of the judgments were the same and 100% were within ±1 scale point. For pitch, 40% of the judgments were the same and 75% were within ±1 scale point.

Recordings of the "Rainbow Passage" were also used to obtain a speech naturalness rating for each participant. A 7-point rating scale, with 1 as natural and 7 as very unnatural, was used (Darley et al., 1975). Three experienced speech-language pathologists who had not participated in the rating of vocal tone, loudness, and pitch served as judges. The order of tape presentation was randomized across participants and recording intervals. Interjudge reliability studies revealed that 62% of the ratings by the three judges were the same and 98% of the ratings were within ±1 scale point.

Communication Effectiveness Each subject completed a questionnaire on communication strategies and communicative effectiveness (Yorkston, Bombardier, & Hammen, 1992) (Table 2). This 100-item questionnaire was developed to investigate how dysarthric individuals experience their disorder in terms of characteristics of the disorder, situational difficulty, compensatory strategies, and the perceived reactions of others.

Exit Interview At the completion of the group speech intervention, the participants and their spouses were interviewed by the first or second author to ascertain their impressions of the experience.

Aerodynamic Measures It was the authors' intent to measure oral air flow and intraoral air pressure in order to estimate subglottal air pressure and glottal resistance using the method described by Smitheran and

Table 2. Sample questions from the Communication Profile for Speakers with Motor Speech Disorders

Situational Difficulty
I find it difficult when I am . . .
1. chatting with someone while riding in a car. A* D DA
2. talking with someone while riding in a car. A D DA
3. explaining a new project to someone at work. A D DA
 *A = Agree, D = Disagree, DA = Doesn't apply

Communication Strategies
Please indicate if you find these techniques useful or not.
1. I don't change topics without letting my listener know. Y* N DN
2. I ask people to be patient when talking with me. Y N DN
3. I tell people not to interrupt until I am finished. Y N DN
 *Y = Yes, N = No, DN = Don't know

Reactions of Others
Please indicate if you agree or disagree with the following statements:
1. My speech will improve if I work hard. A* D DN
2. Others criticize me for the way I talk. A D DN
3. Others get irritated with my speech. A D DN
 *A = Agree, D = Disagree, DN = Don't know

Excerpted from Yorkston, K.M., Bombardier, C., & Hammen, V. (1992). *The Communication Profile for Speakers with Motor Speech Disorders.* Unpublished questionnaire, University of Washington, Seattle; reprinted by permission.

Hixon (1981). The aerodynamic measurement system was similar to that described by Barlow (1989). Initial efforts to obtain these measures were considered unreliable because several of the participants were unable to maintain a consistent lip seal during the production of labial consonants. Others spoke in an atypical manner, including exaggerated articulatory patterns, maximal inhalations, and difficulty initiating speech acts, when aerodynamic measures were attempted.

Information from the aerodynamic studies of two participants was used in the intervention sessions to illustrate increases in oral air pressure associated with increased effort. However, aerodynamic measures were not used as indicators of speech performance as a result of the intervention.

Intervention Procedures

Intervention consisted of eight sessions given twice weekly, with the participant and some spouses interacting in a group therapy session. Each session consisted of a training period to introduce a technique to improve speech intelligibility. Practice of the technique was completed in various activities focusing on functional communication strategies. The sessions were completed with a social time during which coffee and cookies were served to allow the participants to practice their techniques in functional communication interaction to aid in generalization and maintenance of these skills outside the therapy session.

Goals of treatment were to 1) increase breath support for speech; 2) increase voice projection; 3) encourage precise articulation; 4) encourage increased use of intonation and appropriate phrasing; 5) encourage rate reduction, rate control, or both; 6) increase awareness and use of communication-enhancing techniques; 7) increase family awareness of the participants' deficits and ways to assist in improving the communication of the participant; and 8) promote generalization of speech techniques outside of treatment. A videotape was made of the group practicing the various techniques, and written practice materials were provided during treatment and at the completion of the program for continued practice outside of treatment. All participants attended all sessions. All the measures with the exception of the questionnaire were administered at four different times: before treatment, immediately after treatment, and at 5- and 10-month follow-up visits. The questionnaire was completed before treatment and at the 5-month follow-up visit. Follow-up data were collected from everyone in the group except at the 10-month follow-up session, which two individuals were not able to attend.

RESULTS

The two research questions posed in this study are addressed by reviewing the experiences of each of the six participants.

Participant 1

Participant 1 was a 58-year-old woman who had been diagnosed 6 years ago. The severity of her PD was rated as Stage 4.5 (Hoehn & Yahr, 1967) throughout the study. Although she was able to stand and walk with assistance, she used a wheelchair for mobility. She routinely sat with a lateral tilt of her trunk, making it difficult for her to maintain an upright position. When initially tested, her primary speech deficits included a breathy, monotonous voice with reduced loudness and rapid rushes of speech. Articulation precision was compromised during rapid rushes of speech, but she was relatively intelligible in a quiet setting. Although all of the participants utilized each of the treatment techniques, specific intervention goals for this participant were 1) to control her rate through pacing, 2) to increase her vocal loudness through increased breath support and voice projection within the group, and 3) to develop compensatory strategies for her speech deficits outside of treatment.

Although she reportedly did not recognize her speech deficits, her spouse complained of difficulty understanding her. Her spouse, who participated in all of the group treatment sessions, sporadically wore a hearing aid.

Changes in Speech Performance Pre- and posttreatment measures for Participant 1 are summarized in Table 3. Because her initial speech intelligibility measure taken from the sentence portion of the CAIDS was relatively high (90.6%), only a small increase in intelligibility (93%) was measured immediately after treatment. Habitual rate as measured by the CAIDS was rapid prior to treatment (273.9 words per minute [wpm]) and was markedly reduced (143.9 wpm) immediately after rate control treatment with a pacing board.

Improvements in perceptual measures were also noted during all postintervention recordings as compared to the preintervention recording. Using a 5-point perceptual scale, with 1 as the best vocal quality, improvements in vocal tone, pitch, and loudness were all noted immediately after treatment. Using a 7-point scale, with 1 as the most natural, the judges rated this participant's speech naturalness as improved immediately after treatment (pre = 6.4, post = 4.7) using a slow rate with a pacing board.

Evidence of Maintenance of Speech Changes Participant 1 did not demonstrate maintenance of the speech changes recorded immediately after treatment at a 5-month testing interval with the exception that the naturalness of her speech was rated as demonstrating continued improvement (5-month score = 4). Her intelligibility had actually decreased below her baseline measure (baseline = 90.6%, 5-month = 87.4%). Her husband reported that she had not practiced with the video sent home at the end of

Table 3. Data for Participant 1

Background information	
Age:	58 years
Gender:	Female
Marital status:	Married
Residence:	Home
Employment:	Retired housewife
Years postonset:	5
Hoehn & Yahr stage:	4.5
Participant hearing:	PTA[a]: left = 25 dB, right = 16.3 dB
Spouse hearing:	PTA: left = 43.8 dB, right = 42.5 dB

Speech

	Intelligibility (%)	CAIDS rate (wpm)	Naturalness[b]	Tone[c]	Pitch[c]	Loudness[c]
Preintervention	90.6	273.9	6.4	3.0	2.0	2.3
Immediately after	93.0	143.9	4.7	2.0	1.6	1.3
5 months after	87.4	219.6	4.0	3.0	2.3	2.3
10 months after	91.8	237.4	4.0	2.3	2.0	2.3

[a]Pure tone average.
[b]7-point scale (1 = normal).
[c]5-point scale (1 = normal).

treatment and was not using the pacing board outside of treatment. Following the 5-month recording session, Participant 1 was encouraged to practice and use her pacing board. Her husband reported an increase in her compliance at the 10-month testing interval, and her intelligibility measure increased to 91.8%. She was still not using the pacing board outside of treatment, and her habitual rate displayed a continued increase at each testing interval but had not returned to the pretreatment baseline. The perceived improvement in loudness and pitch were not maintained, but the speech naturalness rating remained stable.

More situations were endorsed as difficult on the communication questionnaire (Figure 1) following treatment, possibly related to an increased awareness of her speech deficits according to the situation. A change in her perception of the reaction of others to her speech indicated that, following treatment, she was more aware of the helpfulness of others and considered them to be less solicitous. No change was noted in her perception of the reactions of others as punishing. According to her responses on the questionnaire of her use of communication strategies, she had decreased her use of communication strategies and increased her avoidance of communication situations. Her responses were puzzling to the authors because she and her spouse reported increased use of commu-

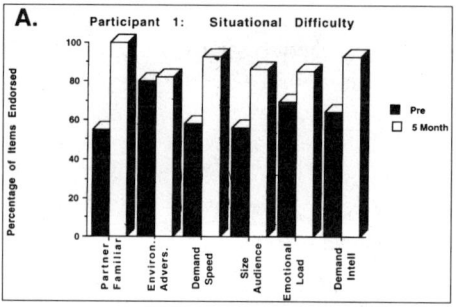
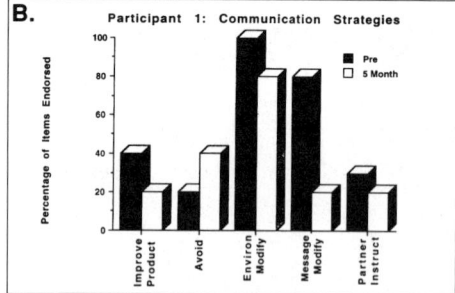
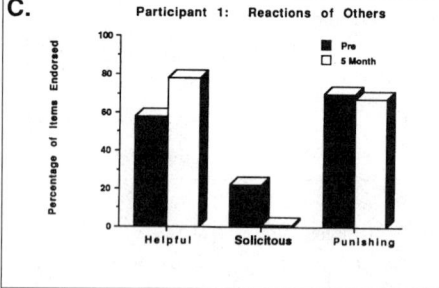

Figure 1. Results from the communication questionnaire before treatment and 5 months after treatment for Participant 1.

nication strategies at home, such as purchasing a remote control for the television so that she could press the mute button to decrease background noise when she wanted to speak.

Although Participant 1 reported an increased awareness of the difficulty of communication situations, she still reported difficulty monitoring the quality of her own speech and needed to use her spouse as a communication partner to encourage her to use communication strategies to improve her speech intelligibility in daily situations. Spouse participation in the group treatment program was considered essential for this participant.

Participant 2

Participant 2 was a 77-year-old man who had been diagnosed 6 years ago. The severity of his PD was rated as Stage 2.0 (Hoehn & Yahr, 1967) at the beginning of treatment. He complained of stiffness and rigidity and displayed a shuffling gait with festination. During the 10-month period of treatment and follow-up testing, Participant 2 was reportedly having more physical difficulties and was placed in a nursing home. His Hoehn and Yahr rating was 3.0 at the conclusion of the study.

His speech was characterized by reduced intelligibility with imprecise articulation. He and his spouse both reported that the participant's speech intelligibility was reduced outside of treatment. Both he and his spouse had hearing impairments (Table 4).

Table 4. Data for Participant 2

Background information	
Age:	77 years
Gender:	Male
Marital status:	Married
Residence:	Home/nursing home at 10 months
Employment:	Retired Navy officer and postal worker
Years postonset:	5
Hoehn & Yahr stage:	2.0
Participant hearing:	PTA[a]: left = 46.3 dB, right = 37.5 dB
Spouse hearing:	PTA: left = 45 dB, right = 41.3 dB

Speech	Intelligibility (%)	CAIDS rate (wpm)	Naturalness[b]	Tone[c]	Pitch[c]	Loudness[c]
Preintervention	75.5	216.0	5.0	2.0	2.0	1.3
Immediately after	90.9	178.0	3.0	2.6	1.6	1.3
5 months after	85.5	210.0	3.0	1.0	1.0	1.0
10 months after	88.2	200.6	3.0	1.3	1.0	1.3

[a]Pure tone average.
[b]7-point scale (1 = normal).
[c]5-point scale (1 = normal).

Changes in Speech Performance All pre- and posttreatment measures for Participant 2 are summarized in Table 4. The primary goal for this participant was to increase the precision of his articulation in order to increase his speech intelligibility. He demonstrated the largest gain in intelligibility of all of the participants in the group. Intelligibility increased immediately after treatment from 75.6% to 90.9%. Habitual rate simultaneously decreased from 216 to 178 wpm.

Unlike many individuals with Parkinson's disease, this participant's voice was judged as being harsh and too loud. On perceptual measures, the quality of his voice was judged to be more harsh immediately after treatment, with an improvement in pitch and with loudness remaining the same.

As with Participant 1, the judges noted an improvement in speech naturalness immediately after treatment (pre = 5, post = 3).

Evidence of Maintenance of Speech Changes Participant 2 maintained increased intelligibility when evaluated at the 5- (85.5%) and 10-month (88.2%) intervals, well above preintervention recordings (75.6%), although not as high as his intelligibility percentage immediately after treatment (90.9%). The maintenance of intelligibility was considered an excellent result in light of a decrease in his physical abilities over the 10-month period. Habitual rate increased from his measure immediately after treatment and may be a factor in the gradual reduction in intelligibility for this participant. Perceptual ratings of vocal tone, pitch, and loudness were higher at follow-up than on either pre- or immediately postintervention measures. The improvement in speech naturalness ratings observed immediately after treatment were maintained at the 5- and 10-month recordings. This participant reported that his speech had improved outside of treatment and reportedly realized that he would need to put into practice what he had learned during the treatment. His spouse also reported improvement outside of treatment, although she felt that she needed to provide reminders for him to decrease his rate.

Participant 2 appeared to increase his confidence in his speaking ability during the treatment. His intelligibility increased, and he received praise from other members of the group for his "loud" voice. He rated all communication situations on the questionnaire (Figure 2) as less difficult following treatment. There was no change in his perceived reaction to others, but he tended to avoid communication situations less.

Participant 3

Participant 3 was a 55-year-old man who had been diagnosed 6 years ago. The severity of his PD was maintained at Stage 1.5 (Hoehn & Yahr, 1967) throughout the study. He reported that he had a mild hand tremor and decreased vocal loudness. On initial testing, his primary speech deficits were

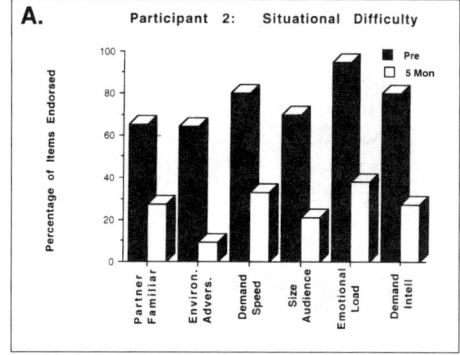
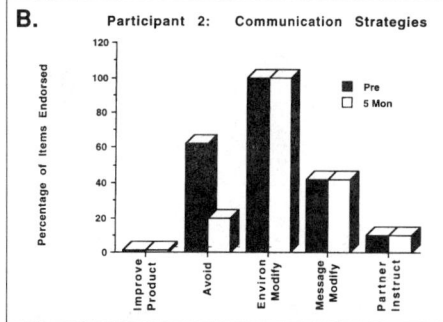
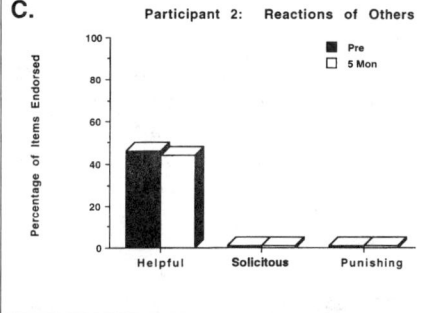

Figure 2. Results from the communication questionnaire before treatment and 5 months after treatment for Participant 2.

reduced vocal loudness and a hoarse vocal quality. He complained of difficulty projecting his voice, and his wife reported that the amount of his communication had decreased since his diagnosis. The primary goal for this participant was to increase vocal loudness and improve vocal quality. Both he and his spouse were active participants in the sessions and provided innovative practice materials for the group.

Changes in Speech Performance All pre- and posttreatment measures for Participant 3 are summarized in Table 5. Pretreatment intelligibility was high at 92.4% and increased to 96.7% immediately after treatment. As with the previous two participants, habitual rate decreased immediately after treatment from 236.1 to 178.8 wpm. The listeners noted an improvement in vocal tone, pitch, and loudness following treatment. The naturalness of this participant's speech was judged to improve with treatment (pre = 4.4, post = 2).

Evidence of Maintenance of Speech Changes Participant 3 maintained a high rate of intelligibility at the 5- (93.5%) and 10-month (93.9%) testing intervals. Habitual rate increased in the months following treatment but did not return to preintervention levels. Improvements in the perceptual

Table 5. Data for Participant 3

Background Information
- Age: 55 years
- Gender: Male
- Marital status: Married
- Residence: Home
- Employment: Management analyst
- Years postonset: 5
- Hoehn & Yahr stage: 1.5
- Participant hearing: PTA[a]: left = 33.8 dB, right = 25.0 dB
- Spouse hearing: PTA: left = 7.5 dB, right = 10.0 dB

Speech

	Intelligibility (%)	CAIDS rate (wpm)	Naturalness[b]	Tone[c]	Pitch[c]	Loudness[c]
Preintervention	92.4	236.1	4.4	3.0	2.3	2.3
Immediately after	96.7	178.8	2.0	2.0	1.6	1.0
5 months after	93.5	219.6	3.0	2.3	1.3	1.0
10 months after	93.9	224.5	2.0	2.6	1.3	1.3

[a]Pure tone average.
[b]7-point scale (1 = normal).
[c]5-point scale (1 = normal).

ratings of vocal tone, pitch, and loudness all were maintained at the testing intervals following treatment. Speech naturalness ratings were maintained for all postintervention recordings.

The participant and his wife both reported an improvement in the loudness of his voice outside of treatment. This participant was observed to successfully project his voice from the back of a large room at a Parkinson's disease support group meeting. He reported that he would not have attempted to talk from the back of the room prior to treatment. His wife also reported that she has noticed that the participant was communicating more outside of treatment.

This participant rated all communication situations on the questionnaire (Figure 3) as more difficult following treatment. He reported less avoidance of communication situations. There was not much change in his ratings of the reactions of others, although he found others to be a little less helpful than at pretreatment. This perception may have been influenced by a change in employment accompanied by a new group of listeners. The participant reported that, although he was unable to maintain increased volume all of the time, he was able to increase volume as necessary for the speaking situation.

Participant 4

Participant 4 was a 75-year-old man who had been diagnosed 16 years ago. The severity of his PD was judged to be Stage 2.5 (Hoehn & Yahr,

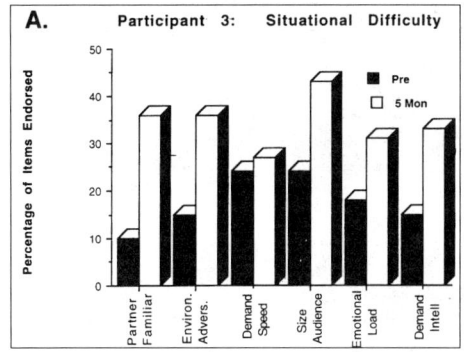
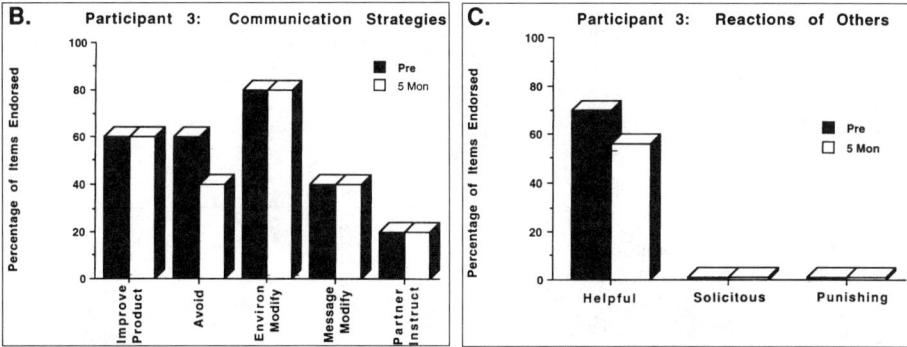

Figure 3. Results from the communication questionnaire before treatment and 5 months after treatment for Participant 3.

1967) throughout the study. He reported increased muscle weakness and tremor. His speech was characterized by hoarseness with phonation breaks and reduced loudness and intelligibility. He and his spouse complained of the participant having difficulty maintaining consistent vocal quality and of intermittent swallowing difficulty. The goals for this participant were to increase speech intelligibility, reduce phonation breaks, and increase loudness. His spouse participated in all of the group sessions.

Changes in Speech Performance All pre- and posttreatment measures for Participant 4 are summarized in Table 6. Intelligibility increased from 85.5% before treatment to 93% immediately after treatment. Habitual speech rate decreased from 205.3 wpm before treatment to 172.1 wpm after treatment.

The tone, pitch, and loudness of Participant 4's voice were judged to improve after treatment. Before treatment, this participant had difficulty maintaining voicing, with interruptions in fluency that were not present on the posttreatment measures. Participant 4 was judged to have a more natural quality to his speech following treatment (pre = 5, post = 3.4).

Evidence of Maintenance of Speech Changes Participant 4 demonstrated increased intelligibility at the 5-month testing interval (96.7%). As

Table 6. Data for Participant 4

Background information
    Age: 75 years
    Gender: Male
    Marital status: Married
    Residence: Home
    Employment: Retired railroad switchman
    Years postonset: 15
    Hoehn & Yahr stage: 2.5
    Participant hearing: PTA[a]: left = 51.3 dB, right = 48.8 dB
    Spouse hearing: PTA: left = 37.5 dB, right = 36.3 dB

Speech

	Intelli-gibility (%)	CAIDS rate (wpm)	Natural-ness[b]	Tone[c]	Pitch[c]	Loudness[c]
Preintervention	85.5	205.3	5.0	3.0	3.0	2.0
Immediately after	93.0	172.1	3.4	2.0	1.6	1.3
5 months after	96.7	217.5	3.3	2.0	1.0	1.0
10 months after	NA	NA	NA	NA	NA	NA

[a] Pure tone average.
[b] 7-point scale (1 = normal).
[c] 5-point scale (1 = normal).

with the previous participants, habitual rate increased during the interval after treatment, but in his case the increase in habitual rate did not interfere with intelligibility. The vocal tone, pitch, and loudness ratings were stable or demonstrated improvement at the 5-month interval. Speech naturalness ratings continued to improve. Participant 4 reported that use of precise articulation and visualizing people as further away to increase loudness were effective techniques for improvement in his speech. He used the group sessions to practice a speech intended for a future audience. His spouse also reported that the participant had attempted to project his voice better outside of treatment but that she felt a need for occasional reminders. This participant was unavailable for testing at the 10-month interval.

Participant 4's responses to the questions on the communication questionnaire were considered invalid because he gave the same response to all of the items.

Participant 5

Participant 5 was a 70-year-old man who had been diagnosed 4 years ago. The severity of his PD was judged to be Stage 2.5 (Hoehn & Yahr, 1967) throughout the investigation. He displayed weakness and tremor. His speech was characterized by reduced volume and a breathy vocal quality. He reported that his wife complained that she could not hear him because he talked too softly, but he was unable to monitor his loudness adequately. The primary goal for this participant was increased vocal loudness. Although his wife accompanied him to the initial testing, she did not participate in the treatment sessions.

Changes in Speech Performance All pre- and posttreatment measures for Participant 5 are summarized in Table 7. Intelligibility was high and remained approximately the same before (96.1%) and after treatment (95.5%) for this participant. Habitual rate decreased immediately after treatment from 190.2 to 182.6 wpm.

Participant 5's voice was judged to improve in tone quality and loudness, with pitch judgments remaining the same. His speech was judged to be more natural immediately after treatment (pre = 3, post = 2.4).

Evidence of Maintenance of Speech Changes Participant 5 maintained his intelligibility and further reduced his habitual rate when tested at 5 months after treatment. Vocal tone and loudness demonstrated continued improvement during the months following treatment, with pitch remaining stable. It was gratifying to note that his ability to increase his loudness was maintained over the 5-month interval because loudness was his primary deficit. Speech naturalness ratings continued to improve. Participant 5 reported that his speech had improved if he took the time to think about the techniques before he spoke. His spouse, who did not actively participate in the group program, reported no change in her partner's speech

Table 7. Data for Participant 5

Background information
Age:	70 years
Gender:	Male
Marital status:	Married
Residence:	Home
Employment:	Semiretired business owner
Years postonset:	3
Hoehn & Yahr stage:	2.5
Participant hearing:	PTA[a]: left = 35.0 dB, right = 37.5 dB
Spouse hearing:	PTA: left = 26.3 dB, right = 18.8 dB

Speech

	Intelligibility (%)	CAIDS rate (wpm)	Naturalness[b]	Tone[c]	Pitch[c]	Loudness[c]
Preintervention	96.1	190.2	3.0	2.3	2.3	2.0
Immediately after	95.5	182.6	2.4	2.0	2.3	1.3
5 months after	97.6	161.2	2.0	1.0	2.3	1.0
10 months after	NA	NA	NA	NA	NA	NA

[a]Pure tone average.
[b]7-point scale (1 = normal).
[c]5-point scale (1 = normal).

outside of treatment. She reported that she needed to "prod" the participant to remember to project his voice. This participant was unavailable for testing at the 10-month interval.

Participant 5 indicated that most communication situations were less difficult following treatment except when he was placed under time pressure (Figure 4). He reported an increased use of the communication strategies of improved speech production, message modification, and partner instruction. He noted that others were less solicitous but much more punishing. This participant remained frustrated by his inability to perceive that he talked with inadequate loudness in some situations. His spouse reported that she has noted an increased awareness of his speech deficits in this participant rather than his placing the blame on her for not listening.

Participant 6

Participant 6 was a 57-year-old man who had been diagnosed 15 years ago. The severity of his PD was judged to be Stage 2.0 (Hoehn & Yahr,

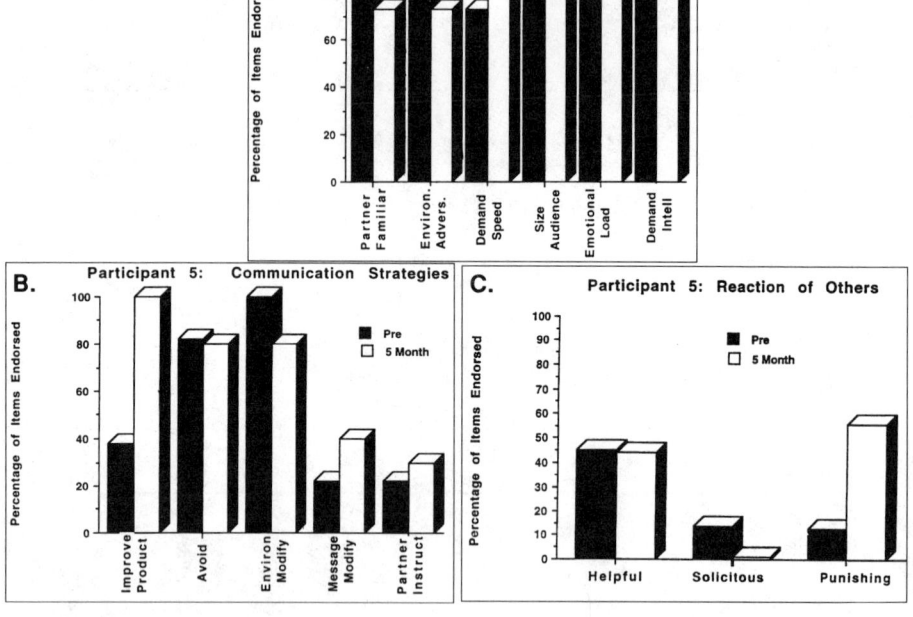

Figure 4. Results from the communication questionnaire before treatment and 5 months after treatment for Participant 5.

1967) and remained at this level through the study. This participant complained of rigidity. His speech was characterized by rapid rushes of speech and dysfluency. His primary complaint was the lack of fluency. The primary goal for this participant was decreased rate. His spouse participated in a few of the treatment sessions.

Changes in Speech Performance All pre- and posttreatment measures for Participant 6 are summarized in Table 8. Intelligibility was high before treatment (97.7%) and remained high after treatment (98.2%). Habitual rate decreased from 208.9 to 178 wpm immediately after treatment.

Improvements in perceptual measures were observed. Vocal tone and pitch were all judged to improve immediately after treatment. Unlike all of the other participants, speech naturalness was judged to be less natural immediately after treatment (pre = 2, post = 2.4).

Evidence of Maintenance of Speech Changes At the 5- and 10-month intervals, Participant 6 improved or maintained posttreatment scores on all of the measures except rate, which was the primary goal of treatment. The participant reported, however, that he is able to control his rate and fluency if he concentrates hard enough. Participant 6 also brought a speech to practice in front of the group. His spouse reported little change in his speech in the home environment. Both thought that individual therapy might have been a better form of treatment for him. The participant

Table 8. Data for Participant 6

Background information
- Age: 57 years
- Gender: Male
- Marital status: Married
- Residence: Home
- Employment: Tax insurance consultant
- Years postonset: 14
- Hoehn & Yahr stage: 2.0
- Participant hearing: PTA[a]: left = 17.5 dB, right = 11.3 dB
- Spouse hearing: PTA: left = 11.3 dB, right = 5.0 dB

Speech

	Intelligibility (%)	CAIDS rate (wpm)	Naturalness[b]	Tone[c]	Pitch[c]	Loudness[c]
Preintervention	97.7	208.9	2.0	1.6	1.3	1.0
Immediately after	98.2	178.0	2.4	1.3	1.6	1.0
5 months after	98.8	199.1	2.0	1.0	1.0	1.0
10 months after	97.4	211.5	1.3	1.0	1.0	1.0

[a]Pure tone average.
[b]7-point scale (1 = normal).
[c]5-point scale (1 = normal).

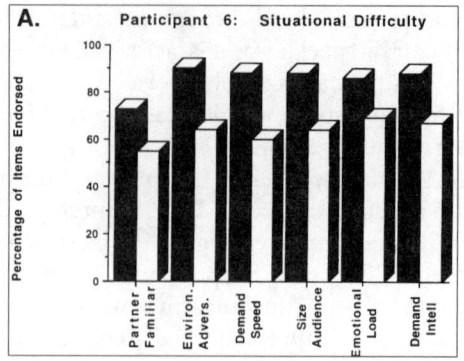
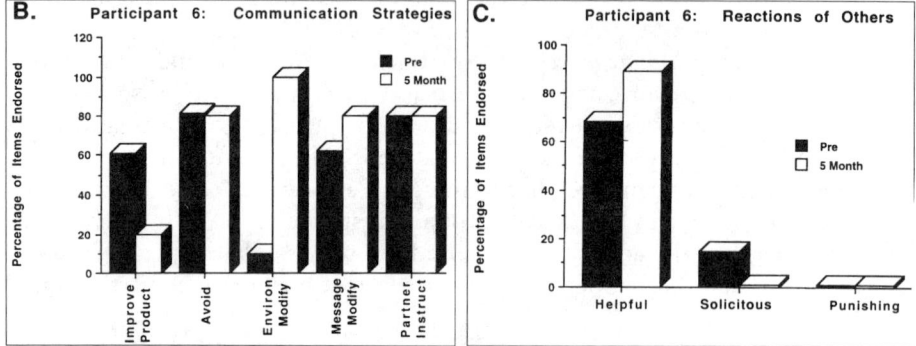

Figure 5. Results from the communication questionnaire before treatment and 5 months after treatment for Participant 6.

expressed pride in his speech and had difficulty relating to other members of the group as peers.

Participant 6 reported that all communication situations were less difficult for him following treatment (Figure 5). He reported no increased use of communication strategies but found others to be more helpful than prior to treatment. Both he and his wife reported a need for him to continue to work on rate control following treatment.

Summary of Spouse and Participant Interviews

The group speech intervention experience received a generally positive review from the participants and their spouses. All of the individuals with PD participated actively in intervention activities. Five of the six participants reported that they enjoyed their involvement in the group and felt accepted as a member of the group. However, Participant 6 frequently commented to project staff that he was not comfortable as a peer with the other participants because he viewed himself as less disabled than they were. All participants expressed the need for ongoing activities to maintain their speech performance.

Four of the spouses participated in all of the sessions. One attended about half of the sessions, and one spouse did not attend any of the sessions beyond the initial assessment. Generally, the spouses who participated in all of the treatment sessions identified more generalized improvement in their partners' speech and actively attempted to assist their partners to maintain the speech performance across settings. Spouses who did not attend or attended infrequently noted little change in their partner's speech.

DISCUSSION

Group Dynamics

As this group intervention progressed, the authors became aware of the importance of group dynamics among the participants and their spouses. With minimal encouragement, participants commented frequently regarding the speech performance of their peers. These evaluations were both positive and negative; however, the evaluations from peers tended to be honest and straightforward. Participants 1 and 5 frequently commented that they were unaware of the extent of their speech disorders and therefore were surprised at the feedback from other members of the group. Rarely did a participant discount or disagree with peer observations, even though their spouses reported frequent disagreement with spouse observations outside of the intervention context.

As the intervention progressed, some participants and their spouses shared strategies with their peers that they had found useful to improve speaking effectiveness. They were most insistent that persons with PD establish daily routines that encourage them to practice effective speaking techniques. Some of the participants developed practice materials and strategies and shared them with the group. They encouraged their peers to think of themselves as *public* speakers rather than *regular* speakers as a way of reminding themselves to utilize speech enhancement strategies. Some participants were able to monitor the effectiveness of their speech performance in a context and adopt the "public speaker" strategy when they considered it useful. Others monitored their speech performance less effectively and were instructed to utilize the strategies in all contexts. Spouses were recruited to remind and encourage the use of the strategies by those participants who monitored their speech less effectively.

Intervention Effectiveness

This clinical research effort addressed the issue of treatment effectiveness for persons with PD. The evaluation of intervention effectiveness for persons with communication disorders has always been difficult, and it is even more so for persons with progressive neurologic diseases. How does one determine the impact of an intervention when disease processes impair the neuromotor basis for speech in a progressive pattern? Obviously, improvement in speech performance by speakers with a progressive neurologic disease in response to an intervention protocol might be viewed as efficacious, if there is no reason to assume there has been a concomitant improvement of the neuromotor impairment. In the face of a progressive condition, such as PD, one would not expect a spontaneous improvement in the underlying impairment.

Following this line of reasoning, a review of the results of the current study reveals that five of the six participants improved their speech performance and maintained improvements for up to 10 months after treatment. Therefore, the authors suggest that the performance of five of the six participants is supportive of the effectiveness of this group speech intervention, while reminding the reader of the contextual constraints of this study. Although speech measures were taken over a number of months, all measures were taken in the clinical setting. Speech performance in other settings was not assessed; therefore, no claims regarding generalization can be made, except for reports of family members and clinician observations at PD support group meetings. Closer inspection of the data reveals that the maintenance of speech rate reductions measured in the immediate postintervention assessments was not maintained as successfully as improvements in other speech parameters.

Participant 6, who maintained few of his speech improvements achieved in treatment, demonstrated primarily a rate control problem. As his habitual speaking rate increased over the months following group intervention, many of his gains were lost. Parenthetically, he was the individual who complained about his involvement with other members of the group because he viewed them as more disabled. One might attempt to make the case that maintaining speech performance at a stable level in the presence of a degenerative disease is also evidence of efficacious intervention. The authors would argue that stable performance cannot be judged as an efficacious result of speech intervention unless there is documented evidence that the neuromotor impairment of the speech mechanism became more extensive during the course of the study. This investigation was not designed to collect such data.

REFERENCES

Barlow, S.M. (1989). A high-speed data acquisition system for clinical speech physiology. In E. Editor (Ed.), *Recent advances in clinical dysarthria* (pp. 39–52). Boston: College-Hill Press.

Darley, F., Aronson, A., & Brown, J. (1975). *Motor speech disorders.* Philadelphia: W.B. Saunders.

Downie, A.W., Low, J.M., & Lindsay, D.D. (1981). Speech disorders in parkinsonism: Usefulness of delayed auditory feedback in selected cases. *British Journal of Disorders of Communication, 16,* 135–139.

Hanson, W., & Metter, E. (1983). DAF speech rate modification in Parkinson's disease: A report of two cases. In W. Berry (Ed.), *Clinical dysarthria* (pp. 321–351). Austin, TX: PRO-ED.

Hanson, W., Metter, E., & Riege, W.H. (1984). *Acoustic variability of hypokinetic dysarthria in Parkinson's disease.* Paper presented at the Annual Convention of the American Speech-Language-Hearing Association, San Francisco, CA.

Hoehn, M.M., & Yahr, M.D. (1967). Parkinsonism: Onset, progression and mortality. *Neurology, 17,* 427–442.

Hull, J.T. (1970). The prevalence and incidence of Parkinson's disease. *Geriatrics, 25,* 128–133.

Johnson, J.A., & Pring, T.R. (1990). Speech therapy and Parkinson's disease: A review and further data. *British Journal of Disorders of Communication, 25,* 183–194.

LeDorze, G., Dionne, L., Ryalls, J., Julien, M., & Ouellet, L. (1992). The effects of speech and language therapy for a case of dysarthria associated with Parkinson's disease. *European Journal of Disorders of Communication, 27,* 313–324.

Logemann, J.A., Fisher, H.B., Boshes, B., & Blonsky, E.R. (1978). Frequency and occurrence of vocal tract dysfunctions in the speech of a large sample of Parkinson's patients. *Journal of Speech and Hearing Disorders, 20,* 58–64.

Ramig, L., Horri, Y., & Bonitati, C. (1991, June). *The efficacy of voice therapy for patients with Parkinson's disease.* NCVS Status & Progress Report (pp. 61–86). Boulder: University of Colorado.

Robertson, S., & Thomson, F. (1984). Speech therapy in Parkinson's disease: A study of the efficacy and long term effectiveness of intensive treatment. *British Journal of Disorders of Communication, 19,* 213–224.

Sarno, M.T. (1968). Speech impairment in Parkinson's disease. *Archives of Physical Medicine and Rehabilitation, 49,* 269–275.

Scott, S., & Caird, F. (1983). Speech therapy for Parkinson's disease. *Journal of Neurology, Neurosurgery, and Psychiatry, 46,* 140–144.

Smitheran, J., & Hixon, T. (1981). A clinical method for estimating laryngeal airway resistance during vowel production. *Journal of Speech and Hearing Disorders, 46,* 138–146.

Solomon, N., & Hixon, T.J. (1993). Speech breathing in Parkinson's disease. *Journal of Speech and Hearing Research, 36,* 294–310.

Yorkston, K.M., Beukelman, D.R., & Traynor, C. (1984). *Computerized Assessment of Intelligibility of Dysarthric Speech* [Computer program]. Tigard, OR: C.C. Publications.

Yorkston, K.M., Bombardier, C., & Hammen, V. (1992). *The Communication Profile for Speakers with Motor Speech Disorders.* Unpublished questionnaire, University of Washington, Seattle.

Yorkston, K.M., Hammen, V., Beukelman, D.R., & Traynor, C. (1990). The effect of rate control on the intelligibility and naturalness of dysarthric speakers. *Journal of Speech and Hearing Disorders, 55,* 550–559.

SECTION VIII

SPASMODIC DYSPHONIA, INSPIRATORY AIRWAY COMPROMISE, AND APRAXIA OF SPEECH

Chapter 18

Abductor Spasmodic Dysphonia
Acoustic Influence of Voicing on Connected Speech

Michael P. Cannito,
Laura S. McSwain, and James P. Dworkin

SPASMODIC DYSPHONIA (SD) may be characterized by intermittently strained–strangled voice (adductor), intermittently breathy voice (abductor), or mixed forms of these primary types (Aronson, 1973; Cannito & Johnson, 1981; Wolfe & Bacon, 1976). Adductor spasmodic dysphonia (ADSD) occurs more frequently, and abductor spasmodic dysphonia (ABSD) tends to be more resistive to treatment (Blitzer & Brin, 1992b; Ford, Bless, & Patel, 1992). Each form, however, is currently viewed by many clinical researchers to be of neurologic origin—sequelae of focal laryngeal dystonia or essential tremor (Aronson & Hartman, 1981; Blitzer & Brin, 1992a, 1992b; Cannito, 1989; Hartman & Aronson, 1981; Rosenfield, 1988; Schaefer, 1983). Psychogenic and idiopathic etiologies are also espoused by some (Aronson, 1990; Cannito, 1991a; Watterson & McFarlane, 1992). Perceptually, ABSD patients generally exhibit intermittent breathiness and arrests of phonation, and voice improves on prolongation of vowels in comparison to ongoing speech. Breathy moments occur in the initial, medial, or final word positions and on words produced in succession and are perceived to occur more frequently in association with voiceless rather than voiced consonant production (Hartman & Aronson, 1981; Izdebski, Shipp, & Dedo, 1989).

In an ongoing effort to more objectively characterize and quantify the distinctive diagnostic features of ABSD, researchers have turned increasingly to acoustic analyses of various types. Although several papers have been published about the characteristics of ABSD, the total number of patients studied remains relatively small, and only limited acoustic data have been reported (see Table 1). For example, Hartman and Aronson (1981) acoustically analyzed sustained vowel productions of 17 ABSD subjects, but connected speech analysis was limited to subjective clinical impressions. Furthermore, acoustic studies have tended to utilize very small control samples or none at all, acoustic analysis procedures varied greatly across investigations, and in many cases acoustic data were not analyzed statistically (Freeman, Cannito & Finitzo-Hieber, 1985; Rontal et. al., 1991; Zwitman, 1979), presumably as a consequence of the small sample sizes involved.

Acoustic characteristics of connected speech, other than intermittent breathiness (Wolfe & Bacon, 1976), that have been reported for ABSD include

- Abnormal fundamental frequency (F_0) or abnormal F_0 fluctuations (Ludlow, Naunton, Terada, & Anderson, 1991; Merson & Ginsberg, 1979; Rontal et al., 1991)
- Abnormally prolonged voice onset time (VOT) for voiceless stop consonants (Freeman et al., 1985; Zwitman, 1979)
- Abnormally prolonged word and sentence durations (Ludlow et al., 1991; Merson & Ginsberg, 1979)

Despite some consistency of observations across earlier reports, different researchers have examined different speech parameters using a variety of acoustic analysis techniques and (with the exception of Ludlow et al., 1991) have included very small numbers of ABSD subects with limited comparative data from appropriate samples of matched normal controls. It is therefore unclear to what extent these speech characteristics may be generalizable to the ABSD population, or whether some acoustic "abnormalities" that have been reported do in fact differ statistically from the range of normal speaking variation.

An adequate understanding of the nature of ABSD requires further acoustic analyses over a range of phonetic variables to evaluate their occurrence across grouped ABSD subjects in comparison with age- and gender-matched nondysphonic normal controls. In addition, despite some evidence of phonetically mediated voicing constraints on spasm elicitation (i.e., greater frequency with voiceless consonant material and lesser frequency on sustained phonation) (Hartman & Aronson, 1981), systematic acoustic studies of the response of ABSD speakers to experimental manipulation of laryngeal coordinative requirements for speech production have not been previously reported. In addition, further decomposition of relatively global acoustic variables is needed. For example, it is not known whether voice pitch seems more variable in ABSD because it fluctuates

Table 1. Review of 20 years of ABSD speech research

Author(s) (year)	N	Speech sample	Measurements	Results
Aronson (1973)	9 AB	Conversational speech	Perceptual voice symptoms	Identified ABSD patients as having abrupt moments of aphonia or breathy dysphonia resulting from a sudden widening of the glottis
Wolfe & Bacon (1976)	2: 1 AB 1 AD	"Rainbow Passage"	Spectrographic description (frequency, intensity, time); voice quality	Data indicated that there are two types of SD. ADSD patient had spectrographic characteristics of irregular vertical striations. ABSD patient exhibited a breakdown in the formant structures, with reduced intensity and turbulence noise.
Zwitman (1979)	3: 2 AB 1 CS	Connected speech; phonetically controlled test sentences (voiced versus voiceless stops)	Spectrographic description; aspiration time; VOT; voice quality	Diagnosed the ABSD speech characteristics as 1) loudness impairment, 2) pitch does not change but the voice is breathier, 3) intermittent phonation, and 4) alteration of voiced/voiceless pattern. Prolonged VOT between the initial consonant and subsequent vowel was the main identifying characteristic.
Merson & Ginsberg (1979)	3: 2 AB 1 CS	Sustained vowel /a/; connected speech; phonetically controlled sentence (all vocalic)	Fundamental frequency (mean, standard deviation); sentence duration; airflow rates	ABSD patients exhibited intermittent breathiness, high airflow rates, drops in pitch, and vowel prolongations without strain–strangle phonation.
Cannito & Johnson (1981)	1 MX	Spontaneous speech; yawn-sigh; sustained vowel /a/	Spectrographic description; speech rate; percent normal; breathy and harsh phonemes	Patient exhibited mixed symptoms of breathiness, strain-strangle, hard glottal attack, and prolonged phoneme durations. Proposed that SD lies on a continuum from breathiness to harshness, rather than being amenable to strict categorization.

(continued)

Table 1. (continued)

Author(s) (year)	N	Speech sample	Measurements	Results
Hartman & Aronson (1981)	17 AB	"Grandfather Passage"; sustained vowel /a/	Vocal amplitude variations for sustained vowel; perceptual analysis of connected speech	Intermittent breathiness showed variability across all conditions. Four variants in voice symptoms were identified, indicating differences between patients. Neurogenic and psychogenic causes of ABSD were evident, indicating that ABSD may not be a single entity.
Freeman, Cannito, & Finitzo-Hieber (1985)	2: 1 AB 1 AD	Sustained vowel /a/; singing; nonspeech vocalizations; phonetically controlled sentences (voiced vs. voiceless consonants)	Spectrographic description (frequency, intensity, time); fundamental frequency variation; segment duration; voice quality	"ABSD with voice tremor" was classified with voice stoppages during speech, occasional good voice, improvement for singing and nonspeech vocalization, intermittent breathiness, intermittent harshness, vocal tremor, prolonged phoneme durations, and voicing errors on voiced and voiceless consonants. Idiopathic ADSD patient exhibited similar vocal symptoms, except with greater predominance of harshness.
Cannito (1989)	36: 18 CS 4 AB 6 AD 8 MX	Sustained vowels produced using an electro-larynx	LPC analysis of variability of the second formant frequency	ABSD, ADSD, and mixed SD subjects all differed significantly from matched control subjects; however, increased variability was based on subjects of the positive tremor category under all three spasm classifications.
Watson et al. (1991)	5: 3 AB 2 AD	Valsalva; sustained vowel /i/; sustained vowel /s/; inhalation against oral resistance	EMG for TA; EMG for PCA	SD subjects had abnormal laryngeal activity when compared to control subjects. TA and PCA activity failed to distinguish between ADSD and ABSD subtypes.

(continued)

Table 1. *(continued)*

Author(s) (year)	N	Speech sample	Measurements	Results
Ludlow, Naunton, Terada, & Anderson (1991)	20: 10 AB 10 CS	Three test sentences (voiceless stops plus fricatives)	EMG for CT before BOTOX; sentence duration; periodic phonation; voice offset time	Pre-BOTOX ABSD speech characteristics were prolonged voiceless consonants, pitch breaks, longer sentence durations, and less proportion of periodic phonation. Post-BOTOX, only sentence duration improved.
Rontal et al., (1991)	6 AB	Spontaneous speech; "Rainbow Passage"; sustained phonation	Spectrographic description; fundamental frequency; perturbation; pitch shifts; syllable durations	Pre-BOTOX ABSD speech characteristics were sudden aphonic episodes, sharp pitch shifts, and syllable prolongations. Post-BOTOX measures indicated reduced perturbation and eliminated ABSD spasms.
Cannito, Ege, Ahmed, & Wagner (1993)	15: 5 AB 5 AD 5 CS	Duration of trisyllables /tukipa/ and /dugiba/; whispered vs. phonated	Interval length between repetitive trisyllable productions	ABSD and ADSD productions had longer and more variable trisyllable durations than the control productions, but only ADSD productions exhibited longer intertrisyllable intervals.

Note: AB, abductor SD subjects; AD, adductor SD subjects; BOTOX, botulinun toxins; CT, cricothyroid muscle; EMG, electromyogram; MX, mixed ADSD and ABSD subjects; CS, normal control subjects; PCA, posterior cricoarytenoid muscle; TA, thyroarytenoid muscle.

more broadly or because it is generally of greater frequency than that of normal speakers. Thus, quantitative measures of average fundamental frequency as well as fundamental frequency variability are presently of interest. Similarly, increased sentence durations reported in ABSD subjects (Ludlow et al., 1991) may be attributable to increases in voiceless consonant duration alone, to an overall decrease in articulation rate, or to more frequent pausing. Finally, the effects of ABSD on subtle acoustic–phonetic variations related to consonant voicing have not been previously explored. These include 1) progressive lengthening of VOT as a function of posterior stop consonant placement (Klatt, 1975; Lisker & Abramson, 1967) and 2) production of greater and more variable F_0 values in vowels following voiceless stop consonants (House & Fairbanks, 1953; Ohde, 1984; Silverman, 1986; Umeda, 1981). Given that ABSD remains controversial and poorly understood, as well as persistently resistant to treatment, additional quantitative information may help elucidate the mechanisms underlying this unusual disorder. It may also have relevance for the identification of diagnostic subgroups within the ABSD population and eventual development of empirically guided behavioral or medical treatment protocols.

The purpose of this study, therefore, was to examine the acoustic characteristics of F_0, VOT, and sentence level duration measurements of ABSD and normal speech in phonetically controlled sentence environments. Specifically, sentences containing all voiced and all voiceless consonants were compared. It was hypothesized that contrastive voicing conditions, which systematically varied laryngeal coordinative demands, would yield differential patterns of performance on the part of ABSD subjects in comparison to control subjects without ABSD. In addition, the potential influence of ABSD on subtle, secondary phonetic cues to consonant place and voicing, which are normally mediated by VOT and F_0, was examined.

METHODOLOGY

Subjects

Ten patients with established diagnoses of ABSD and 10 nondysphonic control (NC) subjects without other disabilities were matched by age and gender. Diagnoses were originally accomplished by consensus of two speech-language pathologists and an otolaryngologist who were familiar with the disorder, in accordance with accepted clinical criteria (Aronson, 1990; Freeman et al., 1985). Each ABSD subject underwent fiberoptic endoscopy as well as a comprehensive speech/voice assessment protocol described in Cannito (1991a). Criteria for inclusion in the patient group were 1) occasional moments of normal-sounding voice, 2) presence of intermittent cessation of phonation during the production of vowels and vowellike speech sounds, 3) frequent intermittent breathy dysphonia, 4) infrequent or no occurrence of strain–strangle dysphonia, 5) absence of perceptual symptoms of the dysarthrias, 6) normal- or near-normal-sounding whispered speech, 7) improved voice quality for nonspeech vocalizations, 8) improved voice quality for phonation at high pitch levels, and 9) reported worsening of dysphonia with increased situational stress. The presence/absence of audible voice tremor was noted but was not considered an exclusionary criterion. Subjects were free of history of psychiatric, neurologic, and communicative disorders other than ABSD. Clinical characteristics of the ABSD subjects are provided in Table 2.

Procedures

High-quality audiotape recordings were obtained of each subject reading the phonetically controlled sentences 1) "Pick up a tasty cake" (voiceless consonant condition), and 2) "Good dogs beg in bed" (voiced consonant condition). Recordings were obtained in a sound-isolated booth with the

Table 2. ABSD subject characteristics

Subject	Gender	Age	Severity[a]	Tremor[a]
1	Female	58	Mild	No
2	Male	50	Severe	Yes
3	Male	52	Severe	No
4	Female	42	Moderate	No
5	Female	42	Severe	Yes
6	Male	29	Moderate	Yes
7	Female	28	Moderate	No
8	Female	47	Moderate	Yes
9	Female	46	Mild	Yes
10	Female	37	Moderate	Yes

[a]Clinical subclassifications were determined by consensus of two certified speech-language pathologists experienced in assessment of spasmodic dysphonia. Severity refers to the clinicians' impression of the severity of dysphonia during oral reading of a standard passage. Tremor refers to the presence/absence of audible voice tremor on sustained phonation.

microphone positioned below the breathstream approximately 10 cm from the subject's mouth. Each sentence was produced twice by each subject. The subjects were instructed to use their usual speaking voice and to try to avoid any compensatory strategies they may have acquired. Both trials of each sentence production were included in the data analyses in order to increase the overall reliability of the findings.

Speech signals were converted from analog to digital using a 10-kHz sampling frequency (with low-pass filtering at 5 kHz) and analyzed using the Kay Elemetrics Computer Speech Laboratory (CSL). Temporal cursor measurements were accomplished using a combination of repeated listening to digitized signal segments (digital-to-analog converted) and visual inspection of waveform and spectrographic displays on the computer monitor. All temporal measures were to the nearest millisecond. F_0 analyses employed CSL's automated pitch extraction subroutines ("CSL Computerized Speech Lab," 1992), which included a peak-picking algorithm that identifies all "positive-going zero crossings that precede the first positive-going amplitude peaks of the voice impulses" in the waveform (p. 199). These locations were then marked, with the distance between adjacent voice impulse marks representing the fundamental periods. F_0 was calculated by taking the reciprocal of each period and was rounded to the nearest Hertz.

Acoustic–phonetic measurements included

- *Average F_0* (arithmetic mean) in Hertz—computed from the first to the last identifiable "pitch periods" within each sentence production
- *F_0 variability* (standard deviation) in Hertz—an index of the degree of variation of the fundamental frequency around its mean (average F_0, above) for each sentence production

- *VOT* for word–initial stop consonants /p,t,k,b,d,g/—measured in milliseconds from the release of the initial stop burst (abrupt onset of aperiodic noise) to the first identifiable occurrence of quasiperiodic glottal pulsing. This was done for each sentence production
- *Sentence pause time*—the duration in seconds (to the nearest millisecond) of the sum of all silent intervals occurring between words that exceeded 10 ms in duration (Picheny, Durlach, & Braida, 1986). This measurement was computed for each sentence production
- *Sentence articulation time*—the duration in seconds (to the nearest millisecond) of each sentence production, measured from onset of aperiodic noise of the initial consonant of the first word to offset of aperiodic noise of the final consonant of the last word within each sentence, minus the sentence pause time. This measurement was computed for each sentence production

Statistical Analysis

Because the research design included five voicing-related dependent variables, a multivariate statistical model was selected to examine the overall significance of the effects of subject groups (NC vs. ABSD), consonant voicing conditions (voiced vs. voiceless), and trials (first vs. second), as well as the Subject Groups × Voicing Condition interaction. The variable of gender was also included in the model as a covariate to control for the potentially confounding influence of male–female differences in laryngeal structure and function (Titize, 1989) on the voicing measures. Thus, a three-way multivariate analysis of covariance (MANCOVA) with repeated measures was employed (Morrison, 1976). Given multivariate significance, univariate multifactorial analysis of covariance (ANCOVA) was used to evaluate the patterning of significance for the individual variables (Neter & Wasserman, 1974).

Reliability

Interexaminer reliability coefficients (Pearson product-moment correlations) for acoustic variables ranged from $r = .898$ (F_0 variability) to $r = .998$ (VOT) for a random sample of 20% of the ABSD and NC data. This was considered to achieve an acceptable level of measurement consistency to permit further statistical analysis of the overall data set.

RESULTS

Descriptive statistics for the acoustic measurements are presented in Table 3. Results of the MANCOVA procedure indicated that there were significant overall effects of the covariate of gender (Wilkes lambda = .241, $F_{5,70}$

Table 3. Acoustic measures of connected speech: means and standard deviations (in parentheses)

Variable	Group[a]	Voiced[b]	Voiceless[b]
Average F_0 (Hz)	ABSD	159 (24)	171 (22)
	CS	148 (36)	153 (31)
F_0 (Hz) variability	ABSD	25 (11)	30 (09)
	CS	26 (07)	33 (12)
Voice onset time[c] (ms)	ABSD	22 (16)	127 (131)
	CS	16 (06)	54 (16)
Articulation time (ms)	ABSD	1,804 (198)	1,719 (326)
	CS	1,600 (235)	1,366 (220)
Pause time (ms)	ABSD	310 (301)	343 (326)
	CS	314 (205)	166 (110)

[a]ABSD, abductor spasmodic dysphonia subjects ($n = 10$); CS, control subjects ($n = 10$).
[b]Consonant voicing classifications for sentence environments.
[c]Averaged across places of articulation.

$= 44.187, p = .0001$). With gender held constant, overall statistical significance was observed for the main effects of subject groups (Wilkes lambda $= .597$, $F_{5,70} = 9.436$, $p = .0001$) and consonant voicing conditions (Wilkes lambda $= .531$, $F_{5,70} = 12.350$, $p = .0001$). The effect of trials was not significant (Wilkes lambda $= .960$, $F_{5,70} = .582, p = .7138$). There was also a significant overall interaction of Subject Groups × Voicing Conditions for the multivariate data set (Wilkes lambda $= .840$, $F_{5,70} = 2.500$, $p = .0385$). Trials did not interact significantly with any other variable.

To further explore the patterns of significance associated with the individual variables, five univariate multifactorial ANCOVAs (Subject Groups × Voicing Conditions × Trials) were computed. These analyses yielded the following results.

Fundamental Frequency Analysis

A three-way, repeated-measures ANCOVA was computed for average F_0. ABSD subjects had significantly greater average F_0 than controls ($F_{1,74} = 13.854$, $p < .0004$), and voiceless consonant sentences employed significantly greater average F_0 than voiced consonant sentences ($F_{1,74} = 5.605$, $p = .0205$), irrespective of subject group. The covariate gender was significantly related to average F_0 ($F_{1,74} = 217.000$, $p = .0001$). No other effects or interactions attained statistical significance. A three-way repeated measures ANCOVA computed for F_0 variability indicated that voiceless consonant sentences evidenced greater variability than voiced consonant sentences ($F_{1,74} = 7.537$, $p = .0076$), irrespective of subject group. The covariate gender was also significantly related to F_0 variability ($F_{1,74} = 4.189$, $p = .0442$). No other effects or interactions attained statistical significance.

VOT Analysis

A three-way repeated-measures ANCOVA was computed for VOT. ABSD subjects exhibited significantly longer VOTs than did control subjects ($F_{1,74} = 10.207, p = .0021$), and voiceless VOTs were longer than voiced VOTs ($F_{1,74} = 33.859, p = .0001$). There was also a significant interaction of Subject Group × Voicing Conditions ($F_{1,74} = 7.596, p = .0074$), wherein the ABSD subjects differed significantly from control subjects only in the voiceless consonant condition. Figure 1 illustrates the highly similar mean VOT values exhibited by the subject groups for voiced stop consonant productions, in contrast to the significant lengthening of VOT values exhibited by the ABSD group in comparison to the control subjects for voiceless stop consonant productions. No other effects or interactions attained statistical significance.

In order to evaluate the effects of articulator placement on VOT, a treatment of relevance only to this variable, an additional analysis was computed in which place of articulation (bilabial, alveolar, velar) was included in the model as a fourth dependent variable. Results demonstrated that the progressive lengthening of VOT across bilabial, alveolar, and velar placements was statistically significant ($F_{2,144} = 12.183, p = .0001$), irrespective of subject group. This phenomenon is illustrated in Figure 2. It is evident that, although ABSD subjects exhibited generally longer VOTs than the control subjects, a consistent increase of VOT across stop consonant placements from bilabial to velar was maintained by both the NC and ABSD groups.

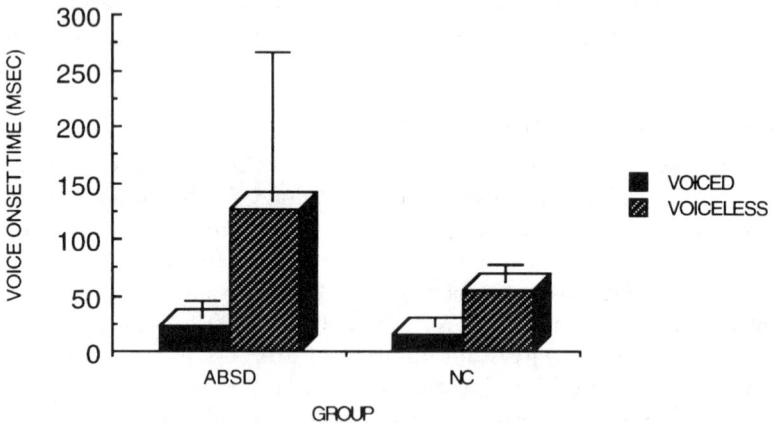

Figure 1. Mean VOT by voicing contexts for two subject groups (bars indicate standard deviations). NC = nondysphonic control.

Sentence Pause and Articulation Times

A three-way repeated-measures ANCOVA was computed for sentence pause time. No statistically significant main or interaction effects were observed ($p > .08$). A three-way repeated-measures ANCOVA was also computed for sentence articulation time, which was longer for the ABSD group than for the controls ($F_{1,74} = 22.660, p = .0001$), irrespective of voicing conditions. It was also longer in voiced than in voiceless consonant sentences ($F_{1,74} = 8.119, p = .0057$), irrespective of subject group.

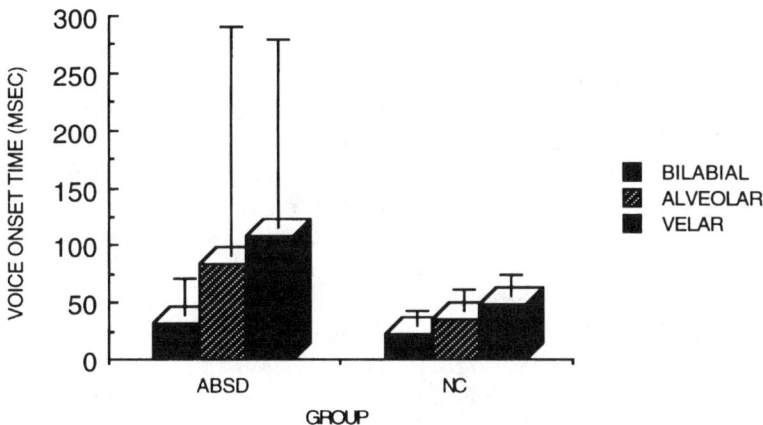

Figure 2. Mean VOT by place of articulation for two subject groups (bars indicate standard deviations). NC = nondysphonic control.

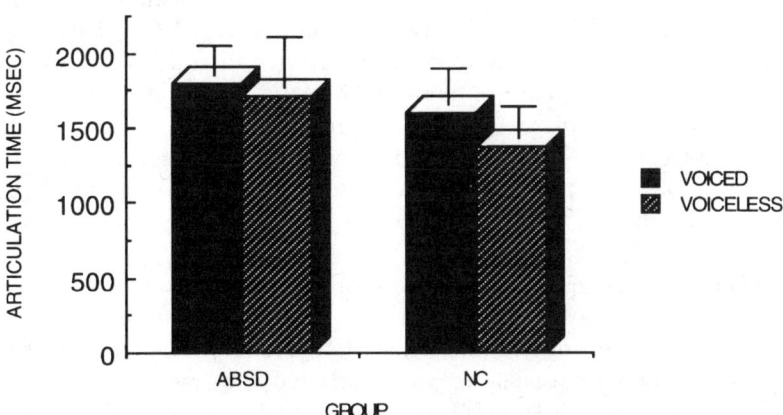

Figure 3. Mean sentence articulation time by voicing contexts for two subject groups (bars indicate standard deviations). NC = nondysphonic control.

Figure 3 depicts these relationships, demonstrating that the ABSD subjects remained generally slower than the controls for both voiced and voiceless consonant sentence productions. No other effects or interactions attained statistical significance.

DISCUSSION

The present findings demonstrate that ABSD subjects differ from control subjects along phonetic characteristics other than "intermittent breathy dysphonia." These dimensions include increased sentence articulation times, prolonged VOTs for voiceless consonants, and elevated average F_0. Increased articulation durations were not restricted to voiceless consonant sentences and, therefore, cannot be explained solely by increased voiceless VOTs. Of interest, despite high levels of symptom variability often attributed to ABSD, the subjects' vocal behaviors were reliable within the context of the experimental session. In no case was a significant effect or interaction involving trials observed for any variable.

Secondary phonetic cues related to voicing remained intact in ABSD subjects, despite significant overall impairments. Specifically, VOT lengthening across posterior consonant placements and elevated average and variability of F_0 in voiceless consonant contexts were preserved. Indeed, these features appeared to have been overlaid on the generally aberrant speaking patterns exhibited by the ABSD group. These unimpaired voicing phenomena may be attributable to biomechanical interactions among articulatory and phonatory mechanisms in normal speakers. Klatt (1975) suggested that decreasing VOTs across posterior-to-anterior consonant placements may be a natural consequence of comparably decreased consonant burst durations across these placements: "If VOT depends on the amount of time available to open the glottis, then the VOT will get shorter as [consonant] closure duration shortens, because the glottis cannot be fully opened before the [consonant] closing command is issued" (p. 701). Klatt (1975) demonstrated that, when VOT is decomposed into burst duration and aspiration time, it is the burst duration and not the aspiration time that varies across articulator placements in speakers without ABSD.

Increased average and variability of F_0 following voiceless consonants, relative to their voiced cognates, has been attributed to both greater vertical and greater longitudinal tension on the larynx as a result of increased suprahyoid muscular activity associated with voiceless consonant articulation (Ohde, 1984). It is hypothesized that this mechanism continues to function in ABSD and is independent of the increased average F_0. Thus, preservation of voicing-related secondary cues in ABSD appears to result from extralaryngeal (i.e., articulatory) as opposed to intralaryngeal factors, further attesting to the focal nature of the disorder (Cannito, 1991b). The present findings did not support previous observations of abnormal pitch fluctuations in ABSD (Ludlow et al., 1991; Rontal et al., 1991). However, it is noteworthy that direct patient-to-normal sample comparisons were not performed specifically regarding pitch fluctuations in the earlier studies.

The pattern of findings obtained in this study appears to be compatible with the interpretation that ABSD is a focal hyperkinetic movement disorder (Blitzer & Brin, 1992a; Karnell, 1992). Watson et al. (1991) have demonstrated generally heightened levels of intrinsic laryngeal muscle electromyographic (EMG) activity in patients with ABSD. Accordingly, increased average F_0 might reflect these heightened levels of muscular activity. Inasmuch as the cricothyroid muscle is a primary determinant of F_0 (Atkinson, 1978), increased EMG activity in that muscle should be associated with elevations of average F_0. Increased cricothyroid muscle EMG activity has been reported in a subset of ABSD patients studied by Ludlow et al. (1991).

In the present sample, between-group differences in average F_0, although statistically significant, remained small, and the group means fell within broad normal limits. Although the variability associated with average F_0 reported in Table 3 appears to be relatively high (e.g., 22–36 Hz), it should be recognized that much of this variation was attributable to gender differences within the subject groups. Employment of a statistical analysis procedure that eliminated the influence of gender (i.e., covariance analysis) considerably reduced this variability and permitted an independent assessment of the between-group difference. The inclusion of gender as a covariate in the statistical design reduced the least squares estimate of the standard deviation for the group effect to 14 Hz, in comparison to a standard deviation of 28 Hz had gender been excluded from the model. Therefore, the actual (i.e., gender-adjusted) mean difference in F_0 between groups was slightly greater than 1 standard deviation.

A neurophysiologic interpretation of this difference, suggesting that increased cricothyroid activity may have yielded increased average F_0, seems plausible. The fact that F_0 for several ABSD subjects fell within 1 standard deviation of the control subjects' mean indicates that significantly increased average F_0 is exhibited only by a subset of the ABSD subjects. This finding is also consistent with Ludlow et al.'s (1991) observation that some ABSD subjects did not exhibit increased cricothyroid EMG activity. It is also possible, however, that pitch raising may have been employed as a compensatory speaking strategy by subjects in the ABSD group (Aronson, 1990; Merson & Ginsberg, 1979).

Prolonged overall sentence durations in ABSD also have been previously observed (Ludlow et al., 1991; Merson & Ginsberg, 1979). In the present study this has been shown to be a consequence of reduced articulation rate rather than of increased pause time. Similarly, increased articulation time without increased intersyllabic transition time in ABSD has been reported for rapid alternating speechlike movements (Cannito, Ege, Ahmed, & Wagner, 1993). Prolonged articulation time may be interpreted to reflect either an underlying motoric slowness or compensation for difficulty coordinating laryngeal with articulatory and respiratory activity. The fact that, in the present study, articulation time increased in the absence of increased interword pause time may indicate that the temporal alterations exhibited by the ABSD subjects were not entirely voluntary. For example, in a study in which subjects without disabilities intentionally slowed their speaking rates as if to compensate for listeners who had hearing impairments, both frequency and duration of pauses were substantially increased, in addition to articulation time being prolonged (Picheny et al., 1986). Longer articulation time in all voiced than in all voiceless consonant sentences, seen in both subject groups, was probably due to phonologically conditioned lengthening of vowels preceding syllable-final voiced stops in English (House & Fairbanks, 1953; Ladefoged, 1993).

Prolonged voiceless VOTs have also been reported in ABSD (Freeman et al., 1985; Zwitman, 1979) and may be a specific instance of the generally prolonged voiceless consonant length observed by Ludlow et al. (1991). An abnormality specific to voiceless (but not voiced) consonants may suggest difficulty with voiceless-to-voiced glottal transitions. Particularly in the intervocalic positions common to connected speech, initial voiceless consonant productions required a complex glottal gesture comprised of an *abduct-and-stiffen* component timed to precede the stop closure as well as an *adduct-and-relax* component following the stop release, whereas for the voiced consonants subjects could simply maintain the vocal folds in an "approximated and slack" state throughout the closure (Klatt, 1975).

Additional evidence that the voiceless-to-voiced transition is the locus of the spasm-triggering mechanism (as opposed to "voicelessness" per se) derives from the relatively small difference between subject groups for VOTs in the bilabial context (see Figure 3). The voiceless bilabial occurred in sentence-initial position in the word "pick." Because /p/ was not preceded by a voiced sound, the required laryngeal adduction gesture may have been less complex (i.e., the abduct-and-stiffen component was unnecessary). Production may also have been facilitated by the fact that, in this position, the word received a reduced level of stress, allowing for production of weakly aspirated or unaspirated stops, which were evident in the spectrograms of both the control and ABSD subjects. The fact that ABSD performance becomes more similar to that of normal speakers under circumstances in which the need for rapid glottal adjustments is minimized (e.g., sustained vowels) suggests that laryngeal timing and coordination difficulty may be integral components of this disorder. The present observation of normal VOTs in all-voiced environments is consistent with this view.

It should be acknowledged that, in themselves, the present data may not clearly differentiate between neurogenic and psychogenic interpretations of the etiology of ABSD. It is known that fundamental frequency may increase as a function of situationally induced emotional stress (Hecker, Stevens, von Bismark, & Williams, 1968; Streeter, Macdonald, Apple, Krauss, & Galotti, 1983; Williams & Stevens, 1972). It is also known that clinically depressed patients speak with abnormally slow speaking rates (Godfrey & Knight, 1984; Greden, Albala, Smokler, Gardner, & Carroll, 1981). Given that clinically significant elevations of anxiety and depression are not uncommon among SD patients exhibiting either abductor or adductor type symptomatology (Cannito, 1991a), findings of elevated F_0 and reduced speaking rate may also be compatible with a psychogenic model. However, comparison of the present findings with existing literature reveals that ABSD speech is not a good fit of speech produced by depressed or anxious individuals. Although depressed patients slow their speaking rate, they do so by increasing interword pause time without increasing actual speaking time (Greden et al., 1981). This pattern is precisely opposite that exhibited by the ABSD subjects in the present study. In contrast to depressed patients, individuals with anxiety disorders tend to increase rather than decrease their speaking rate (Pope, Blass, Siegman, & Raher, 1970). In addition, studies of individuals speaking under conditions of situationally induced stress often exhibit increased F_0 variability in association with either elevated or decreased average F_0 (Hecker et al., 1968; Streeter et al., 1983; Williams & Stevens, 1972). Although Hecker et al. (1968) described "devoicing and aspiration" of "certain portions of speech" along with other indications of "inadequate control of the laryngeal musculature" when the speaker is stressed (p. 999), it remains difficult to envision an affective disorder whose effects on speech would be selective for voiceless consonant environments. Perhaps future comparisons of ABSD speech to that of known affectively disordered subjects may help clarify these concerns. Taken together with earlier literature, the present findings appear to be more consistent with a neurogenic interpretation of the etiology of ABSD. Confirmation of this hypothesis, however, awaits direct simultaneous observation of dynamic myoelectric and kinematic activity in addition to acoustic analysis (see Roark et al., 1990).

Apart from etiologic considerations, acoustic analyses of the type employed in the present study may be useful for identifying diagnostic subtypes of ABSD, in order to better characterize differential patterns of initial impairment and monitor responses to specific treatments. For example, Hartman and Aronson (1981) observed very favorable responses to psychotherapy in one patient and to voice therapy in another out of 17 ABSD patients studied. Although acoustic analyses of sustained phonation did not differentiate the two successfully treated cases from the majority of subjects who remained resistant to therapy, it is possible that acoustic analyses of connected speech may have provided additional information that would have characterized these unusual individuals. Ludlow et al. (1991) employed acoustic analysis to document improvement in 6 of 10 ABSD patients treated by botulinum toxin injection of the cricothyroid muscle. For those who benefited from the treatment, acoustic analysis revealed that, although there was no posttreatment improvement in percentage of periodicity for phonated segments, overall sentence duration and voiceless consonant time did decrease substantially. Not surprisingly, the patients who benefited were also the patients exhibiting cricothyroid muscle abnormalities during the preinjection EMG assessment. Although the present study did not address treatment directly, the findings highlight the utility of acoustic analysis techniques to quantitatively profile relative degrees of impairment versus nonimpairment of a variety of voicing-related variables in ABSD connected speech. Measurements of this type may provide a useful basis for future pre- to post-treatment comparisons.

REFERENCES

Aronson, A.E. (1973). *Audio seminars in speech pathology—psychogenic voice disorders.* Philadelphia: W.B. Saunders.
Aronson, A.E. (1990). *Clinical voice disorders.* New York: Thieme, Inc.
Aronson, A.E., & Hartman, D.E. (1981). Adductor spastic dysphonia as a sign of essential (voice) tremor. *Journal of Speech and Hearing Disorders, 46,* 52–58.
Atkinson, J.E. (1978). Correlation analysis of the physiological factors controlling fundamental voice frequency. *Journal of the Acoustical Society of America, 63,* 211–222.
Blitzer, A., & Brin, M.F. (1992a). The dystonic larynx. *Journal of Voice, 6,* 294–297.
Blitzer, A., & Brin, M. (1992b). Treatment of spasmodic dysphonia (laryngeal dystonia) with local injections of botulinum toxin. *Journal of Voice, 6,* 365–369.
Cannito, M.P. (1989). Vocal tract steadiness in spasmodic dysphonia. In K.M. Yorkston & D.R. Beukelman (Eds.), *Recent advances in clinical dysarthria* (pp. 243–262). Boston: Little, Brown and Co.
Cannito, M.P. (1991a). Emotional considerations in spasmodic dysphonia psychometric quantification. *Journal of Communication Disorders, 24,* 313–329.
Cannito, M.P. (1991b). Neurobiologic interpretations of spasmodic dysphonia. In D. Vogel & M.P. Cannito (Eds.), *Treating disordered speech motor control* (pp. 275–317). Austin, TX: PRO-ED.
Cannito, M.P., Ege, P., Ahmed, F., & Wagner, S. (1993). Diadochokinesis for complex trisyllables in individuals with spasmodic dysphonia and nondisabled subjects. In J.A. Till, K.M. Yorkston, & D.R. Beukelman (Eds.), *Motor speech*

disorders: Advances in assessment and treatment (pp. 91–100). Baltimore: Paul H. Brookes Publishing Co.

Cannito, M.P., & Johnson, J.P. (1981). Spastic dysphonia: A continuum disorder. *Journal of Communication Disorders, 14*, 215–223.

CSL Computerized Speech Lab: Operations manual. (1992). Pine Brook, NJ: Kay Elemetrics Corporation.

Ford, C.N., Bless, D.M., & Patel, N.Y. (1992). Botulinum toxin treatment of spasmodic dysphonia: Techniques, indications, efficacy. *Journal of Voice, 6*, 370–376.

Freeman, F.J., Cannito, M.P., & Finitzo-Hieber, T. (1985). Classification of spasmodic dysphonia by perceptual-acoustic-visual means. In G. Gates (Ed.), *Spasmodic dysphonia: The state of the art, 1984* (pp. 5–18). New York: The Voice Foundation.

Godfrey, H.P., & Knight, R. (1984). The validity of actometer and speech activity measures in the assessment of depressed patients. *British Journal of Psychiatry, 146*, 159–163.

Greden, J.F., Albala, A., Smokler, F.A., Gardner, R., & Carroll, B.J. (1981). Speech pause time: A marker of psychomotor retardation among endogenous depressives. *Biological Psychiatry, 16*, 851–859.

Hartman, D.E., & Aronson, A.E. (1981). Clinical investigations of intermittent breathy dysphonia. *Journal of Speech and Hearing Disorders, 46*, 428–432.

Hecker, M.H.L., Stevens, K.N., von Bismark, G., & Williams, C.E. (1968). Manifestations of task-induced stress in the acoustic speech signal. *Journal of the Acoustical Society of America, 44*, 993–1001.

House, A.S., & Fairbanks, G. (1953). The influence of consonant environment upon the secondary acoustical characteristics of vowels. *Journal of the Acoustical Society of America, 25*, 105–113.

Izdebski, C., Shipp, T., & Dedo, H. (1979). Predicting post-operative voice characteristics for spastic dysphonia patients. *Otolaryngology—Head and Neck Surgery, 87*, 428–434.

Karnell, M. (1992). Adductor and abductor spasmodic dysphonia: Related until proven otherwise. *American Journal of Speech-Language Pathology, 1*, 17–18.

Klatt, D.H. (1975). Voice onset time, frication, and aspiration in word-initial consonant clusters. *Journal of Speech and Hearing Research, 18*, 686–705.

Ladefoged, P. (1993). *A course in phonetics.* Fort Worth, TX: Harcourt, Brace and Jovanovich.

Lisker, L., & Abramson, A.S. (1967). Some effects of context on voice onset time in English stops. *Language and Speech, 10*, 1–28.

Ludlow, C.L., Naunton, R.F., Terada, S., & Anderson, B.J. (1991). Successful treatment of selected cases of abductor spasmodic dysphonia using botulinum toxin injection. *Otolaryngology—Head and Neck Surgery, 104*, 849–855.

Merson, R., & Ginsberg, A. (1979). Spasmodic dysphonia: A clinical report of acoustic, aerodynamic, and perceptual characteristics. *Laryngoscope, 89*, 129–139.

Morrison, D.F. (1976). *Multivariate statistical methods.* New York: McGraw-Hill.

Neter, J., & Wasserman, W. (1974). *Applied linear statistical models.* Homewood, IL: Richard D. Irwin, Inc.

Ohde, R. (1984). Fundamental frequency as an acoustic correlate of stop consonant voicing. *Journal of the Acoustical Society of America, 75*, 224–230.

Picheny, M., Durlach, N., & Braida, L. (1986). Speaking clearly for the hard of hearing. II: Acoustic characteristics of clear and conversational speech. *Journal of Speech and Hearing Research, 29*, 434–446.

Pope, B., Blass, T., Siegman, A.W., & Raher, J. (1970). Anxiety and depression in speech. *Journal of Consulting and Clinical Psychology, 35*, 128–133.

Roark, R.M., Schaefer, S.D., Kondraske, G., Watson, B., Freeman, F., Butsch, R.W., & Dembowski, J. (1990). Systems architecture for quantification of dynamic myoelectric and kinematic activity of the human vocal tract. *Annals of Otology, Rhinology, and Laryngology, 99*, 902–910.

Rontal, M., Rontal, E., Rolnick, M., Merson, R., Silverman, B., & Truong, D.D. (1991). A method for the treatment of abductor spasmodic dysphonia with botulinum toxin injections: A preliminary report. *Laryngoscope, 101*, 911–914.

Rosenfield, D.B. (1988). Spasmodic dysphonia. *Advances in Neurology, 49*, 317–327.

Schaefer, S. (1983). Neuropathology of spasmodic dysphonia. *Laryngoscope, 93*, 1183–1204.

Silverman, K. (1986). F_0 segmental cues depend on intonation: The case of the rise after voiced stops. *Phonetica, 43*, 46–91.

Streeter, L.A., MacDonald, N.H., Apple, W., Krauss, R.M., & Galotti, K.M. (1983). Acoustic and perceptual indicators of emotional stress. *Journal of the Acoustical Society of America, 73*, 1354–1360.

Titze, I.R. (1989). Physiologic and acoustic differences between male and female voices. *Journal of the Acoustical Society of America, 85*, 1699–1707.

Umeda, N. (1981). Influence of segmental factors on fundamental frequency in fluent speech. *Journal of the Acoustical Society of America, 70*, 350–355.

Watson, B., Schaefer, S., Freeman, F., Dembowski, J., Kondraske, G., & Roark, R. (1991). Laryngeal electromyographic activity in adductor and abductor spasmodic dysphonia. *Journal of Speech and Hearing Research, 34*, 473–482.

Watterson, T., & McFarlane, S. (1992). Adductor and abductor spasmodic dysphonia: Different disorders. *American Journal of Speech-Language Pathology, 1*, 19–20.

Williams, C.E., & Stevens, K.N. (1972). Emotions and speech: Some acoustical correlates. *Journal of the Acoustical Society of America, 52*, 1238–1250.

Winer, B.J. (1971). *Statistical principles in experimental design*. New York: McGraw-Hill.

Wolfe, V.I., & Bacon, M. (1976). Spectrographic comparison of two types of spasmodic dysphonia. *Journal of Speech and Hearing Disorders, 41*, 325–332.

Zwitman, D. (1979). Bilateral cord dysfunctions: Abductor type spastic dysphonia. *Journal of Speech and Hearing Disorders, 44*, 373–378.

Chapter 19

Effects of Inspiratory Airway Impairment on Continuous Speech

*James A. Till, Mehdi Jafari,
Roger L. Crumley, and Cindy B. Law-Till*

FROM AN AERODYNAMIC perspective, continous speech may be viewed as a series of adjacent breath groups each composed of 1) inspiration; 2) valved expiration during production of speech; and, optionally, 3) one or more pauses. The larynx performs important valving functions associated with each of these three partitions of a breath group. Bilateral vocal fold abduction is required for optimum speech inspiration between successive breath groups. In normal speakers, speech inspiration is accomplished in about 0.6 s at airflow rates slightly above 1 L/s. This results in approximately 0.7 L of average inspired volume for each breath group (Horii & Cooke, 1978; Till, Crumley, Jafari, & Law-Till, 1994).

Laryngeal valving during speech requires both vocal fold abduction and adduction gestures for transitions between voiced and voiceless speech segments. In addition, phonated portions of speech require an appropriate laryngeal muscular set to maintain voicing and to allow for fine adjustments in intensity and frequency necessary for prosodic variations. Combined with valving by the upper airway articulators, laryngeal valving during speech typically results in average airflow rates of 100–200 ml/s during conversational speech (Horii & Cooke, 1978; Till et al., 1994). Finally, there may be important laryngeal valving functions during linguistically motivated pauses. Studies of pause loci have been completed (Grosjean & Collins, 1979; Henderson, Goldman-Eisler, & Skarbek, 1965), but

---

This work was partially supported by Rehabilitation Research and Development Grant 468RA, Department of Veterans Affairs, Washington, D.C., and by National Institutes of Health Grant RO1-DC01147. This work is in the public domain.

aerodynamic characteristics have seldom been reported. One study reports that normal speakers expire 50–100 ml of air during noninspiratory pauses (Till & Alp, 1991).

A variety of pathologies and structural deviations can disrupt the normal pattern of vocal tract valving for speech. Laryngeal defects have potential to cause intended and unintended alterations in aerodynamic and temporal characteristics of connected speech because specific laryngeal actions are required during inspiration as well as during speaking and pausing. During inspiration, the major determinant of upper airway resistance is related to changes in the cross-sectional area of the glottis (Baier, Wanner, Zarzecki, & Sackner, 1977; Stanescu, Pattijn, Clement, & Van De Woestijne, 1972). In normal speakers, glottic aperture increases during inspiration and decreases during voiced segments of speech. However, vocal fold paralysis and sequelae of surgical treatments for vocal fold paralysis can result in mild to moderate degrees of inspiratory airway obstruction. For some patients, one or both of the vocal folds may adduct appropriately for voice but fail to abduct sufficiently for efficient inspiration. In extreme cases, abnormal audible noise on inhalation (stridor) may be present (George, O'Connell, & Batch, 1990). Other vocal fold paralysis patients may have abnormal laryngeal valving for both inspiration and speech expiration. Temporal and aerodynamic irregularities in this latter group may be particularly likely because members of the group have difficulty efficiently inspiring for speech and difficulty controlling excess expiration during speech. However, little attention has been given to potential effects of inspiratory airway compromise on patterns of speech production.

This chapter presents data for two groups of patients with documented inspiratory airway compromise at the laryngeal level and varying degrees of stridor. One patient group had normal expiratory laryngeal valving during speech production. The other patient group had abnormally large expiratory airflows during speech production. We hypothesized that both patient groups would have reduced airflow during inspiration relative to a normal control group. We expected at least some patients to acquire normal inspiratory volumes by extending the duration of inspiration. We also expected more severe disruption of speech temporal and aerodynamic patterns in the group that had both impaired inspiration and impaired expiration than in the group with only impaired inspiration.

METHODOLOGY

Subjects

Two groups of patients with a diagnosis of mild to moderate inspiratory airway compromise were studied. One group was composed of 10 subjects who had dysphonia and abnormally large expiratory speech flows in addition to the inspiratory airway impairment. The second group was composed of five subjects with inspiratory airway impairment with relatively normal vocal quality and speech expiratory airflows within normal limits. The patients had been referred for diagnostic assessment related to complaints of voice problems, stridor, or both. Each was subsequently diagnosed as having inspiratory airway compromise after examination by a laryngologist that included videoendoscopy. Speech problems, when present, were limited to dysphonia. Demographic information and etiology appear in Table 1. The results for each patient group were compared to results obtained from 20 normal subjects described previously (Till & Alp, 1991). Both patient subjects and normal-speaking subjects were native speakers of American English and had sufficient unaided hearing to follow conversational level instructions. No subject had a medical history of past or current pulmonary or neurologic disease.

Procedures

Each patient was seated in a quiet examination room and completed two tasks. The first task was a 1-minute monologue that allowed collection of simultaneous airflow and acoustic data. Subjects were instructed to speak continuously on a single topic for 1 minute at a conversational effort level without laughing or coughing. A "live listener" was present to help ensure use of conversational effort levels. The subjects wore a single-chamber pneumotachographic mask (Glottal Enterprises Model MA-1) connected to a differential pressure transducer and electronics system (Glottal Enterprises Model MA-2) that provided voltage linearly proportional to airflow

Table 1. Description of subjects

Subject	Sex	Age	IAC severity	Stridor noted	Expiratory valve integrity	Physical findings
HK	M	78	Moderate	Y	Hypo	Bilateral TVC fixation
JS	M	60	Mild	Y	Hypo	Left TVC paralysis
LP	F	35	Mild	Y	Hypo	Left TVC paralysis, right TVC paresis
SA	M	17	Moderate	Y	Hypo	Bilateral TVC paralysis
KC	F	56	Moderate	Y	Hypo	Bilateral paralysis
GF	F	62	Moderate	Y	Hypo	Left TVC paralysis
AD	M	43	Moderate	Y	Hypo	Bilateral TVC paralysis
NV	F	28	Mild	Y	Hypo	MVA—laryngeal crush
BT	F	57	Moderate	Y	Hypo	MVA—tracheal stenosis
KC	F	37	Moderate	Y	Hypo	Functional
ML	F	55	Severe	Y	WNL	Bilateral TVC paralysis
IS	F	57	Moderate	Y	WNL	Bilateral TVC fixation
LD	F	53	Mild	N	WNL	Left TVC paralysis
DB	F	44	Mild	N	WNL	Left TVC paralysis
MT	F	75	Mild	N	WNL	Left TVC paralysis

Note: IAC, inspiratory airway impairment; MVA, motor vehicle accident; TVC, true vocal cord; WNL, within normal limits.

over the range measured. The transducer electronics included a 30-Hz low-pass filter module for the airflow channel. The airflow system was calibrated prior to each subject's test session using a rotameter and airflow meter system (Glottal Enterprises Model MCU-2) which delivered known quantities of airflow through the pneumotachographic mask. Subjects also wore a head-mounted microphone (Telex Model Ph-91). The microphone element was located 7 cm from the subject's mouth at approximately 45 degrees azimuth to midline. Figure 1 shows representative raw waveform airflow data obtained from the 1-min monologue task from a patient subject (upper panel) and from a normal subject (lower panel). The vertical cursor line is positioned to provide readout of inspiratory airflow (shown in the lower left of each panel).

The acoustic and airflow signals were amplified (SA Instrumentation Model SA-410), connected to the analog-to-digital interface of an 80486 laboratory computer, and digitized at 1 kHz with 12-bit quantization (RC Electronics Model IAC-16). Because our pilot work had shown the initial inspiration for the monologue tasks to be significantly different from subsequent inspirations (Till & Goff, 1987), data collection was not initiated until after the initial inspiration.

Data Analysis

The CASPER automated speech diagnostic system (Till, 1990, 1993) was used for acoustic and aerodynamic feature extraction. The software initially partitioned the data into breath groups, each composed of an inspiratory period followed by speech expiratory and pause periods. Data collected prior to the onset of the initial inspiration and after the onset of the

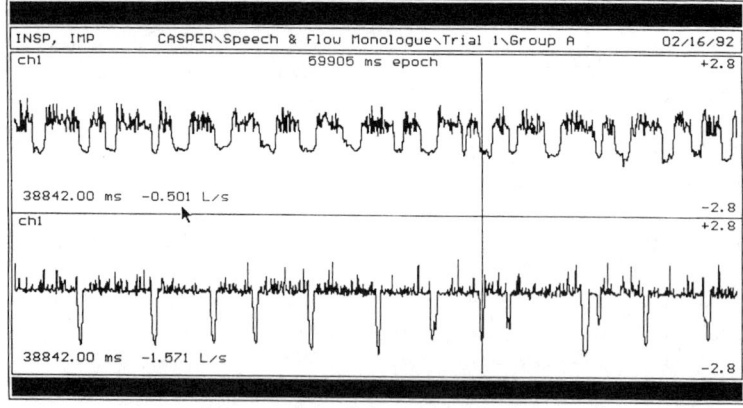

Figure 1. Sixty-second display of digitized airflow signals for a subject with inspiratory airway impairment (upper panel) and a normal-speaking subject (lower panel). Note that inspirations are longer in duration and lower in peak airflow for the subject with inspiratory airway impairment compared to the normal-speaking subject.

last inspiration were excluded. Inspirations were defined as negative airflow events exceeding 300 ms in duration and with integrated volume greater than 50 ml. Our pilot investigations had shown that short-duration negative flow events less than 50 ml in volume were produced by buccal and lingual movements and were not pulmonary in nature. All records were inspected to confirm accurate marking of inspiratory onsets and offsets. No software errors were detected.

The expiratory period of a breath group was further partitioned into speech segments and noninspiratory pause segments by locating the pauses in the acoustic signal. Pauses were defined as periods of "silence" that exceeded 200 ms in duration (Canter, 1965). Silence was detected by the software on the basis of a root-mean-square (rms) reference voltage automatically calculated from a sample of ambient noise prior to the monologue sample. Specifically, silent periods were portions of the record in which the rms voltage on the acoustic channel remained below 4/3 of the rms silence reference voltage for greater than 200 ms. The speech portions of a breath group were the remaining data that were not identified as inspiration and exceeded th 4/3-rms silence threshold. Figure 2 shows a plot of a representative breath group for a patient subject with both inspiratory airway compromise and expiratory hypovalving. The software marked inspiration onset and offset as numbers 1 and 2, respectively; pause onset and offset were marked by numbers 3 and 4, respectively.

Twelve specific measures were extracted by the CASPER software for the monologue task. The 1-minute summary measures—breaths per minute, pauses per minute, and minute volume—were based on observed rates and volumes extrapolated to a full minute of speaking. Minute vol-

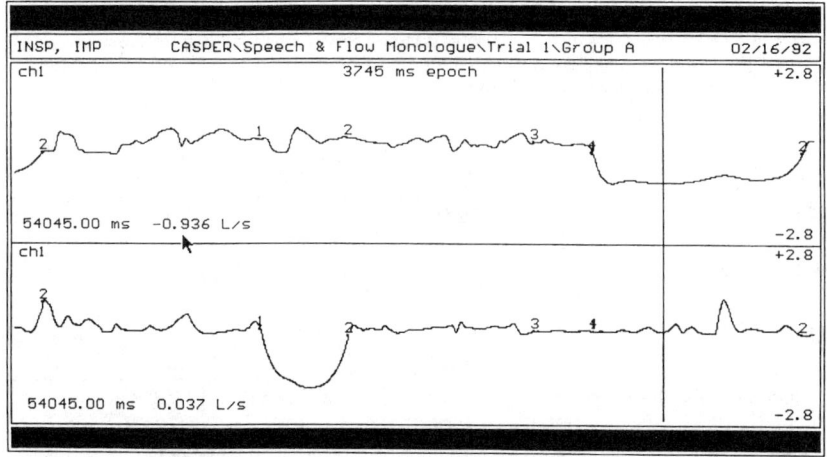

Figure 2. Four-second display of airflow signals for a subject with impaired inspiratory airway showing software partitioning into inspiration onset and offset (1 and 2) and pause onset and offset (3 and 4).

ume was calculated by multiplying mean inspiratory volumes by breaths per minute. For each breath group, mean airflow rate and duration were measured for the inspiration, speech, and pause epochs. Air volumes for inspiration, speech, and pause epochs were calculated by multiplying the corresponding mean airflow rates and durations. These values were then averaged across breath groups in the 1-min sample and expressed as means per breath group. Comparisons between the patient group and normal group were accomplished for all measures using a one-way analysis of variance (ANOVA). An alpha level of .01 was used to infer significant group difference.

RESULTS AND DISCUSSION

Group Comparisons

Inspiration Group means, standard deviations, F ratios, and post hoc contrasts of means for the inspiratory measures appear in Table 2. The F ratio was derived from a single-factor (groups) ANOVA that partitioned the variance into between-group variance and error variance. The table shows that the patient groups had significantly smaller mean inspiratory airflows than did the normal group. Moreover, mean inspiratory durations for the patient groups were significantly larger than those observed for the normal group. However, mean inspiratory volumes were not significantly different among the three groups. This suggests that, as a group, the patients increased inspiratory duration sufficiently to acquire near-normal inspiratory volumes despite reduced inspiratory airflow rates. For example, the patient whose airflow is displayed in Figure 1 acquired nearly nor-

Table 2. Descriptive statistics and group comparison F ratios for inspiratory measures for normal (N) group and patient groups with both inspiratory and expiratory abnormality (IE) and only inspiratory airway abnormality (I)

		Measures				
Group (n)		MV (L)	BPM	Flow (ml)	Duration (ms)	Volume (L)
N (20)	Mean	7.47	12.09	1036.4	610.5	623.3
	SD	1.62	2.55	215.0	111.1	128.2
IE (10)	Mean	11.9	18.83	679.1	982.3	640.8
	SD	2.85	5.63	172.3	300.5	178.5
I (5)	Mean	7.14	14.78	529.0	912.0	474.1
	SD	2.33	4.21	210.6	173.6	203.1
F ratio (df = 2,32)		16.05	10.15	18.11	14.48	2.20
p		.0001	.0004	.0001	.0001	.13
Sheffé contrasts (p = .01)		IE > N,I	IE > N	N > IE,I	N < IE,I	NS

Note: BPM, breaths per minute; MV, minute volume; NS, not significant; SD, standard deviation.

mal mean inspiratory volumes (609 ml) using increased mean inspiratory durations (1.07 s) at reduced (or limited) mean inspiratory airflows (579 ml/s).

The results reported for minute volume suggest that it is conditioned by expiratory airflow rate rather than inspiratory airflow rate. That is, the patient group with abnormally high expiratory airflows had significantly greater minute volume than did either group with normal expiratory valving. The patient group with higher expiratory airflows also had significantly larger mean breaths per minute relative to the other two groups. Despite the trend toward increased mean breaths per minute shown for the patient group with normal expiratory valving, there was not a significant difference between this group and the other patient group or the normal group.

Speech Expiration Group means, standard deviations, F ratios, and post hoc contrasts of means for the speech expiratory measures appear in Table 3. As noted previously, one patient group was composed of subjects with dysphonia and insufficient vocal fold contact. As we expected, the average expiratory airflow during speech was significantly larger for this group relative to the other two groups. Because this patient group did not have abnormally large inspiratory volumes (Table 2), the significant reduction in mean speech duration shown in Table 3 would be expected unless the patients encroached on pulmonary reserve volume. Although there was a trend toward reduced speech duration in the patient group with normal speech valving, this contrast failed to reach statistical significance. There were no significant differences among the three groups regarding mean expiratory volume.

Table 3. Descriptive statistics and group comparison F ratios for expiratory measures for normal (N) group and patient groups with both inspiratory and expiratory abnormality (IE) and only inspiratory airway abnormality (I)

		Measures		
Group (n)		Flow (ml)	Duration (ms)	Volume (ml)
N (20)	Mean	144.9	4073	581.4
	SD	32.8	991	157.3
IE (10)	Mean	313.2	2170	659.1
	SD	72.2	811	211.5
I (5)	Mean	142.8	2992	449.1
	SD	40.8	1182	273.7
F ratio (df = 2,32)		43.88	13.21	2.01
p		.0001	.0004	.15
Sheffé contrasts (p = .01)		IE > N,I	N > IE	NS

Note: NS, not significant; SD, standard deviation.

Pauses Group means, standard deviations and F ratios for the pause measures are shown in Table 4. There were no significant group differences for any of the pause measures. The trend toward lower airflow rates and lower pause volumes in the patient group with normal speech valving will be discussed later.

Compensatory Behaviors in Inspiratory Airway Compromise

Relative to the normal group, the patient groups had significantly reduced mean inspiratory airflow values and significantly increased inspiratory duration. There was no significant difference among the three groups in inspiratory volume. Taken together, this pattern of findings suggests that the patients increased duration of inspiration sufficiently to acquire normal inspiratory volumes. However, other findings suggest that not all patients uniformly followed this strategy. If normal inspiratory volumes were to be acquired by patients with varying inspiratory airflow rates using duration adjustments only, the inspiratory duration would have to be increased in proportion to the decrease in inspiratory airflow rate. Figure 3 shows the bivariate plot and Pearson r value for these two variables. Although Figure 3 suggests there is a trend toward this behavior, clearly there is substantial dispersion in inspiratory durations among the subjects at low, medium, and high inspiratory airflow rates. The subjects in the patient groups did not uniformly increase their inspiratory durations sufficiently to achieve normal volumes.

In fact, 6 of the 15 patients had inspiratory volumes that deviated from mean inspiratory volume for the normal subjects by a magnitude greater than 1.5 times the normal group standard deviation. Two of the patient subjects with expiratory hypovalving had increased mean inspira-

Table 4. Descriptive statistics and group comparison F ratios for pause measures for normal (N) group and patient groups with both inspiratory and expiratory abnormality (IE) and only inspiratory airway abnormality (I)

Group (n)		Measures			
		Flow (ml)	Duration (ms)	Volume (ml)	PPM
N (20)	Mean	166.1	395.0	69.9	15.06
	SD	110.0	77.2	55.2	6.94
IE (10)	Mean	205.0	339.4	65.3	15.00
	SD	92.7	72.8	22.9	19.11
I (5)	Mean	88.3	578.2	39.2	13.98
	SD	78.8	344.1	29.9	9.6
F ratio (df = 2,32)		2.19	4.92	0.92	0.017
p		.12	.014	.41	.98

Note: PPM, pauses per minute; SD, standard deviation.

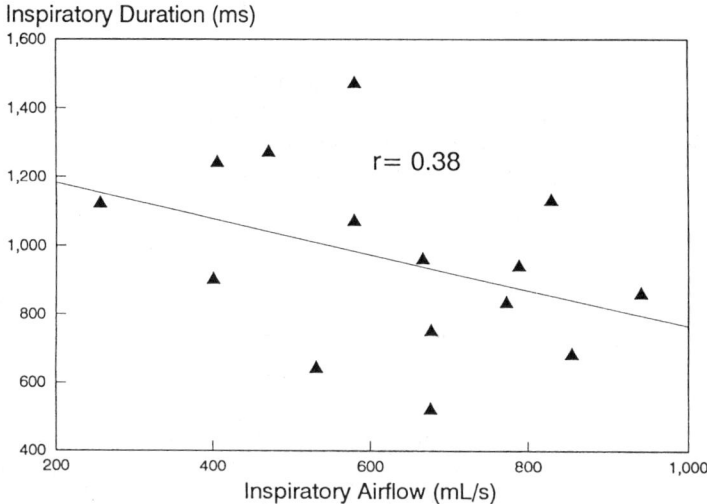

Figure 3. Bivariate plot and Pearson *r* value for mean inspiratory duration and mean inspiratory airflow for the 15 subjects with impaired inspiratory airway.

tory volumes (850–950 ml). Four other patient subjects, three with normal expiratory valving and one with expiratory hypovalving, had abnormally low mean inspiratory volumes (<400 ml). As might be expected, these subjects required more frequent inspirations as their individual inspiratory volumes decreased.

Finally, examination of this latter subgroup of patients with low inspiratory volumes leads to the conjecture that one other adaptive behavior might have occurred in some patients with normal laryngeal expiratory valving. Unlike the patients with expiratory hypovalving, these subjects had the physiologic capability to voluntarily restrict *expiratory* airflow during speech. Therefore, it is possible that subjects in this group with particularly low lung volumes available for speech voluntarily hyperconstricted the larynx in order to conserve their relatively meager lung volume and produce longer, more normal speech epochs. Whether any of the current subjects employed this "dope smoker's strategy" cannot be determined on the basis of the current experiment. Low expiratory airflow rates may have been caused by lower lung volumes alone. However, it is interesting to note that mean expiratory flow values during speech were less than 120 ml/s for two of the subjects who also had mean inspiratory volumes less than 350 ml. Of course, such reasoning is also complicated by absence of subglottal driving pressure measures in the current experiment. Still, the notion may be worthy of additional investigation.

SUMMARY

This chapter has presented data describing effects of mild to moderate inspiratory airway impairment at the laryngeal level. As expected, there was a reduction in group mean inspiratory airflow for the patient groups relative to the normal group. The patient groups had increased mean inspiratory duration during speech, which for some subjects resulted in near-normal mean inspiratory volumes. However, the patients were not uniformly successful in achieving normal inspiratory volumes. For patients with near-normal inspiratory volumes and without expiratory valving deficits, mean speech duration, minute volume, and inspiratory rate (breaths per minute) were approximately normal in magnitude. Other patients failed to compensate fully for abnormally low inspiratory airflows by increasing duration of inspiration. For these patients, mean speech durations were reduced from normal expectations and breaths per minute were increased. Speculation was offered regarding another potential compensatory behavior related to reduced lung volumes for speech. For individuals with normal speech valving capabilities and reduced inspiratory volumes, the dope smoker's strategy might have been employed. That is, the patient might have volitionally constricted the larynx to limit speech airflow in order to conserve the relatively meager lung volume and extend time available for syllable production. Two subjects were observed to display less than normal speech expiratory airflows in the presence of reduced inspiratory air volumes.

The results reported illustrate that laryngeal inspiratory airway impairment can affect both inspiratory and expiratory speech functions. In planning treatment for these patients, it is important to consider more than just restoration of ventilatory function or restoration of voice in isolation. The larynx does serve as the vibratory sound source for phonated speech; however, it also serves other valving functions during inspiratory and expiratory portions of a speech breath group. This perspective implies the need to attend to the inspiratory, voiced/voiceless transition and pausing functions of the larynx as well as phonatory functions when planning treatments.

REFERENCES

Baier, H., Wanner, A., Zarzecki, S., & Sackner, M. (1977). Relationships among glottis opening, respiratory flow, and upper airway resistance in humans. *Journal of Applied Physiology, 43,* 603–611.

Canter, G.J. (1965). Speech characteristics of patients with Parkinson's disease. II: Physiological support for speech. *Journal of Speech and Hearing Disorders, 30,* 44–49.

George, M., O'Connell, J., & Batch, A. (1990). Paradoxical vocal cord notion: An unusual cause of stridor. *Journal of Laryngology and Otology, 109,* 312–314.

Grosjean, F., & Collins, M. (1979). Breathing, pausing and reading. *Phonetica, 36,* 98–114.

Henderson, A., Goldman-Eisler, F., & Skarbek, A. (1965). The common value of pausing time in spontaneous speech. *Quarterly Journal of Experimental Psychology, 17,* 343–345.

Horii, Y., & Cooke, P.A. (1978). Some airflow, volume, and duration characteristics of oral reading. *Journal of Speech and Hearing Research, 21,* 470–481.

Stanescu, D., Pattijn, J., Clement, J., & Van De Woestijne, K. (1972). Glottis opening and airway resistance. *Journal of Applied Physiology, 32,* 460–466.

Till, J.A. (1990). Computer-assisted speech evaluation: Rationale and direction for the future. *Journal for Computer Users in Speech and Hearing, 6,* 134–148.

Till, J.A. (1993). CASPER: Computer Assisted Speech Evaluation Expert System. In B. Granstrom, S. Hunnicutt, & K. Spens (Eds.), *Speech and language technology for disabled persons* (pp. 141–144). Stockholm: ESCA & KTH.

Till, J.A., & Alp, A.L. (1991). Aerodynamic and temporal measures of continuous speech in dysarthric speakers. In C. Moore, K. Yorkston, & D. Beukelman (Eds.), *Dysarthria and apraxia of speech: Perspectives on management* (pp. 185–204). Baltimore: Paul H. Brookes Publishing Co.

Till, J.A., Crumley, R.L., Jafari, M., & Law-Till, C. (1994). Aerodynamic and temporal disruptions of speech in laryngeal insufficiency. *Archives of Otolaryngology—Head Neck Surgery, 120,* 317–325.

Till, J.A., & Goff, A.M. (1987, November). *Lung volumetric characteristics of phrase initiation and termination.* Paper presented at the annual meeting of the American Speech-Language-Hearing Association, New Orleans.

Chapter 20

Phonemic Retrieval in Apraxia of Speech
Is There More Than One Type of Impairment?

Monica Strauss Hough and Salvatore DeMarco

WORD RETRIEVAL IS an interactive process constrained by the specific nature of a task. Information retained for short periods is dependent on a multicomponent short-term memory system known as working memory. Some researchers have suggested that this system has a phonologic basis (Baddeley, 1986, 1992; Baddeley, Vallar, & Wilson, 1987). This working memory network is composed of a controlling central executive system, consisting of attentional components, and several subordinate slave systems. In the recall of verbal information, the most prominent subsidiary system is the phonologic loop. The loop comprises two components: 1) a passive phonologic store and 2) an articulatory control and rehearsal process (Baddeley, 1986, 1992; Baddeley et al., 1987; Daneman & Tardif, 1987). The phonologic loop is involved in the process of constructing stable phonologic representations. Information is registered in the phonologic store either auditorily or through subvocal rehearsal. Baddeley (1986, 1992) has hypothesized that the phonologic representation within the store will fade in 2 s unless it is refreshed by rehearsal.

Models of speech production and repetition, which comprise some of the components of working memory such as the adapted representation in Figure 1 (Caramazza, Miceli, & Villa, 1986; Margolin, 1991), have been proposed to account for retrieval of real and nonsense words by normal adults and adults with brain damage. Route 1 (spoken input to acoustic-to-phonologic transcoding to phonologic buffer) is utilized for nonword pro-

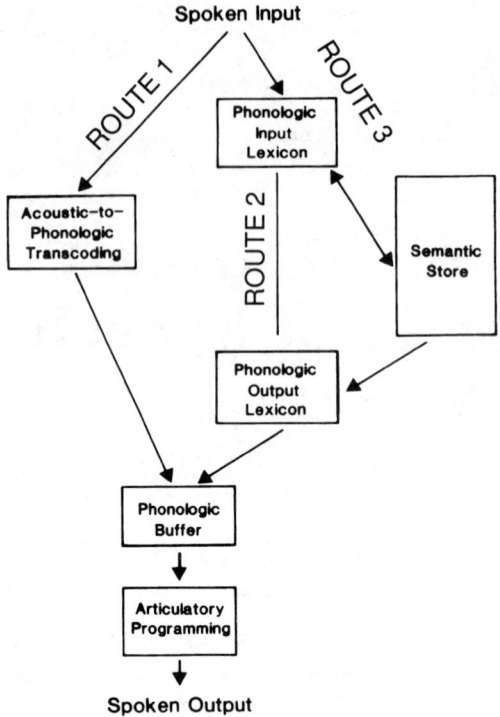

Figure 1. Model of speech production and repetition. (Adapted from Caramazza, Miceli, & Villa, 1986; Margolin, 1991.)

ductions for which there is no permanent underlying phonologic representation on which to draw. Route 2 (spoken input to phonologic input lexicon to phonologic output lexicon to phonologic buffer) is principally used for real words out of context for which the underlying phonologic representation of the word is permanently stored in the phonologic lexicon. Some level of activation of the semantic store probably occurs for familiar words used out of context. Route 3 (spoken input to phonologic input lexicon to semantic store to phonologic output lexicon to phonologic buffer) is used for semantically based real words.

In the present study, a delayed repetition paradigm was utilized to investigate the retrieval of real words and nonwords by two adults with apraxia of speech. Previous studies have involved the immediate repetition of real and nonsense words. In these studies, it is possible that some of the errors produced were due in part to random error, inattention, misperception, misarticulation, and/or lexical biasing. With deferred repetition, the likelihood of random error is reduced because an individual's accurate immediate repetition of the word ensures that the word is initially encoded in memory. Thus, errors in deferred repetition are more likely due to interference or rapid decay of information, although random error is never totally eliminated.

In the current study, the deferred repetition paradigm involved the retrieval of real and nonsense target words after the presentation of real and nonsense distractor words. The paradigm allows for systematic manipulation of the degree of phonetic and lexical contrast between target words and distractor words. Thus, the magnitude of a phonetic similarity effect and the interaction between real and nonsense words can be analyzed by manipulating the phonetic feature relationship and lexicality of the target and the distractor words, respectively. Furthermore, the paradigm permits examination of the interactive effects of these two relationships for a more systematic study of phonetic and lexical interference on deferred short-term retrieval.

Apraxia of speech has been considered a disorder of motor programming for speech (Canter, Trost, & Burns, 1985; Kent & McNeil, 1987; Kent & Rosenbek, 1983; Pierce, 1991). Some researchers have identified apraxia of speech more specifically as a deficit in motor planning, sequencing, control, and/or timing (Itoh et al., 1982; Kelso & Tuller, 1981; Lebrun, 1989). Apraxia of speech usually occurs as the result of a lesion to the left frontal lobe, often involving the third frontal convolution and the adjacent subcortical regions (Kertesz, 1984, 1985; Rosenbek, Kent, & LaPointe, 1984). Behavioral symptomatology in apraxia of speech includes but is not limited to disordered articulation, reduced speech rate, scanning speech, speech initiation difficulties, prosodic disturbance, audible groping, oral posturing, and labored articulatory productions (Lebrun, 1989, 1990; Odell, McNeil, Rosenbek, & Hunter, 1990; Wertz, LaPointe, & Rosenbek, 1984). Many of these behaviors have been attributed to a breakdown in articulatory programming, as presented in Figure 1. However, there has not been complete agreement regarding lesion localization as well as behavioral symptomatology in apraxia of speech, resulting in the hypothesis that there are subtypes of this phenomenon (Kertesz, 1985; Lebrun, 1989; Square-Storer & Apeldoorn, 1991; Square-Storer & Roy, 1989), with different underlying bases for these deficits.

Phonemic retrieval deficits have been observed to underlie some of the speech production errors of aphasic adults, particularly in the immediate repetition of real and nonsense words (Favreau, Nespoulous, & Lecours, 1990; Kohn, 1988). It also is possible that phonemic retrieval impairments may be the basis for some of the production errors in apraxia of speech. As previously mentioned, apraxia has been considered a deficit in motor programming. The role of cognitive functions, such as attention, memory, and retrieval, relative to motor control and motor functions has been generally discussed in the literature (MacKay, 1985; Peters, 1990;

Roy, 1982). Work by Roy (1981) and Jason (1983) in which the sequencing of limb movements was examined in adults with left frontal brain damage revealed significant deficits in sequencing hand movements, particularly when these had to be generated from memory. The influence of cognitive functions specifically on the motor programming of articulatory speech gestures has been minimally considered. Roy and Square (1985; Roy & Square-Storer, 1990) identified the importance of cognitive processes such as attention and memory on motor speech control. Square-Storer, Roy, and Hogg (1990) suggested that apraxic speech errors may reflect cognitive selection disorders in which there is a misselection, inaccessibility to memory files of stored motor programs, or both. That is, in some cases, the motor program may be intact but the difficulty lies in control and/or retrieval of the program or movement sequence (Roy & Square-Storer, 1990). The current study examines the influence of working memory on articulatory programming through the investigation of phonemic retrieval abilities of two adults with apraxia of speech (AOS). In word repetition, we sought to determine whether retrieval of real and nonsense target words was influenced by several factors, including 1) lexicality (real vs. nonsense) of the target, 2) phonetic similarity of the distractor to the target, and/or 3) lexical nature of the distractor word.

METHODOLOGY

Subjects

Apraxia of speech Subjects 1 and 2 were an 80-year-old man and a 67-year-old woman, respectively. Clinical characteristics for the subjects are presented in Table 1. Both had suffered single-episode, left hemisphere middle cerebral artery cerebrovascular accidents resulting in AOS with minimal aphasic involvement. AOS was their primary communication deficit. Brain damage was verified by reported neurologic examination and clinical reports. Lesion site information, as determined by computed tomography, also is presented in Table 1. AOS was diagnosed based on performance on the verbal and oral subtests of the Boston Diagnostic Aphasia Examination (BDAE) (Goodglass & Kaplan, 1983) and an oral–motor test examining oral movement during speech and nonspeech tasks (Hough & Klich, 1987). The criteria for diagnosis of AOS included the following: 1) effortful trial-and-error, groping articulatory behavior; 2) dysprosody throughout segmentally fluent and dysfluent productions; 3) sound distortions and substitutions; 4) difficulty in initiating utterances; and 5) imitation better than spontaneous speech (Rosenbek, 1985; Wertz et al., 1984). On the BDAE, both subjects had an Aphasia Severity Rating of 2, indicating that "Conversation about familiar subjects is possible with help from

Table 1. Clinical characteristics for subjects 1 and 2

Characteristics	Subject 1	Subject 2
TAWF SS[a]	80	80
BDAE Subtests[b]		
Word discrimination	75	100
Body part identification	100	100
Oral commands	65	90
Word repetition	40	70
Phrase repetition		
High probability	50	55
Low probability	70	50
Automatized sequences	70	70
Word reading	75	80
Responsive naming	75	70
Confrontation naming	65	60
Oral sentence reading	65	70
Animal naming	80	85
Verbal fluency[c]		
Words per minute	29	32
Average phrase length	2.8	2.9
Longest phrase[d] (phrase length)	4 (40+)	4 (40)
Melodic line[d] (intonational contour)	3 (25)	3 (25)
Articulatory agility[d]	3 (25)	3 (25)
Lesion site	Broca's area, anterior insula, inferior premotor area	Broca's area, superior premotor area

[a] Test of Adolescent/Adult Word Finding, standard score (German, 1990).
[b] Percentile ranks for Boston Diagnostic Aphasia Examination subtests (Goodglass & Kaplan, 1983).
[c] Verbal fluency measures were obtained in a conversational speech sample.
[d] Ratings based on the BDAE Rating Scale Profile of Behavioral Characteristics.

the listener. There are frequent failures to convey the idea, but patient shares the burden of communication with the examiner" (Goodglass & Kaplan, 1983, p. 84).

Both subjects had a 10th grade education, and both had had a cerebrovascular accident approximately 7 months previously. They were both native English speakers and were right handed by self-report. Both subjects passed a modified pure-tone hearing screening bilaterally across the speech frequencies (1, 2, and 4 kHz) at a 40-dB hearing level (Weinstein, 1989). Both subjects had speech discrimination scores of at least 80% at a 40-dB hearing level in each ear. Both subjects achieved 100% accuracy on the Boston University Speech Sound Discrimination Picture Test (Pronovost & Dombleton, 1955).

Materials

The experimental task (deferred repetition paradigm) consisted of 70 randomized pairs (target and distractor) of consonant–vowel–consonant (CVC) stimuli, samples of which are presented in Table 2. Fifty pairs were 10 target words paired with five different types of distractor words. The distractors included 1) a word phonetically similar to the target word, differing in one phonetic feature; 2) a word phonetically similar to the target word, differing by two or three phonetic features; 3) a word phonetically dissimilar to the target word; 4) a nonsense word phonetically similar to the target word; and 5) a nonsense word phonetically dissimilar to the target word. As can be seen in Table 2, the other 20 pairs of CVC stimuli consisted of 10 nonsense target words paired with two different types of distractors. The distractors included a phonetically similar real word and a phonetically similar nonsense word distractor.

A nonsense word has been defined as a plausible phonologic sequence that does not exist in an adult's phonologic lexicon. A real word is a word that is part of the adult's phonologic lexicon; in this paradigm, the semantic store should be minimally accessed for the word's realization because of the imitative nature of the task. A semantically based real word would be one that exists within the adult's semantic store that receives contextual elaboration. All real words used in the task had a word frequency of less than 1 per 30,000 of the most frequently used words in the American English language (Carroll, Davies, & Richman, 1971).

Procedures

For each stimulus pair, each subject was instructed to repeat the target word after the examiner while the examiner pointed to a nonsense geometric shape ("Say _____"). Following a 1-s pause after the subject's response, the examiner pointed to a second shape and produced the distractor word ("Now say _____"), which the subject repeated. After another 1-s pause after the subject's response, the subject was asked to reproduce

Table 2. Stimulus examples

Target word	Distractors[a]				
	A	B	C	D	E
bat	back	bag	phone	bap	shuve
pibe	pipe			pige	

[a] A, phonetically similar real word differing in one feature; B, phonetically similar real word differing in two or more features; C, phonetically dissimilar real word; D, phonetically similar nonsense word; E, phonetically dissimilar nonsense word.

the target word ("What is this?") while the examiner pointed to the first geometric shape.

The task was broken up into three parts: Items 1–25, Items 26–50, and Items 51–70. A 2-min break separated each part of the task. During the task, 5 s were provided for subjects to respond after both the initial presentation of the target word and the presentation of the distractor. Five seconds also were provided for deferred retrieval of the target word. If subjects misproduced the initial presentation of the target word or misproduced the distractor word, the examiner presented the appropriate production of the word and moved on to presentation of the next word pair. The examiner presented these misproduced items at the end of the presentation of each group of stimuli and scored them in the same manner as the other stimuli.

A 5-s pause separated the presentation of each stimulus pair. Three word pairs were provided as practice items to ensure the subject's understanding of the task. These words were not part of the experimental stimuli but were representative of target/distractor pairings presented during the experimental task. The stimuli were all presented through live voice. All responses were phonetically recorded and audiotaped for later verification.

Data Analysis

The intent of the original study was to examine the deferred repetition of real and nonsense words in a group of adults with apraxia of speech as well as particular aphasic subtype groups. However, on analysis of the data, it was observed that some apraxic adults demonstrated good immediate repetition while having difficulty with deferred repetition, whereas other adults with apraxia of speech had extensive difficulty with immediate repetition. Subject 1 had difficulty with immediate repetition of both real and nonsense words. In contrast, Subject 2 had good immediate repetition but impaired deferred repetition. The number of errors on immediate repetition of the target words based on error type and lexicality of the target (nonsense vs. real word) were determined for Subject 1. The number of errors on deferred repetition of the target words based on error type, distractor type, and lexicality of the target word were determined for Subject 2.

Both intraexaminer and interexaminer reliability were determined. For intraexaminer reliability, the examiner listened to audiotape recordings and scored each of the subjects' responses at least 2 weeks after their participation in the study. Percentage of agreement was 100%. For interexaminer reliability, another speech-language pathologist independently listened to audiotape recordings and scored each of the subjects' responses. Percentage of agreement was 93%.

RESULTS

Error performance for Subject 1 based on lexicality of the target words is presented in Table 3. As can be seen, the results revealed that the percentage of errors was much greater for nonsense (85%) than for real (18%) target words. Error patterns based on specific error types are presented in Table 4. The findings revealed that the most frequently produced error by Subject 1 was no response (69%). This result was observed regardless of whether the target was a nonsense or real word but, as seen in Table 3, more no-response errors occurred on nonsense than real words. No-response errors accounted for 76% and 56% of the errors produced on nonsense and real words, respectively.

For Subject 2, error performance based on lexicality of the target words and distractor type is presented in Table 5. The percentage of errors was greater for the nonsense (30%) than real (18%) target words. However, the percentage of error discrepancy between nonsense and real words was not as large as what was observed for Subject 1. Error pattern performance, presented in Table 4, revealed that errors mainly consisted of repetition of the distractor and one or two feature changes. As can be seen in Table 5, distractor repetition errors were produced primarily on retrieval of nonsense target words; furthermore, four of the five errors occurred when the distractor was a real word. One or two feature change errors occurred only when retrieving real target words. Additionally, error occurrence for the real target words was not influenced by the lexical nature or phonetic similarity of the distractor to the target. Further analysis

Table 3. Number of errors on immediate recall based on lexicality and error type for Subject 1

Lexicality	Error type[a]						Overall errors[b]
	1	2	3	4	5	6	
Real words	5	0	0	NA	3	1	18
Nonsense words	13	1	0	3	0	0	85

[a]1, no response; 2, reduce CVC to CV; 3, perseveration; 4, change nonsense word to real word; 5, one or two feature changes; 6, other.

[b]Numbers signify the percentage of errors based on the total possible responses.

Table 4. Number of errors per error type for both subjects

	Error type[a]						
	1	2	3	4	5	6	7
Subject 1[b]	18	1	0	NA	3	3	1
Subject 2[c]	2	0	0	6	1	6	0

[a]1, no response; 2, reduce CVC to CV; 3, perseveration; 4, repetition of the distractor; 5, change nonsense word to real word; 6, one or two feature changes; 7, other.

[b]Errors are for immediate repetition.

[c]Errors are for deferred repetition.

Table 5. Number of errors on deferred recall per target/distractor pairing and error type for Subject 2

Lexicality	Error type[a]							Overall errors[b]
	1	2	3	4	5	6	7	
Real/real +1	0	0	0	1	0	1	0	
Real/real +2–3	1	0	0	0	0	1	0	
Real/dissimilar real	0	0	0	0	0	1	0	18%
Real/similar nonsense	0	0	0	0	0	1	0	
Real/dissimilar nonsense	1	0	0	0	0	2	0	
Nonsense/similar real	0	0	0	4	1	0	0	30%
Nonsense/similar nonsense	0	0	0	1	0	0	0	

[a] 1, no response; 2, reduce CVC to CV; 3, perseveration; 4, repetition of the distractor; 5, change nonsense word to real word; 6, one or two feature changes; 7, other.
[b] Numbers signify the percentage of errors based on the total possible responses.

of the specific feature changes in the one or two feature change errors for the real target words was conducted by examining the particular distractor with which the real target word was paired. This analysis, presented in Table 6, revealed that, for five of the six word pairs, production of the distractor interfered with retrieval of the target word in a unique manner. Specifically, the feature errors consisted of substituted segments or particular features that were retained or perseverated from the distractor during deferred retrieval of the target.

DISCUSSION

One variable that influences the ability to retrieve phonologic information from working memory in AOS appears to be the lexical nature of the target word (real vs. nonsense). Real target words were easier for both subjects to retrieve than nonsense words. This finding also has been observed for normal adults (Caplan, 1987; Hough, DeMarco, & Farler, 1994), indicating that, for real words, the underlying phonologic representation needed to construct the surface representation of the word is permanently stored in memory because of its lexical basis. The nature of this represen-

Table 6. Specific one or two feature change errors for Subject 2

Lexicality	Target	Distractor	Error
Real/real +1	rope	robe	/rot/
Real/real +2–3	bat	bag	/bæd/*
Real/dissimilar real	bat	phone	/bæn/*
Real/similar nonsense	comb	cos	/kon/*
Real/dissimilar nonsense	bone	veet	/bot/*
	cape	zad	/ked/*

*Errors involving perseveration of feature or segment from distractor to deferred retrieval of target.

tation allows for easier access to real words (Favreau et al., 1990; Jackendorf, 1987). However, for nonsense words, there is no permanent underlying representation on which to draw. In Figure 1, Route 1 (spoken input to acoustic-to-phonologic transcoding to phonologic buffer) is activated for nonreal words where there is no permanent underlying representation on which to draw because the word is novel or unfamiliar. Route 2 (spoken input to phonologic input lexicon to phonologic output lexicon to phonologic buffer) is activated primarily for real words in which the underlying phonologic representation needed to construct the surface representation of the word is permanently stored in the phonologic lexicon; however, the word is not contextually realized. For adults, it is probable that repetition of single real words also activates Route 3 (spoken input to phonologic input lexicon to semantic store to phonologic output lexicon to phonologic buffer) to some extent, but to a lesser degree than Route 2. Route 3 is mainly activated for real words that have been contextually realized.

Patterns of Error Production

Patterns of error production based on specific error types were different for the two subjects. Subject 1 displayed a much higher percentage of errors on nonsense than real targets. There was a high predominance of no-response errors on both real and nonsense targets; however, this pattern was more significant for nonsense targets. Subject 2's error type pattern was definitely influenced by the lexical nature of the target, producing repetition of the distractor errors primarily during retrieval of nonsense target words, and, interestingly, mainly on nonsense target–real distractor word pairs. One or two feature change errors occurred only during the recall of real target words. Subject 2's error performance was not influenced by the lexical nature of the distractor or phonetic similarity of the distractor for real target words; that is, errors were distributed throughout all the real target–distractor pair combinations. However, specific one or two feature change errors during retrieval involved perseveration of segments or features of the distractor to the target.

The unique patterns of error type production for Subjects 1 and 2 suggest different underlying bases for their impairments. Returning to Figure 1, the poor immediate repetition performance of Subject 1, with a high percentage of errors on nonsense targets and the frequent occurrence of no-response errors, may be accounted for by a breakdown in articulatory programming. Information from the phonologic buffer (phonologic store component of working memory) in the form of word images is not consistently acted on by articulatory programming. This appears to proportionately occur much more often when retrieving nonsense than real words and results in many no-response errors. This profile suggests one type of apraxia of speech, which is characterized primarily by difficulty in initiating production, particularly for nonsense words. The very significant lexical influence on error performance exhibited by Subject 1, characterized by a much higher percentage of errors on nonsense than real words, suggests that initiation of novel utterances is much more difficult for the adult with this type of AOS than is initiation of utterances that are permanently stored in the phonologic lexicon. Additionally, it is possible that the strength of word images in the phonologic buffer is highly dependent on storage permanence in the phonologic lexicon itself (Friedrich, 1990), with real words having greater strength than nonsense words because of their permanent underlying phonologic representation in the lexicon. Consequently, this results in higher error percentages for nonsense words that do not have permanent phonologic representations on which to draw. As mentioned, Subject 1 exhibited a dramatic lexical effect with extensive difficulty in the immediate retrieval of nonsense words. The strength of word images for real and nonsense words in the phonologic buffer may be proportionately the same for Subject 1 as for normal speakers; however, he may not appropriate the cognitive resources or articulatory strategies needed for immediate repetition of nonsense words that are novel or unfamiliar. Subject 1's phrase repetition performance on the BDAE and his verbal fluency profile lend some support to this conclusion because he was able to produce real words with some success.

Waters, Rochon, and Caplan (1992) have suggested that initiation difficulties in AOS may be indicative of impaired access to the articulatory rehearsal mechanism of working memory. This hypothesis also was suggested by Rochon, Caplan, and Waters (1990) and by Martin (1987, 1990) in regard to other nonfluent adults. Martin (1987, 1990) indicated that, in general, these individuals had very slow inner speech rates on a covert articulation task relative to fluent aphasic and normal adults. Feher (1987) found no effect of articulatory properties on memory span task performance for nonfluent adults. These individuals had difficulty rehearsing during delays on these tasks, regardless of the articulatory properties of the stimuli. Feher also administered a recognition memory probe that did not draw on inner rehearsal for adequate performance. The nonfluent adults performed within the normal range on this latter task, whereas fluent aphasic patients, who were identified as having a phonologic store deficit, performed poorly on the recognition task. Thus, for the nonfluent patients, the deficit appeared to involve difficulty in using the articulatory rehearsal process rather than an impairment in the phonologic store.

The good immediate but impaired deferred repetition of Subject 2 suggests that a deficit in central executive control over articulatory programming may be responsible for the error performance. This subject's performance pattern may reveal a second type of apraxia of speech. For

Subject 2, the deferred nature of the task appears to influence function of articulatory programming. During immediate repetition of the target and then distractor, disengagement from previous articulatory sets is possible as a result of the total activation of Routes 1 and 2 in Figure 1. During deferred repetition, there is less activation of Routes 1 and 2. Consequently, the more recent activation of the distractor word may inhibit or block the production of the previously produced target word. As mentioned previously, Subject 2 produced repetition of distractor errors primarily when attempting to retrieve nonsense targets paired with real-word distractors. Thus, with nonsense targets, she appears to have a problem with lexical disengagement, perseverating on the real-word distractor.

As indicated, Subject 2 produced one or two feature change errors only during retrieval of real target words. Production of the distractor appeared to interfere with completely accurate retrieval of the real target words in a particular way; features or segments of the distractor were carried over or perseverated to the deferred retrieval of the real target word. Thus with real targets, Subject 2 appears to have a problem with segment and feature disengagement. That is, she displays difficulty with articulatory disengagement, perseverating only particular aspects of the distractor. Overall, Subject 2's impairment is characterized by problems in the central control of disengagement from previously produced articulatory sets. Subject 2 appears to have difficulty regulating shift, focus, and/or control from one articulatory set of speech gestures (distractor) to the next (target). The performance pattern indicates problems in switching out of articulatory programs designed for circumstances that no longer apply (Mayes, 1988). Thus, our observations suggest that, for Subject 2, central executive control over articulatory programming may be disrupted (Baddeley, 1990), particularly impeding lexical, segmental, and feature disengagement.

Implications for Treatment

The deficits displayed by both subjects appeared to interfere with the adequate functioning of working memory. The interaction between articulatory programming and the various components of working memory should be considered when devising treatment tasks. For Subject 1, factors such as the ability to initiate speech production, the strength of word images in working memory, and the allocation of cognitive resources should be explored in relation to their therapeutic influence. In particular, the influence of the strength of word images for real words should be further examined in treatment, specifically in regard to their frequency in the language, concreteness, length, and personal familiarity. For Subject 2, factors such as lexical and articulatory disengagement may need to be evaluated regarding their interference in speech production as well as their treatment value. In particular, therapeutic approaches that specifically control or facilitate disengagement from antecedent articulatory sets should be considered for use with this type of apraxic speaker. Techniques such as reading, pacing boards, and direct approaches to treating perseveration may be more appropriate and especially beneficial for patients similar to Subject 2. These particular methods provide patients with a definitive framework regarding the beginning and termination of stimuli.

REFERENCES

Baddeley, A.D. (1986). *Working memory.* Oxford, England: Clarendon Press.
Baddeley, A.D. (1990). The development of the concept of working memory: Implications and contributions of neuropsychology. In G. Vallar & T. Shallice (Eds.), *Neuropsychological impairments of short-term memory* (pp. 54–73). New York: Cambridge University Press.
Baddeley, A.D. (1992). Working memory. *Science, 255,* 556–559.
Baddeley, A., Vallar, G., & Wilson, B. (1987). Sentence comprehension and phonological memory: Some neuropsychological evidence. In M. Coltheart (Ed.), *The psychology of reading* (pp. 509–530). London: Lawrence Erlbaum Associates.
Canter, G.J., Trost, J.E., & Burns, M.S. (1985). Contrasting speech patterns in apraxia of speech and phonemic paraphasia. *Brain and Language, 24,* 204–222.
Caplan, D. (1987). Phonological representations in word production. In E. Keller & M. Gopnik (Eds.), *Motor and sensory processes of language* (pp. 111–124). Hillsdale, NJ: Lawrence Erlbaum Associates.
Caramazza, A., Miceli, G., & Villa, C. (1986). The role of the output phonological buffer in reading, writing, and repetition. *Cognitive Neuropsychology, 3,* 37–76.
Carroll, D., Davies, R., & Richman, A. (1971). *American Heritage word frequency book.* New York: American Heritage Publishing Company.
Daneman, M., & Tardif, T. (1987). Working memory and reading skill reexamined. In M. Coltheart (Ed.), *The psychology of reading* (pp. 491–508). London: Lawrence Erlbaum Associates.
Favreau, Y., Nespoulous, J., & Lecours, A. (1990). Syllabic structure and lexical frequency effects in the phonemic errors of four aphasics. *Journal of Neurolinguistics, 5,* 165–187.
Feher, E. (1987). *An examination of short-term memory deficits in nonfluent aphasics.* Unpublished doctoral dissertation, University of Houston, Houston, TX.
Friedrich, F.J. (1990). Multiple phonological representations and verbal short-term memory. In G. Vallar & T. Shallice (Eds.), *Neuropsychological impairments of short-term memory* (pp. 74–93). New York: Cambridge University Press.
German, D. (1990). *The Test of Adult/Adolescent Word Finding.* Austin, TX: DLM Publishers.
Goodglass, H., & Kaplan, E. (1983). *The assessment of aphasia and related disorders.* Philadelphia: Lea & Febiger.
Hough, M.S., DeMarco, S., & Farler, D. (1994). Phonemic retrieval in conduction aphasia and Broca's aphasia with apraxia of speech: Underlying processes. *Journal of Neurolinguistics, 8,* 235–246.
Hough, M.S., & Klich, R. (1987). Effects of word length on lip EMG activity in apraxia of speech. In R. Brookshire (Ed.), *Clinical aphasiology conference proceedings* (pp. 271–276). Minneapolis: BRK Publishers.

Itoh, M., Sasanuma, S., Tatsumi, I., Murakami, S., Fukusako, Y., & Suzuki, T. (1982). Voice onset time characteristics in apraxia of speech. *Brain and Language, 17*, 193–210.
Jackendorf, R. (1987). *Consciousness and the computational mind.* Cambridge, MA: MIT Press.
Jason, G. (1983). Hemispheric asymmetries in motor function: I. Left hemisphere specialization for memory but not performance. *Neuropsychologia, 21*, 35–46.
Kelso, J.A.S., & Tuller, B. (1981). Toward a theory of apractic syndromes. *Brain and Language, 12*, 224–245.
Kent, R.D., & McNeil, M.R. (1987). Relative timing of sentence repetition in apraxia of speech and conduction aphasia. In J.H. Ryalls (Ed.), *Phonetic approaches to speech production in aphasia and related disorders* (pp. 181–220). Boston: College-Hill Press.
Kent, R.D., & Rosenbek, J.C. (1983). Acoustic patterns of apraxia of speech. *Journal of Speech and Hearing Research, 26*, 231–249.
Kertesz, A. (1984). Subcortical lesions and apraxia of speech. In J.C. Rosenbek, M.R. McNeil, & A.E. Aronson (Eds.), *Apraxia of speech: Physiology–acoustics–linguistics–management* (pp. 73–90). San Diego: College-Hill Press.
Kertesz, A. (1985). Apraxia and aphasia: Anatomical and clinical relationship. In E.A. Roy (Ed.), *Neuropsychological studies of apraxia and related disorders* (pp. 163–178). Amsterdam: North Holland.
Kohn, S. (1988). Phonological production deficits in aphasia. In H.A. Whitaker (Ed.), *Phonological processes and brain mechanisms* (pp. 93–117). New York: Springer-Verlag.
Lebrun, Y. (1989). Apraxia of speech: The history of a concept. In P. Square-Storer (Ed.), *Acquired apraxia of speech in aphasic adults* (pp. 3–19). London: Taylor & Francis.
Lebrun, Y. (1990). Apraxia of speech: A critical review. *Journal of Neurolinguistics, 5*, 379–406.
MacKay, D.G. (1985). A theory of representation, organization and timing of action with implications for sequencing disorders. In E.A. Roy (Ed.), *Neuropsychological studies of apraxia and related disorders* (pp. 267–308). Amsterdam: North Holland.
Margolin, D. (1991). Cognitive neuropsychology: Resolving enigmas about Wernicke's aphasia and other higher cortical disorders. *Archives of Neurology, 48*, 751–765.
Martin, R.C. (1987). Articulatory and phonological deficits in short-term memory and their relation to syntactic processing. *Brain and Language, 32*, 159–192.
Martin, R.C. (1990). Neuropsychological evidence on the role of short-term memory in sentence processing. In G. Vallar & T. Shallice (Eds.), *Neuropsychological impairments of short-term memory* (pp. 390–427). New York: Cambridge University Press.
Mayes, A.R. (1988). *Human organic memory disorders.* New York: Cambridge University Press.
Odell, K., McNeil, M., Rosenbek, J.C., & Hunter, L. (1990). Perceptual characteristics of consonant production by apraxic speakers. *Journal of Speech and Hearing Disorders, 55*, 345–359.
Peters, M. (1990). Interaction of vocal and manual movements. In G.E. Hammond (Ed.), *Cerebral control of speech and limb movements* (pp. 535–574). Amsterdam: North Holland.

Pierce, R.S. (1991). Apraxia of speech versus phonemic paraphasia: Theoretical, diagnostic, and treatment considerations: In M. Cannito & D. Vogel (Eds.), *Treating disordered speech motor control: For clinicians by clinicians* (pp. 185–216). Austin, TX: PRO-ED.
Pronovost, W., & Dombleton, C. (1955). *The Boston University Speech Sound Discrimination Picture Test.* Boston: Boston University Press.
Rochon, E., Caplan, D., & Waters, G. (1990). Short-term memory processes in patients with apraxia of speech: Implications for the nature and structure of the auditory verbal short-term memory system. *Journal of Neurolinguistics, 5,* 237–264.
Rosenbek, J.C. (1985). Treating apraxia of speech. In D.F. Johns (Ed.), *Clinical management of neurogenic communicative disorders* (2nd ed., pp. 267–312). Boston: Little, Brown.
Rosenbek, J.C., Kent, R.D., & LaPointe, L.L. (1984). Apraxia of speech: An overview and some perspectives. In J.C. Rosenbek, M.R. McNeil, & A.E. Aronson (Eds.), *Apraxia of speech: Physiology–acoustics–linguistics–management* (pp. 1–72). San Diego: College-Hill Press.
Roy, E.A. (1981). Action sequencing and lateralized cerebral damage: Evidence for asymmetries in control. In J. Long & A.D. Baddeley (Eds.), *Attention and performance IX* (pp. 487–498). Hillsdale, NJ: Lawrence Erlbaum Associates.
Roy, E.A. (1982). Action and performance. In A. Ellis (Ed.), *Normality and pathology in cognitive function* (pp. 265–298). New York: Academic Press.
Roy, E.A., & Square, P.A. (1985). Common considerations in the study of limb, verbal and oral apraxia. In E.A. Roy (Ed.), *Neuropsychological studies of apraxia and related disorders* (pp. 111–162). Amsterdam: North Holland.
Roy, E.A., & Square-Storer, P. (1990). Evidence for common expressions of apraxia. In G.E. Hammond (Ed.), *Cerebral control of speech and limb movements* (pp. 477–502). Amsterdam: North Holland.
Square-Storer, P., & Apeldoorn, S. (1991). An acoustic study of apraxia of speech with different lesion loci. In C.A. Moore, K.M. Yorkston, & D.R. Beukelman (Eds.), *Dysarthria and apraxia of speech: Perspectives on management* (pp. 216–227). Baltimore: Paul H. Brookes Publishing Company.
Square-Storer, P., & Roy, E.A. (1989). The apraxias: Commonalities and distinctions. In P. Square-Storer (Ed.), *Acquired apraxia of speech in aphasic adults* (pp. 20–63). Hillsdale, NJ: Lawrence Erlbaum Associates.
Square-Storer, P., Roy, E.A., & Hogg, S.C. (1990). The dissociation of aphasia from apraxia of speech, ideomotor limb, and buccofacial apraxia. In G.E. Hammond (Ed.), *Cerebral control of speech and limb movements* (pp. 452–476). Amsterdam: North Holland.
Waters, G.S., Rochon, E., & Caplan, D. (1992). The role of high-level speech planning in rehearsal: Evidence from patients with apraxia of speech. *Journal of Memory and Language, 31,* 54–73.
Weinstein, B.E. (1989). Guidelines for the identification of hearing impairment/handicap in adult/elderly persons. *ASHA, 31,* 59–62.
Wertz, R.T., LaPointe, L.L., & Rosenbek, J.C. (1984). *Apraxia of speech in adults.* Orlando, FL: Grune & Stratton.

Index

Page numbers followed by "t" or "f" indicate tables or figures, respectively

Abduct-and-stiffen transitions, 324
Abductor spasmodic dysphonia
  (ABSD), 311–316
  acoustic characteristics of connected
    speech for, 312
  speech research review, 311–312,
    313t–315t
  voicing contrasts in, 311–328
    statistical analysis, 318
    study methodology, 316–318
    study procedures, 316–318
    study reliability, 318
    study results, 318–322, 319t,
      320f–321f
    study subjects, 316, 317t
ABSD, *see* Abductor spasmodic
  dysphonia
Acoustic-phonetic measurements,
  317–318
Acoustics
  analyses, 128–129
  connected speech characteristics,
    312
  connected speech measures,
    318–319, 319t
  selection patterns
    criteria of, 46
    in primates, 49–50
  speech motor programming goals,
    32–38
Acquisition
  repertoire
    criteria of, 46
    in primates, 49–50
  skill, feedback during, 13–16, 15f
Acquisition performance, 5–7
Acquisition phase, 4
Acquisition phenomena, 7–8

Adduct-and-relax transitions, 324
Adductor spasmodic dysphonia, 311
Aerodynamic assessment
  measures, 290–291
  procedure, 211–212
Airway impairment, inspiratory
  compensatory behaviors in,
    336–337, 337f
  effects on continuous speech,
    329–339
ALS, *see* Amyotrophic lateral sclerosis
Amyotrophic lateral sclerosis (ALS),
  193–195
  respiratory symptoms of
    clinical assessment of, 195–196,
      196t
    progression of, 193–202
    study methods, 195–198
    study questions, 195
    study results, 198–201, 199f, 199t,
      200f–201f
    study subjects, 196–198, 197t, 198f
  Amyotrophic Lateral Sclerosis Severity
    Scale, 195–196, 196t
Animal models of speech
  candidate characteristics, 45–47
  developing, 43–63
AOS, *see* Apraxia of speech
Aphonia, 125
Apraxia of speech (AOS), 342f, 343
  criteria for diagnosis, 344
  phonemic retrieval in, 341–355
    data analysis, 347
    implications for treatment,
      352–353
    patterns of error production,
      350–352
    study materials, 346, 346t

Apraxia of speech (AOS)—*continued*
  study methodology, 344–347
  study procedures, 346–347
  study results, 348–349, 348*t*, 349*t*
  study subjects, 344–345, 345*t*
Articulation
  criteria of, 46–47
  in primates, 50–57, 51*f*, 54*f*–57*f*
  times of extraction data, 38
Articulation rate, 161
  of dysarthric speakers, 167, 168*f*
Articulation/pause time ratio, 162
Articulatory-to-acoustic motor equivalence findings
  differences among subjects, 36–38, 37*f*
  effects of times of articulatory data, 38
  factors underlying, 35–38
  preliminary, 33–35, 33*f*, 34*f*
  strength of correlations, 38
  in subsets of data, 35*t*, 36
Assessment
  aerodynamic measures, 290–291
  aerodynamic procedure, 211–212
  electrolaryngographic procedure, 209–210
  instrumental, of laryngeal function after closed head injury, 209–219, 215*t*, 215*f*
  listeners' ability, 84–85
  effects of syntactic and semantic context on, 79, 79*f*
  perceptual
    by dysarthric speakers, 275–286
    of laryngeal impairment after closed head injury, 207–209, 212–213, 213*t*–214*t*, 217*t*
    by primary communication partners, 275–286
  prosodic, of dysarthria, 155–178
  reliability and validity issues in, 121–178
  see also Ratings; Scaling
Audience, size of, 279
Audio presentation format experiment, 99–100
  listening subjects, 99
  methodology, 99
  procedure, 99
  results and discussion, 99–100

Audio+video presentation format experiment, 92–98
  listening format and procedures, 95
  listening subjects, 95
  methodology, 93–95
  recording procedure, 94
  reliability, 95
  results and discussion, 95–98, 96*t*, 97*f*–98*f*
  speaker, 94
  speaking conditions, 95
  stimulus material development, 93–94
Auditory-perceptual scaling, of dysarthria
  rating procedure, 147–148
  recorded samples of dysarthric speech, 147
  reliability of, 145–154
  study methods, 147–148
  study results, 148–149, 148*t*, 149*t*–150*t*
  study subjects, 147
Avoidance, 279

Behavior
  compensatory, in inspiratory airway compromise, 336–337, 337*f*
  compensatory strategies, 279, 282–283, 337
  dope smoker's strategy, 337
  primate communicative, 47–60
  propositional vocal
    criteria of, 47
    in primates, 59–60
  validation of putative vocal contrasts
    criteria of, 47
    in primates, 57–59
  validation of vocal feature production and detection
    criteria of, 47
    in primates, 57–59, 58*f*
Brain injury, traumatic, 229–231
  laryngeal airway resistance after, 229–240
  tongue function in, 241–256
  tongue strength and endurance in, 249–254
Breath(s)
  concurrence of, 184, 188–190, 189*f*

location of, 184, 187–188, 187f
Breath group, words per, 185, 185t
Breath group length, 184–185, 185t
  frequency of occurrence, 184–187, 186f
Breathiness, 123–126
  perceptual spaces for, 126–135
  multidimensional scaling analyses, 128, 128t
  multidimensional scaling solutions, 131, 132f
  study method, 126–130
  study results, 130–135
Breathiness ratings
  independence of, 130
  multidimensional scaling solutions, 135, 137f
  perceptual spaces of, 135–136, 136t
  scaling solutions for listeners, 135–139
  unidimensional vs multidimensional, 131–133, 133t
Bulbar Cumulative Scale score, 197

CAIDS, see Computerized Assessment of the Intelligibility of Dysarthric Speech
CHI, see Closed head injury
Closed head injury (CHI), 205–207
  laryngeal impairment after, 205–227
  instrumental assessment of, 209–212
  instrumental data analysis, 213–219, 215t, 215f
  perceptual analysis of, 212–213, 213t–214t, 217t
  perceptual assessment of, 207–209
  study methods, 207–212
  study results, 212
  study subjects, 207, 208t
  speech samples, 207–209
Communication ability, measures of, 289–291
Communication disability, of Parkinson's disease, 275–286
  analysis, 280
  dependent variables, 279–280
  descriptive statistics, 280, 281t
  multivariate and univariate tests, 280–281, 282f–284f
  study methodology, 277–280

study participants, 277–278
study procedures, 278–279, 278t
study results, 280–281
study scoring, 280
suggestions for future research, 285–286
Communication effectiveness, measures of, 290
Communication partners, perceptions of, 275–286
Communication Profile for Speakers with Motor Speech Disorders, 290, 291t
Communicative behavior, primate, 47–60
Communicative intent indices, 46
  in primates, 47–48
Compensatory behaviors, in inspiratory airway compromise, 336–337, 337f
Compensatory strategies, 279, 282–283
  dope smoker's, 337
Computerized Assessment of the Intelligibility of Dysarthric Speech (CAIDS), scores with Parkinson's disease, 278, 278t
Conference on Motor Speech, 1994, 3
Connected speech
  acoustic characteristics for abductor spasmodic dysphonia, 312
  acoustic influence of voicing on, 311–328
  acoustic measures of, 318–319, 319t
Continuous speech, 329–330
  effects of inspiratory airway impairment on, 329–339
  data analysis, 332–334, 333f
  group comparisons, 332f, 334–336, 334t, 335t–336t
  study methodology, 330–334
  study procedures, 331–332, 332f
  study results and discussion, 334–337
  study subjects, 330–331, 331t
Contrasts
  putative vocal, perceptual and behavioral validation of
    criteria of, 47
    in primates, 57–59
  voicing, in abductor spasmodic dysphonia, 311–328

Conversation, reading vs, 163–166

Digital manipulation, of experimental speech samples, 110–111
Distinguishability
  criteria of, 46
  in primates, 49–50
Dope smoker's strategy, 337
Drills, 9
Dysarthria, 67–68, 275–277
  auditory-perceptual scaling of, 145–154
  hypokinetic, group treatment for, 287–307
  intervention strategies for, 89
  perceptual features, 151, 152t
  perceptual scaling, 145–147
  prosodic assessment of, 155–178
  respiratory involvement in, 179–202
  shared deviant dimensions for, 149, 150t
  treatment of, 116–117
  treatment research, 118–119
Dysarthric speakers, 72–73, 73t
  articulation rates, 167, 168f
  F_0 envelopes, 167, 169f
  intensity envelopes, 167, 169f
  laryngeal impairment after closed head injury, 205–227
  perceptions of, 275–286
  primary communication partners, 275–286
  prosodic impairment in, 166–171
    etiology of, 167
    severity of, 168–170, 170t
  prosodic ratings, 107–109, 109t
  range of intensity variation in, 167, 168f
  reading vs conversation, 163–166
  top-down influences on, 89–103
Dysarthric speech
  characteristics of, 280, 285
  intelligibility of, 80–84, 105
    effects of interword pauses on, 105–120
    effects of natural gestures and situational context on, 89–103
    effects of semantic and syntactic context on, 67–87
    top-down influences on, 89–103
  prosodic assessment measures, 161–163
  respiratory patterning and variability in, 181–192
    data analysis, 184, 185f
    experimental task, 183–184
    study methods, 183–184
    study questions, 182
    study results and discussion, 185–190
    study subjects, 183, 183t
  samples
    acquisition of, 106–107
    recorded, 147
    transcriptions, 107t, 107–109
Dysphonia, spasmodic, 311
  abductor, 311–328
  adductor, 311

Effort, sense of, 252
Electrolaryngographic assessment procedure, 209–210
Electromagnetic midsagittal articulometer (EMMA), 33
EMMA, see Electromagnetic midsagittal articulometer
Emotional load, 279
Endurance, tongue
  in Parkinson's disease, 259–274
  after traumatic brain injury, 241–242, 244, 246–248, 247t, 248f, 249–253, 250f–251f
  and speaking ability, 253–254
Environmental adversity, 279
Environmental manipulation, 279
Error production patterns, 350–352
Evaluation
  listeners' ability, 84–85
    effects of syntactic and semantic context on, 79, 79f
  see also Assessment
Exit interview, 290
Experiments
  audio presentation format, 99–100
  audio+video presentation format, 92–98
  with motor tasks, 9–10, 10f, 14–15, 15f, 17–18, 17f
  with verbal tasks, 10–13, 12f, 15–16, 18

see also Speech samples; *specific studies*
Expiration, speech, 334*t*, 335, 335*t*

Feedback
  faded, 14–15
  during skill acquisition, 13–16, 15*f*
Fundamental frequency (F_0), 319
  average, 317
  envelope, 163, 167, 169*f*
  mean, 163
  range, 163
  variability, 317

Gestural score, 28
Gestures, effects on intelligibility of dysarthric speakers, 89–103
  audio presentation format experiment, 99–100
  audio+video presentation format experiment, 92–98
Group dynamics, 305
Group treatment
  for hypokinetic dysarthria, 287–307
    intervention effectiveness, 305–306
    intervention procedures, 291–292
    spouse and participant interviews, 304–305
    study methodology, 287–292
    study participants, 287–288
    study questions, 287–288
    study results, 292–304, 293*t*, 294*f*–295*t*, 298*t*, 300*t*–301*t*
    speech changes after, 293, 293*t*, 295*t*, 296–297, 298*t*, 299, 300*t*, 301, 301*t*, 303, 303*t*
    evidence of maintenance of, 293–304, 294*f*, 297*f*, 299*f*, 302*f*, 304*f*

Hard palates, 37–38, 37*f*
Head injury
  closed, 205–207
    laryngeal impairment after, 205–227
    traumatic, motor speech involvement in, 203–256
    traumatic brain injury, 229–231
    laryngeal airway resistance after, 229–240
    tongue function after, 241–256
Hoarseness, 123–126
Hoehn and Yahr scale, of clinical disability in Parkinson's disease, 289, 289*t*
Huskiness, 125
HyperCard cards, 111, 111*f*–112*f*
Hypokinetic dysarthria, group treatment for, 287–307
  intervention effectiveness, 305–306
  intervention procedures, 291–292
  spouse and participant interviews, 304–305
  study methodology, 287–292
  study participants, 287–288
  study questions, 287–288
  study results, 292–304, 293*t*, 294*f*, 295*t*, 298*t*, 300*t*–301*t*

Inflected primate vocalizations, 43–63
Injury
  closed head, 205–207
    laryngeal impairment after, 205–227
  traumatic brain, 229–231
    laryngeal airway resistance after, 229–240
    tongue function in, 241–256
    tongue strength and endurance in, 249–254
  traumatic head, motor speech involvement in, 203–256
Inspiration, group comparisons, 332*f*, 334–335, 334*t*
Inspiratory airway impairment
  compensatory behaviors in, 336–337, 337*f*
  effects on continuous speech, 329–339
    data analysis, 332–334, 333*f*
    group comparisons, 332*f*, 334–336, 334*t*–336*t*
    study methodology, 330–334
    study procedures, 331–332, 332*f*
    study results and discussion, 334–337
    study subjects, 330–331, 331*t*
Instruction, partner, 279

Instrumental assessment, of laryngeal
function after closed head
injury, 209–219, 215t, 215f
instrumentation for, 209
subgroups, 213t, 216–219
Intelligibility, 65–120
demand for, 279
of dysarthric speech, 80–84, 105
effects of interword pauses on,
105–120
effects of natural gestures and situational context on, 89–103
effects of semantic and syntactic
context on, 67–87
top-down influences on, 89–103
sentence
nonverbal predictiveness, 93–94,
93t
verbal predictiveness, 94
Intensity envelope, 162–163
for dysarthric speakers, 167, 169f
Intensity range, 162
in dysarthric speakers, 167, 168f
Interpause speech rate, 264
Interviews
exit, 290
spouse and participant, 304–305
Interword pauses, effects on intelligibility of dysarthric speech,
105–120
acquisition of experimental samples,
106–107
digital manipulation of samples,
110–111
implications for future research,
118–119
implications for listener training,
117–118
implications for treatment,
116–117
listener judgments, 111
statistical analysis, 112–113, 113t
study method, 106–111
study results, 113–116, 113t–114t
transcriptions and prosodic ratings,
107–109
Intrajudge reliability, 148, 148t
IOPI, see Iowa Oral Performance
Instrument
Iowa Oral Performance Instrument
(IOPI), 263

Language sound patterns theories,
28–29
Laryngeal airway resistance, after traumatic brain injury, 229–240
study instrumentation, 234
study methodology, 231–234
study results, 234–237, 235t,
236f–237f
study subjects, 231, 232t–233t
Laryngeal impairment, after closed
head injury, 205–227
instrumental assessment of, 209–212
instrumental data analysis, 213–219,
215t, 215f
perceptual analysis of, 212–213,
213t–214t, 217t
perceptual assessment of, 207–209
study methods, 207–212
study results, 212
study subjects, 207, 208f
Learner difficulties, enhancement of
training by introducing, 8–18
Learning
acquisition performance indicator,
5–7
acquisition view of, 5–8
motor, 1–23
processes of, 7
Length of utterance, mean, 162
Listener-oriented reduced speech, variability in, 29–30
Listeners, 75, 76t
evaluation ability, 84–85
effects of syntactic and semantic
context on, 79, 79f
judgments of altered and unaltered speech samples, 111
orientation for, 75–76
scaling solutions for, 135–139
training of, 75–76, 117–118
Listening tasks, 75–77
Literature, addressing prosodic assessment of dysarthria, 155–158
Lx waveform analysis, 210–211

Mann-Whitney test, of reading vs conversation data, 164–165, 165t
Mean F_0, 163
Message modification, 279
Motor control

normal speech, 25–63
speech, goal-based, 27–32
Motor equivalence, 32
    articulatory-to-acoustic findings
        factors underlying, 35–38
        preliminary, 33–35, 33f–34f
        for vowel /u/, 33, 33f
Motor learning, issues in, 1–23
Motor speech
    control
        goal-based, 27–32
        normal, 25–63
    programming, acoustic goals in, 32–38
    in traumatic head injury, 203–256
Motor tasks, experiments with, 9–10, 10f, 14–15, 15f, 17–18, 17f
Multidimensional scaling
    analyses, 128, 128t
    solutions for dissimilar breathiness ratings, 135, 137f
    solutions for dissimilar roughness ratings, 135, 138f, 139
    unidimensional ratings vs, 131–133, 133t

Name recall, on tests, 11, 12f
Natural gestures, effects on intelligibility of dysarthric speakers, 89–103
    audio presentation format experiment, 99–100
    audio+video presentation format experiment, 92–98
Neuroimaging, advancements in, 43–44
Nonverbal predictiveness, 93–94, 93t

Orientation, for listeners, 75–76

Palate, hard, 37–38, 37f
Parkinsonian speakers
    articulation rates, 167, 168f
    F_0 envelopes, 167, 169f
    intensity envelopes, 167, 169f
    range of intensity variation in, 167, 168f
    severity of prosodic impairment in, 170, 170t

Parkinson's disease, 257–307
    CAIDS scores for patients with, 278, 278t
    communication disability of, 275–286
        analysis, 280
        descriptive statistics, 280, 281t
        multivariate and univariate tests, 280–281, 282f–284f
        study methodology, 277–280
        study participants, 277–278
        study procedures, 278–279, 278t
        study results, 280–281
        study scoring, 280
        suggestions for future research, 285–286
    disability level, 276
    functional limitation level, 276
    Hoehn and Yahr scale of clinical disability in, 289, 289t
    hypokinetic dysarthria of, group treatment for, 287–307
    impairment level, 276
    incidence of, 287
    pathology of, 276
    tongue strength and endurance in, 259–274
        statistical analysis, 264
        study methods, 261–264
        study procedures, 263–264
        study results, 265–268, 265t, 266f, 267t–268t, 269f
        study subjects, 261–262, 262t
Partner familiarity, 279
Partner instruction, 279
Pathologic vocal qualities, 123–126
    multidimensional nature of, 123–144
Pause-altered sentences, rules for creating, 110–111
Pauses
    effects on intelligibility of dysarthric speech, 105–120
    group comparisons, 336, 336t
    mean duration of, 162
    number of, 162
    sentence time, 318
    speech rate, 264
Perceived reactions of others, 280, 284, 284f
Perceptual assessment
    by dysarthric speakers, 275–286

Perceptual assessment—*continued*
 judgments, 290
 of laryngeal impairment after closed
   head injury, 207–209, 212–213,
   213*t*–214*t*, 217*t*
 by primary communication partners,
   275–286
 scaling of dysarthria, 145–147
 spaces, interpretation of, 135–139,
   136*t*, 137*f*–138*f*
 spaces for breathiness and roughness, 126–135
 strategies, 133–134, 133*t*, 139–141,
   140*t*
 unidimensional measures of vocal
   quality, 129–130
Perceptual validation
 of putative vocal contrasts
  criteria of, 47
  in primates, 57–59
 of vocal feature production and
   detection
  criteria of, 47
  in primates, 57–59, 58*f*
Phonation
 criteria of, 46–47
 in primates, 50–57, 51*f*, 54*f*,
   56*f*–57*f*
Phonemic retrieval, in apraxia of
 speech, 341–355
 data analysis, 347
 implications for treatment, 352–353
 patterns of error production, 350–352
 study materials, 346, 346*t*
 study methodology, 344–347
 study procedures, 346–347
 study results, 348–349, 348*t*–349*t*
 study subjects, 344–345, 345*t*
Practice
 common assumptions about, 4–8
 induced variability of, 16–18
 new conceptualizations, 3–23
 scheduling of tasks during, 9–13
Precision, improved, 279
Primates
 acquisition repertoire in, 49–50
 communicative behavior, 47–60
 distinguishability, 49–50
 indices of communicative intent,
   47–48

 perceptual and behavioral validation
   of putative vocal contrasts,
   57–59
 perceptual and behavioral validation
   of vocal feature production and
   detection, 57–59, 58*f*
 phonation, 50–57, 51*f*, 54*f*, 56*f*–57*f*
 propositional vocal behavior, 59–60
 selection of acoustic patterns, 49–50
 vocal syntax, 59–60, 60*f*
 vocalizations, 50–55, 52*f*–54*f*
  articulated and inflected, 43–63
  structural diversification of,
    47–48
Propositional vocal behavior
 criteria of, 47
 in primates, 59–60
Prosodic assessment, of dysarthria,
   155–178
 literature addressing, 155–158
 measures, 161–163
 reading vs conversation data,
   163–166, 164*t*–165*t*
 study apparatus, 161
 study design, 160–161
 study methodology, 158–163
 study results, 163–171
 study subjects, 158–160, 159*t*
Prosodic impairment, in dysarthric
   speakers, 166–171
 etiology of, 167
 severity of, 168–170, 170*t*

Range of intensity, 162
 variation in dysarthric speakers, 167,
   168*f*
Ratings
 breathiness
  independence of, 130
  multidimensional scaling solutions
    for, 135, 137*f*
  perceptual spaces of, 135–136,
    136*t*
 procedure, 147–148
 reliability of, 130–131
 roughness
  independence of, 130
  multidimensional scaling solutions
    for, 135, 138*f*, 139

perceptual spaces of, 136–139, 136t
unidimensional vs multidimensional, 131–133, 133t
see also Scaling
Reading, vs conversation, 163–166
Recall, name, 11, 12f
Recorded samples, of dysarthric speech, 147
Reduced speech, listener-oriented, 29–30
Reliability, 77, 95, 318
of auditory-perceptual scaling of dysarthria, 145–154
interjudge, 148, 149t
interrater, 139–141
intrajudge, 148, 148t
issues in assessment, 121–178
rating, 130–131
Repertoire acquisition
criteria of, 46
in primates, 49–50
Research
literature addressing prosodic assessment of dysarthria, 155–158
suggestions for, 285–286
in treatment of dysarthric speakers, 118–119
Respiration
adequate support, 181–182
control, 182
involvement in dysarthria, 179–202
patterning and variability in dysarthric speech, 181–192
data analysis, 184, 185f
experimental task, 183–184
study methods, 183–184
study questions, 182
study results and discussion, 185–190
study subjects, 183, 183t
symptoms of amyotrophic lateral sclerosis, progression of, 193–202
Retention
posttraining, 6
processes of, 7
Retention phenomena, 7–8

Roughness, 123–126
perceptual spaces for, 126–135
acoustic analyses, 128–129
multidimensional scaling analyses, 128, 128t
multidimensional scaling solutions, 131, 132f
study method, 126–130
study results, 130–135
scaling solutions for listeners, 135–139
Roughness ratings
independence of, 130
multidimensional scaling solutions for, 135, 138f, 139
perceptual spaces of, 136–139, 136t
unidimensional vs multidimensional, 131–133, 133t

Scaling
auditory-perceptual, 145–154
rating procedure, 147–148
study methods, 147–148
study results, 148–149, 148t–150t
study subjects, 147
multidimensional
analyses, 128, 128t
of breathiness, 128, 128t
solutions for breathiness ratings, 131, 132f, 135, 137f
solutions for roughness ratings, 135, 138f, 139
unidimensional ratings vs, 131–133, 133t
perceptual, 145–147
solutions for listeners, 135–139
study method, 135
study results, 135–139
variance accounted for by, 135
see also Ratings
Scheduling of tasks, 9–13
common principles, 13
SDDs, *see* Shared deviant dimensions
Semantic context, 74
effects on sentence intelligibility of dysarthric speakers, 67–87
analysis of data, 77
clinical implications, 85
experimental procedure, 76–77

Semantic context—*continued*
  listening tasks, 75–77
  study methodology, 72–77
  study questions, 71–72
  study results, 77–79, 78f–79f
Sentence articulation time, 318, 321–322, 321f
Sentence intelligibility
  effects of semantic and syntactic context on, 67–87
  nonverbal predictiveness, 93–94, 93t
  verbal predictiveness, 93–94, 93t
Sentence pause time, 318, 321–322, 321f
Sentences, pause-altered, 110–111
Shared deviant dimensions (SDDs), 149, 150t
Situational context, effects on intelligibility of dysarthric speakers, 89–103
  audio presentation format experiment, 99–100
  audio+video presentation format experiment, 92–98
Situational difficulty, 279, 283–284, 283f
Skill acquisition, feedback during, 13–16, 15f
Sound patterns theories, 28–29
SoundEdit waveform, 110, 110f
Spacing effects, 10
Spasmodic dysphonia, 311
  abductor, 311–316
    voicing contrasts in, 311–328
  adductor, 311
Speakers, dysarthric, 72–73, 73t
  articulation rates, 167, 168f
  F_0 envelopes, 167, 169f
  intensity envelopes, 167, 169f
  laryngeal impairment after closed head injury, 205–227
  perceptions of, 275–286
  primary communication partners, 275–286
  prosodic impairment in, 166–171
  prosodic ratings, 107–109, 109t
  range of intensity variation in, 167, 168f
  reading vs conversation, 163–166
  top-down influences on, 89–103

Speaking ability, relation between strength/endurance and, 253–254
Speech
  animal models
    candidate characteristics, 45–47
    developing, 43–63
  apraxia of, 342f, 343
    criteria for diagnosis, 344
    phonemic retrieval in, 341–355
    changes after group treatment, 293, 293t, 295t, 296–297, 298t, 299, 300t, 301, 301t, 303, 303t
    evidence of maintenance of, 293–304, 294f, 297f, 299f, 302f, 304f
  connected
    acoustic characteristics of, 312
    acoustic influence of voicing on, 311–328
    acoustic measures of, 318–319, 319t
  continuous, 329–330
    effects of inspiratory airway impairment on, 329–339
  dysarthric
    characteristics of, 280, 285
    effects of interword pauses on, 105–120
    effects of natural gestures and situational context on, 89–103
    effects of semantic and syntactic context on, 67–87
    intelligibility of, 80–84, 105
    prosodic assessment measures, 161–163
    respiratory patterning and variability in, 181–192
    samples, 106–107, 147
    top-down influences on, 89–103
    transcriptions, 107–109, 107t
  interpause rate, 264
  listener-oriented reduced, 29–30
  measures of intelligibility, 289–290
  model of production and repetition, 341–342, 342f
  motor programming, 32–38
  see also Motor speech
Speech expiration, group comparisons, 334t, 335, 335t

Speech research, abductor spasmodic
    dysphonia, 311–312, 313t–315t
Speech samples
  acquisition of, 106–107
  after closed head injury, 207–209
  digital manipulation of, 110–111
  listener judgments of, 111
  recorded dysarthric, 147
  after traumatic brain injury, 244–245
Speech Scale, 195–196, 196t
Speed, demand for, 279
Spouse and participant interviews,
    304–305
Strength and endurance, tongue
  in Parkinson's disease, 259–274
  after traumatic brain injury,
    241–242, 244, 246–253, 247t,
    248f, 250f–251f
  and speaking ability, 253–254
Syntactic context, 74–75
  effects on sentence intelligibility of
    dysarthric speakers, 67–87
  analysis of data, 77
  clinical implications, 85
  experimental procedure, 76–77
  listening tasks, 75–77
  reliability, 77
  study methodology, 72–77
  study questions, 71–72
  study results, 77–79, 78f–79f
Syntax, vocal
  criteria of, 47
  in primates, 59–60, 60f

Tasks
  listening, 75–77
  motor, experiments with, 9–10, 10f,
    14–15, 15f, 17–18, 17f
  during practice, scheduling of,
    9–13
  shared deviant dimensions across,
    149, 150t
  verbal, experiments with, 10–13, 12f,
    15–16, 18
TBI, see Traumatic brain injury
Tests, name recall on, 11, 12f
Tongue
  function after traumatic brain injury,
    241–256

  perceptual judgments, 245–246,
    245t
  statistical analyses, 246
  study method, 242–245
  study questions, 242
  study results, 246–249, 247t, 248f,
    249t, 250f–251f
  study subjects, 242–244, 243t
strength and endurance after traumatic brain injury, 241–242,
    244, 246–253, 247t, 248f,
    250f–251f
  and speaking ability, 253–254
strength and endurance in Parkinson's disease, 259–274
  statistical analysis, 264
  study methods, 261–264
  study procedures, 263–264
  study results, 265–268, 265t, 266f,
    267t–268t, 269f
  study subjects, 261–262, 262t
Tongue-body raising, correlations with
    upper-lip protrusion, 35, 35t
Training
  criteria for evaluation, 7–8
  enhancement by introducing difficulties for learner, 8–18
  for listeners, 75–76, 117–118
  new concepts for, 3–23
  real-world, 6–7
  retention and transfer after, 6
Transfer, posttraining, 6
Traumatic brain injury (TBI), 229–231
  laryngeal airway resistance after,
    229–240
  study instrumentation, 234
  study methodology, 231–234
  study results, 234–237, 235t,
    236f–237f
  study subjects, 231, 232t–233t
  speech samples, 244–245
  tongue function, 241–256
  perceptual judgments, 245–246,
    245t
  statistical analyses, 246
  study method, 242–245
  study questions, 242
  study results, 246–249, 247t, 248f,
    249t, 250f–251f
  study subjects, 242–244, 243t

Traumatic brain injury (TBI)—*continued*
  tongue strength and endurance, 244,
    246–248, 247*t*, 248*f*, 249–253,
    250*f*–251*f*
  and speaking ability, 253–254
Traumatic head injury, motor speech
  involvement in, 203–256

Unidimensional ratings, vs multidimensional ratings, 131–133,
  133*t*
Unstressed vowels
  duration, 162
  time percentage, 162
Upper–lip protrusion, correlations
  with tongue–body raising, 35,
  35*t*
Utterance duration, mean, 162
Utterance length, mean, 162

Validity, issues in assessment, 121–178
Variability of practice, induced, 16–18
Verbal predictiveness, 94
Verbal tasks, experiments with, 10–13,
  12*f*, 15–16, 18
Vocal behavior, propositional
  criteria of, 47
  in primates, 59–60
Vocal contrasts, putative, perceptual
  and behavioral validation of
  criteria of, 47
  in primates, 57–59
Vocal features, perceptual and behavioral validation of production
  and detection
  criteria of, 47
  in primates, 57–59
Vocal qualities
  pathologic, 123–126

multidimensional nature of,
  123–144
unidimensional perceptual measures of, 129–130
Vocal syntax
  criteria of, 47
  in primates, 59–60, 60*f*
Vocalizations
  in primates, 50–55, 52*f*–54*f*
  articulated and inflected, 43–63
  structural diversification of, 47–48
structural diversification of
  criteria of, 46
  in primates, 47–48
Voice onset time (VOT), 318, 320,
  320*f*–321*f*
Voicing
  acoustic influence on connected
    speech, 311–328
  contrasts in abductor spasmodic dys-
    phonia, 311–328
  statistical analysis, 318
  study methodology, 316–318
  study procedures, 316–318
  study reliability, 318
  study results, 318–322, 319*t*,
    320*f*–321*f*
  study subjects, 316, 317*t*
VOT, *see* Voice onset time
Vowel /u/, motor equivalence findings,
  33–34, 33*f*–34*f*
Vowels, unstressed
  duration of, 162
  time percentage, 162

Wheezing, 125
Wilcoxon test, of reading vs conversa-
  tion data, 164, 164*t*
Word retrieval, 341–342, 342*f*
Words per breath group, 185, 185*t*

Nagi p286.